KU-472-964

Multiple Sclerosis

Advances in Clinical Trial Design, Treatment and Future Perspectives

Springer
London
Berlin
Heidelberg
New York
Barcelona
Budapest
Hong Kong
Milan
Paris
Santa Clara
Singapore
Tokyo

D.E. Goodkin and R.A. Rudick (Eds)

Multiple Sclerosis

Advances in Clinical Trial Design, Treatment and Future Perspectives

With 28 Figures
including 5 Colour Plates

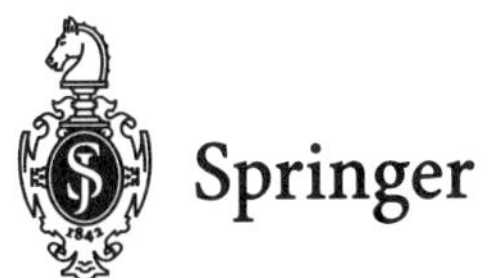

Springer

Donald E. Goodkin, MD
University of California at San Francisco, The UCSF/Mount Zion Multiple Sclerosis Center, 1600 Divisadero Street, San Francisco, CA 94115, USA

Richard A. Rudick, MD
Cleveland Clinic Foundation, Mellen Center for Multiple Sclerosis Treatment and Research, 9500 Euclid Avenue, Cleveland, OH 44195-5244, USA

Cover illustration: The background design shows part of an illustration prepared by Jerry Wolinsky MD (Current Neurology 1993, Volume 13, Chapter 7, Multiple Sclerosis, page 180, Figure 3) and adapted by the editors, illustrating a typical clinical course of multiple sclerosis and the relationship between clinical events and brain MRI activity.

ISBN 3-540-76018-0 Springer-Verlag Berlin Heidelberg New York SPIN 10518518

British Library Cataloguing in Publication Data
Multiple sclerosis : advances in trial design, treatment and future perspectives
1. Multiple sclerosis
I. Goodkin, Donald E., 1946– . II. Rudick, Richard A., 1950–
616.8'34
ISBN 3540760180

Library of Congress Cataloging-in-Publication Data
Multiple sclerosis : advances in trial design, treatment and future perspectives
p. cm.
Includes bibliographical references and index.
ISBN 3-540-76018-0 (hardcover : alk. paper)
1. Multiple sclerosis--Treatment. 2. Clinical trials.
I. Goodkin, Donald E., 1946– . II. Rudick, Richard A.
[DNLM: 1. Multiple Sclerosis--therapy. 2. Clinical Trials--methods.
WL 360 M95365 1996]
RC377.M8435 1996
616.8'3406--dc20
DNLM/DLC 96-12736
for Library of Congress CIP

Printed and bound by Maple-Vail Book Manufacturing Group, York, PA.
Printed in the United States of America.
9 8 7 6 5 4 3 2

Typeset by Richard Powell Editorial and Production Servs, Basingstoke, Hants RG22 4TX
28/3830-543210 Printed on acid-free paper

Preface

Multiple sclerosis (MS) is estimated to affect between one million and one and a quarter million persons worldwide. Prevalence rates in the United States and Europe are 15–145/100 000 population. Disease susceptibility appears to be influenced by genetic determinants and distance of a person's residence from the equator, and possibly by age of exposure to certain infectious agents. Persons with MS often experience a variety of neurologic symptoms, including disturbances of vision, co-ordination, sensation, gait and endurance, and bowel, bladder, cognitive and sexual functions. The clinical course is unpredictable and is characterized by recurrent attacks or "exacerbations", which are often punctuated or followed by more insidious progression of functional impairment. The socioeconomic consequences of the disease are significant, considering that between 1981 and 1992, 75%–85% of MS patients in the USA, UK and Australia were unemployed and at high risk of social isolation.

In 1992, with the help of recognized experts in the field, we published the first edition of *Treatment of multiple sclerosis: trial design, results and future perspectives.* Since that time, unprecedented advances have occurred in the development of disease-modifying therapies and the design of clinical trials in MS. In July 1993, interferon beta-1b (Betaseron®) became the first biological drug approved by the United States Food and Drug Administration (FDA) for treatment of ambulatory patients with relapsing–remitting MS. New drug applications have subsequently been filed with the FDA for interferon beta-1a (Avonex™) and copolymer 1 (Copaxone™), which also showed efficacy in Phase III studies in ambulatory patients with relapsing MS. Phase II studies of methotrexate and 2-chlorodeoxyadenosine (cladribine) reported promising results in patients with chronic progressive MS. A post-hoc analysis of the data from the Optic Neuritis Treatment Trial suggested that intravenous methylprednisolone delayed the onset of MS in patients with isolated idiopathic optic neuritis. Conventional magnetic resonance imaging (MRI) scans were shown to have predictive validity for patients experiencing monosymptomatic attacks of the type seen in MS, in that the presence and extent of brain MRI abnormality was linked to the development of MS and to subsequent disability. Furthermore, MRI is now accepted as the most sensitive primary outcome measure in preliminary trials of promising new therapies. New imaging techniques, such as magnetic transfer imaging and proton spectroscopy, have been applied to patients with MS and promise to improve our understanding of the immunology, pathology and natural history of MS lesions. To spur progress in the field, an international workshop including more than 100 clinical investigators, statisticians, representatives of academic medicine, private practice, regulatory agencies and the pharmaceutical industry was convened in 1994 to review critically the elements of current MS therapeutic trials and to identify the most important aspects of clinical evaluation, study design and data analysis that would allow agents for MS to be tested as accurately, rapidly and economically as possible. As a result of this international workshop, task forces were organized to develop specific guidelines for clinical outcome instruments and MRI imaging. These and other advances relevant to clinical trials in MS prompted us to organize this second volume.

The book centers around the following themes: an overview and assessment of the significance of major advances in MS experimental therapeutics since 1992 (Chapter 1); an updated review of our current understanding of the pathogenesis of MS (Chapter 2) and consequent therapeutic strategies (Chapter 3); new statistical approaches to improve the design and analysis of MS clinical trials (Chapter 4); current clinical and imaging outcome measures and strategies for improving their sensitivity (Chapters 5–8); the role of MRI in defining the prognosis in patients with isolated optic neuritis, brainstem syndromes and acute myelopathy (Chapter 9) and therapeutic strategies to delay the onset of MS in these patients (Chapter 10); disease-modifying therapies, recently approved or likely to gain widespread use in patients with MS (Chapters 11–14); ethical considerations related to the conduct of clinical trials in MS (Chapter 15); and a concluding discussion on the influence of clinical trials on the treatment of MS (Chapter 16).

We thought it appropriate to begin with an overview of the most significant advances in clinical trial design since our last volume. George Ellison's review of this topic provides an interesting overview of the remarkable progress that has been made in this field in the last 3 years. Oksenberg and Hauser provide a scholarly review of the putative immunopathogenic mechanisms in MS. This chapter is complemented by Sriram's review of rational therapeutic approaches developed to target these putative pathogenic mechanisms. Petkau presents a detailed discussion of emerging strategies for improved design and analysis of future clinical trials in MS. Many of the statistical approaches discussed by Petkau will be new to MS clinical investigators and deserve focused attention. Weinshenker's experience and contributions to the MS clinical outcomes assessment task force positioned him to review rigorously the state of current clinical outcome measures and strategies for developing more informative clinical outcomes for future trials. Fischer's important contributions to the application of neuropsychologic testing to multicenter clinical trials enabled her to review this topic with considerable personal experience. The challenges associated with defining and measuring quality of life in MS patients are reviewed by LaRocca and colleagues, who suggest appealing methods for quantifying this relevant clinical outcome. Grossman has contributed a definitive review of current and emerging MRI techniques relevant to MS clinical trials. His comments on strategies for improving sensitivity, specificity and predictive validity of these imaging measures are uniquely insightful. Miller's highly regarded experience with serial MRI of patients with isolated optic neuritis, brain stem syndromes and acute myelopathy made him our logical choice comprehensively to review this topic. Beck's experience as principal investigator of the Optic Neuritis Treatment Trial enabled him to discuss thoughtfully the strategies to delay the onset of MS in patients with optic neuritis. Rudick, Sibley and Durelli present the results of their experiences with various type I interferons, which have emerged through the results of controlled clinical trials as standard therapy for relapsing-remitting MS patients. Goodkin and Fischer review the clinical, imaging and neuropsychologic outcomes from a Phase II study of low dose, weekly, oral methotrexate. This study made use of a composite outcome measure that included quantitative tests of upper extremity function. Such a composite may effectively improve the sensitivity of the Expanded Disability Status Scale (EDSS) for detecting change reliably in MS patients who require assistance to walk. Johnson reviews the data from the recently completed Phase III trial of copolymer 1, which offers a new therapeutic option for ambulatory patients with relapsing MS. Sipe's experience with cladribine enables him authoritatively to review experience in the Phase II clinical trial with this drug in patients with chronic progressive MS. His description of toxicity associated with the use of cladribine will be helpful to those seeking better to define its potential as a future therapy for patients with chronic progressive MS. Foa has provided a thoughtful review of the ethical considerations raised by clinical trials in MS and the approval of new partially effective therapies for this disease. To the best of our knowledge, this is the first published chapter on this topic. McDonald is one of the world's leading authorities on MS. His enormous experience and widely regarded opinion made him our logical choice to provide the concluding historical perspective on the emergence of MS, after 160 years, as a treatable condition.

Our recent advances now prompt us to focus on the following important issues and questions:

1. Obviously relevant clinical change in groups of MS patients occurs over a time frame of 10 or more years, yet our clinical trials occur during a time frame of 2–3 years. Therefore, we need to know the validity of short-term change in current

clinical outcome measures (e.g. exacerbation rates, change in EDSS) in predicting longer-term clinical change. Additionally, as we try to improve on partially effective therapies, we will need more sensitive clinically-based outcomes for detecting change in targeted functions. How can we demonstrate predictive validity of short-term change in these more sensitive outcome measures? Will the use of composite outcome measures improve the sensitivity and precision for detecting treatment effects?

2. What is the validity of conventional MRI scans in predicting future clinically relevant change? What evidence for predictive validity would be adequate to accept MRI as the primary outcome measure in a Phase III controlled clinical trial in MS?
3. How can we best protect the different interests of clinical investigators and representatives of the pharmaceutical industry, who combine forces to conduct important research initiatives in MS? How can we best identify and minimize bias due to intellectual and financial conflicts of interest on the part of the investigators? How can we best assure the publication rights of academic clinical investigators yet protect the marketing interests of the pharmaceutical companies that are funding clinical trials? Is there a role for an external monitoring committee in this regard? How should such a committee be constituted?
4. How can we reconcile the requirements of clinical care with the often conflicting demands of clinical research? Now that partially effective therapies are available for patients with the relapsing form of MS, is it ethical to maintain patients in controlled clinical trials after they have met criteria for treatment failure defined by the study primary outcome measure? Should patients who meet criteria for treatment failure be released from a controlled clinical trial to seek available partially effective therapies or participate in alternative clinical trials? Can or should we continue to conduct placebo-controlled trials involving patients with relapsing MS?
5. How will we address issues of study feasibility that arise when comparing the efficacy of promising new therapies with that of a partially effective therapy instead of a placebo? Will trials that compete for similar patients jeopardize our ability to answer the same question asked in both studies? Can monitoring committees play a useful role in this regard?

As in our previous volume, the contents of this book reflect our concept of MS as a tissue-specific autoimmune disease. Should the actual etiology differ, we expect that future therapeutic trials will move in the appropriate direction. Furthermore, we focused on developments related to MS pathogenesis, clinical trial design and implementation, results of recently approved therapies or therapies that are likely to gain widespread acceptance in the immediate future, and the practical and ethical considerations arising from recently completed trials. We did not cover an important area in MS therapeutics: trials of drugs aimed at ameliorating symptoms of the disease; nor have we exhaustively covered every individual therapeutic modality of potential interest. We did not attempt to develop consensus within the field by dealing directly with areas of controversy, of which there are many. We did not deal directly with the economics of clinical trials, the composition and role of advisory and external monitoring committees, or guidelines for identification and protection of the different interests of academic clinical investigators and the pharmaceutical industry that increasingly provides the main source of funding for MS clinical trials. We expect in future revisions of this book to deal with some of these additional important issues.

We are grateful that so many busy colleagues, all recognized experts in their fields, were again willing to provide comprehensive reviews or ground-breaking chapters, submitted on time, for this effort. We hope that we have achieved our collective goal to extend the scope and succinctly update our 1992 volume on the current state of affairs of MS clinical trial design, results and future perspectives. Most importantly, we hope that the current volume will contribute in some small way to future progress in this field.

September 1995 DEG
San Francisco, California RAR
Cleveland, Ohio

Acknowledgements

We wish to acknowledge the courage, patience and conviction of MS patients participating in clinical trials.

We greatly appreciate the expertise and hard work of Lynda Douglas Hill, who compiled the manuscript for this book.

Contents

Contributors

Howard Andrews, PhD
New York State Psychiatric Institute
Epidemiology of Mental Disorders Research Department
722 West 168th Street
New York, NY 10032
USA

Roy W. Beck, MD, PhD
Jaeb Center for Health Research
3010 East 138th Avenue
Suite 9
Tampa, FL 33613
USA

E. Beutler
Scripps Clinic and Research Foundation
10666 North Torrey Pines Road
La Jolla, CA 92037
USA

M.B. Bornstein, MD
PO Box 1054
Norwich, VT 05055
USA

Luca Durelli, MD
Clinica Neurologica
Via Cherasco, 15
I-10126 Torino
Italy

George W. Ellison, MD
A-125 Reed Neurological Research Center/UCLA
Box 951769
Los Angeles, CA 90095-1769
USA

Jill S. Fischer, PhD
Mellen Center – U10
Cleveland Clinic Foundation
9500 Euclid Avenue
Cleveland, OH 44195-5244
USA

Richard Foa, MD, MA (Ethics)
Virginia Medical Associates
5510 Alma Lane
Springfield, VA 22151
USA

Donald E. Goodkin, MD
UCSF/Mount Zion Multiple Sclerosis Center
1600 Divisadero Street
San Francisco, CA 94115
USA

Robert I. Grossman, MD
Hospital of the University of Pennsylvania
Department of Neuroradiology
Founders Building Ground Floor
3400 Spruce Street
Philadelphia, PA 19104
USA

Stephen L. Hauser, MD
Department of Neurology
University of California, San Francisco
San Francisco, CA 94143-0114
USA

Kenneth P. Johnson, MD
University of Maryland Hospital
Department of Neurology, Room M4W46
22 South Greene Street
Baltimore, MD 21201
USA

Nicholas G. LaRocca, PhD
St Agnes Hospital
303 North Street
Suite 203
White Plains, NY 10605
USA

W. Ian McDonald, MB, PhD, FRCP
University Department of Clinical Neurology
National Hospital for Neurology and Neurosurgery
Queen Square
London WCIN 3BG
UK

David Miller, MD
University Department of Clinical Neurology
National Hospital for Neurology and Neurosurgery
Queen Square
London WCIN 3BG
UK

Deborah M. Miller, PhD
Mellen Center – U10
Cleveland Clinic Foundation
9500 Euclid Avenue
Cleveland, OH 44195-5244
USA

Jorge R. Oksenberg, PhD
University of California San Francisco
Department of Neurology
505 Parnassus Avenue
San Francisco, CA 94143-0435
USA

Donald W. Paty, MD
Vancouver Hospital and Health Services Center
UBC Site Room S195
2211 Wesbrook Mall
Vancouver, BC V6T 2B5
Canada

John Petkau, PhD
University of British Columbia
Department of Statistics
333–6356 Agricultural Road
Vancouver, BC V6T 1Z2
Canada

Paul G. Ritvo, PhD
Department of Psychology
The Toronto Hospital
College Wing 2-332
200 Elizabeth Street
Toronto, Ontario M5G 2C4
Canada

J.S. Romine, MD
Scripps Clinic and Research Foundation
10666 North Torrey Pines Road
La Jolla, CA 92037
USA

Richard A. Rudick, MD
Mellen Center – U10
Cleveland Clinic Foundation
9500 Euclid Avenue
Cleveland, OH 44195-5244
USA

William Sibley, MD
Arizona Health Sciences Center
Department of Neurology
1501 North Campbell
Tucson, AZ 85724
USA

Jack C. Sipe, MD
Scripps Clinic and Research Foundation
10666 North Torrey Pines Road
La Jolla, CA 92037
USA

Subramaniam Sriram, MD
Department of Neurology
Medical Center South
Vanderbilt University
2100 Pierce Avenue
Nashville, TN 38212
USA

Brian G. Weinshenker, MD, FRCP(C)
Department of Neurology
Mayo Clinic
200 First Street Southwest
Rochester, MN 55905
USA

J. Zyroff, MD
Scripps Clinic and Research Foundation
10666 North Torrey Pines Road
La Jolla, CA 92037
USA

1 Recent Advances and Future Challenges in Multiple Sclerosis Clinical Trial Design

George W. Ellison

Introduction

Tore Broman lay down the desiderata for multiple sclerosis (MS) therapeutics in 1970 (Broman 1970):

1. Complete cure of the patient;
2. Success in preventing further relapses;
3. Success in preventing further progress;
4. An acceptable risk that the treatment will be less harmful than the disease.

I feel I am blessed to be living in such awesome times as we (those struck by the scourge, family, friends and researchers) achieve Broman's desiderata and close in on effective treatment(s) for MS. The advances in the design of therapeutic trials just since the completion of the first version of *Treatment of Multiple Sclerosis* (Rudick and Goodkin 1992) are quite impressive.

We can recognize a treatment that works! Despite the extraordinary variability of the course of MS, with current "pivotal" or "full" trial designs, we have been able to detect partially effective palliative treatments for reducing the frequency (by around 30% rather than 100%) and severity of relapses, and for delaying "progression" (IFNB Multiple Sclerosis Study Group 1995; Jacobs et al. 1994; Johnson et al. 1995).

Early on, we can recognize a treatment that does not work (Myers et al. 1995)! Designs for "preliminary" trials, in which we ostensibly seek safety, tolerance and regimen data, have advanced to where we can declare that a potential agent is unlikely to be efficacious – with as few as six volunteers!

What advances account for such firm statements in the quicksands of MS therapeutic trial design?

Advances

Magnetic Resonance Imaging (Table 1.1)

Table 1.1. Advances in magnetic resonance imaging since 1990

Year	Reference
1991	Quantitative MRI changes in gadolinium-DTPA enhancement after high-dose intravenous methylprednisolone in multiple sclerosis (Barkhof et al. 1991)
1991	Magnetic resonance imaging in monitoring the treatment of multiple sclerosis: concerted action guidelines (Miller et al. 1991)
1992	High dose steroids in acute relapses of multiple sclerosis: MRI evidence for a possible mechanism of therapeutic effect (Miller et al. 1992)
1992	Gadolinium-pentetic acid magnetic resonance imaging in patients with relapsing–remitting multiple sclerosis (Capra et al. 1992)
1993	Interferon beta-1b is effective in relapsing–remitting multiple sclerosis. II. MRI analysis results of a multicenter, randomized, double-blind, placebo-controlled trial (Paty and Li 1993)
1994	Magnetic resonance in monitoring the treatment of multiple sclerosis (Miller 1994)
1994	Magnetic resonance imaging in monitoring the treatment of multiple sclerosis patients: statistical power of parallel-groups and crossover designs (Nauta et al. 1994)
1994	Longitudinal MRI in multiple sclerosis: correlation between disability and lesion burden (Khoury et al. 1994)
1994	Are magnetic resonance findings predictive of clinical outcome in therapeutic trials in multiple sclerosis? The dilemma of interferon-beta (McDonald et al. 1994)

Using Magnetic Resonance Imaging to Detect Treatment Efficacy

I think magnetic resonance imaging (MRI) of the cranium (brain) has had the greatest impact upon efficacy trials by the detection of intergroup differences in parallel group designs (placebo and active agent are given to separate groups of patients during the same period) (Miller et al. 1991). MRI can also provide "hints of efficacy" in early preliminary trials for safety and tolerance. If the treatment is effective, MRI "lesions" decrease or cease; if the treatment is not effective, the lesions continue.

Initially, T2-weighted images (frequency of "lesions", area, volume and new or enlarging lesions) were used. Usually several years of follow-up would be required to detect differences in the populations investigated. Paty et al. (1993) performed yearly MRI analyses on 327 of 372 patients in a full (pivotal) 2–3-year trial of interferon beta-1b (Betaseron®, Berlex). With the percentage change in total disease burden (mm^2) the placebo treated patients' group median change increased by 10.9% by the end of the first year, 16.5% by the end of the second year, and 15.0% by the end of the third year. The values for patients receiving 8 MIU were –6.2% for year 1, –0.8% for year two, and –9.3% at the end of the third year. Mean (average) group change values from baseline gave almost identical results. Patients taking 1.6 MIU showed intermediate results. In a subgroup who had MRI every 6 weeks, the disease activity as measured by the number of active scans (an active scan was any scan showing any new, recurrent or enlarging lesion) revealed similar differences. The median percentage of scans active for the placebo group was 29.4; it was 11.8 for 1.6 MIU, and 5.9 for 8 MIU ($P = 0.0062$, placebo versus 8 MIU). Paty's later analysis of the interferon beta-1b trial concluded there was a 70% median reduction of MRI activity over a 2-year trial period in patients receiving the interferon (Paty 1994).

Other investigators also have found serial MRI to be useful. Durelli and colleagues showed that systemic high dose recombinant interferon alpha-2a reduced MRI "signs of disease activity", as well as relapse rate and gamma interferon production by lymphocytes (Durelli et al. 1994). A "pilot" trial of cladribine, a potent lympholytic drug, in patients in the progression phase of MS revealed a drop in "demyelinated volume" compared with baseline by the recipients, but not those receiving placebo (Sipe et al. 1994). Kurtzke's and Scripp's scores and concentrations of cerebrospinal fluid oligoclonal bands also improved. Stone et al. found interferon-beta-1b (IFN-β1b; Beraseron® (Berlex)) treatment reduced total lesion frequency from 3.06/month during 7 months' pretreatment to 0.48/month during 6 months' treatment ($P = 0.002$, Wilcoxon signed-rank test) (Stone et al. 1995).

Paty recently concluded that current MRI techniques are at least five times more sensitive to disease activity than clinical measurements. In the interferon-beta-1b trial, he opined that the MRI was approximately twice as sensitive to treatment effects as the clinical measurements (Paty 1994).

Areas of increased signal intensity in T1-weighted images using gadolinium enhancement correlate better with clinical phenomena and appear to be more responsive (sensitive to change) more quickly than T2-weighted "lesions". Gadolinium may enable us to gain some idea of efficacy in a preliminary trial with only 2 or 3 months of follow-up (McFarland et al. 1992). If MRI changes continue in the face of treatment, we deduce that the intervention is not likely to be effective (efficacious).

In a study of nine patients with mild relapsing–remitting MS, Smith and colleagues recorded neurologic examination results, Expanded Disability Status Scale (EDSS) scores and 24–37-monthly gadopentetate dimeglumine-enhanced lesion numbers and areas. Using logistic regression, they found that an increase in the number and area of enhancing lesions occurred in association with onset and continuation of clinical worsening (Smith et al. 1993). Frank and colleagues found that a "burst" of enhancing lesion number and area above an individual's mean lesion frequency was correlated with an increase ≥0.5 steps in the EDSS (Frank et al. 1994). Kidd and colleagues found that 11 patients with early relapsing–remitting MS (average disease duration 3.5 years) had more new, enlarging or enhancing MRI lesions than those with benign MS (average disease duration 22 years) (Kidd et al. 1994).

Miller and colleagues found that 3 days of high dose intravenous methylprednisolone reduced the blood–brain barrier abnormality in 96% of enhancing lesions. Nevertheless, many lesions re-enhanced and new abnormalities occurred when the steroid was stopped (Miller et al. 1992). Barkhof et al. reported that steroid treatment was followed by clinical improvement in 15 of 20 courses, decreased the gadolinium enhancement in 12 of 16 scans, and returned the cerebrospinal fluid myelin basic protein to reference levels. They concluded methylprednisolone reduced inflammation and myelin breakdown (Barkhof et al. 1992). Subsequently, they reported that high dose intravenous methylprednisolone treatment temporarily (average 9.7 weeks) reduced enhancement as well as the duration and severity of clinical relapses (Barkhof et al. 1994). Since lesions detected on T2-weighted scans were minimally changed, the investigators concluded that the effect of the steroid was primarily on the blood–brain barrier and inflammation rather than on demyelination.

Preliminary Therapeutic Trials: Detecting Agents that are Not Likely to be Beneficial

MRI can help to demonstrate that an intervention is unlikely to be efficacious early in the development process. Using a pre-post treatment design (patients who have outcome variables available for some time before the experimental treatment is begun continue to have the same variables recorded during and after the treatment) Kinnunen et al. found four of six patients with chronic progressive disease who were treated with recombinant interferon alpha-2b 3 MIU subcutaneously daily for 6 months, had new or enlarging MRI lesions and worsened clinically; they had decreased natural killer cells (CD16+), increased intrathecal IgG synthesis and oligoclonal bands (Kinnunen et al. 1993). Even without MRI, we can detect ineffective therapies. It just takes longer.

In early trials for safety and tolerance, we have continued to use "historical controls". To our chagrin, we demonstrated that the outcome with an experimental therapy (gold sodium thiomalate) was worse than treatment with placebo (Ellison et al. 1992a).

Pilot and Full Trials (Table 1.2)

A major clinical advance came, perhaps inadvertently, when investigators stratified (e.g. limited entry criteria to those with an EDSS score ≤5.5 or ≥6.0) patients. This maneuver decreased the variability (and hence the standard deviations) and should have reduced the sample size necessary to detect dramatically effective therapies. In practice, what has really happened is that we can detect treatments that are only partially effective rather than curative.

Past, Present and Future Difficulties in Clinical Trial Design

Generic Problems

I think the most serious past, present and future problem we must overcome is the mismatch between the expectations of those struck by MS and the reality of the trial results. I believe that all of us – investigators, patients and significant others – hope so desperately for a cure that we do not digest emotionally the real limitations of current treatments for MS that we so clearly agree upon

Table 1.2. Milestones in therapeutic trials since 1990

Year	Reference
1991	The Canadian cooperative trial of cyclophosphamide and plasma exchange in progressive multiple sclerosis (Canadian Cooperative Multiple Sclerosis Study Group 1991)
1991	Overview of azathioprine treatment in multiple sclerosis (Yudkin et al. 1991)
1991	The natural history of multiple sclerosis: a geographically based study. 4. Application to planning and interpretation of clinical therapeutic trials (Weinshenker et al. 1991)
1991	A placebo-controlled, double-blind, randomized, two-center pilot trial of Cop 1 in chronic progressive multiple sclerosis (Bornstein et al. 1991)
1992	Effect of age on response to chronic progressive multiple sclerosis patients to cyclophosphamide booster therapy (Weiner et al. 1992)
1993	Interferon beta-1b is effective in relapsing–remitting multiple sclerosis: I. Clinical results of a multicenter, randomized, double-blind, placebo-controlled trial (IFNB Multiple Sclerosis Study Group 1993)
1993	Expanded clinical trials of treatments for multiple sclerosis (Whitaker et al. 1993)
1993	Clinical trials in multiple sclerosis: a critical review (1970–1990) (Bergamaschi et al. 1993)
1994	Multiple sclerosis: approaches to management (Silberberg 1994)
1994	The impact of blinding on the results of a randomized, placebo-controlled multiple sclerosis clinical trial (Noseworthy et al. 1994)
1994	Magnetic resonance imaging in monitoring the treatment of multiple sclerosis patients: statistical power of parallel-groups and crossover designs (Nauta et al. 1994)
1994	Time series for modeling counts from a relapsing–remitting disease: application to modeling disease activity in multiple sclerosis (Albert et al. 1994)
1994	Cladribine in treatment of chronic progressive multiple sclerosis (Sipe et al. 1994)
1994	Results of Phase III trial of intramuscular recombinant beta interferon as treatment for multiple sclerosis (Jacobs et al. 1994)
1995	Low-dose (7.5 mg) oral methotrexate reduces the rate of progression in chronic progressive multiple sclerosis (Goodkin et al. 1995)
1995	Copolymer 1 reduces relapse rate and improves disability in relapsing–remitting multiple sclerosis: Results of a Phase III multicenter, double-blind, placebo-controlled trial (Johnson et al. 1995)
1995	Defining the clinical course of multiple sclerosis: results of an international survey (F. D. Lublin and S. C. Reingold, in press)
1995	Interferon beta-1b in the treatment of multiple sclerosis: Final outcome of the randomized controlled trial (IFNB Multiple Sclerosis Study Group et al. 1995)

intellectually. Please recognize that, when the results of a trial are not those for which we hoped, the designs are not faulty; the agents just are not as effective as all of us want! On the other hand, do not lose sight of the advances occurring incrementally. Ultimately, we may administer combination therapies, such as the oncologists use, rather than a single "cure".

Another thorny problem has arisen: who controls or owns the trial data? Pharmaceutical companies have legitimate proprietary interests in controlling access and reporting. However, the data have great value for future trial design, since untreated and placebo treated patients will be increasingly more difficult to find. I think parallel analysis by the pharmaceutical firm and the investigative team, as was done in the interferon beta-1a trial, is the way to go (Jacobs et al. 1994). Fortunately, since the National Multiple Sclerosis Society (NMSS) (USA) has recently started a registry and database, several pharmaceutical firms are co-operating and releasing their data to the Society.

We desperately need a better clinical or laboratory measure; a "gold standard" that summarizes the changes over time of the neurologic state of the person with the syndrome of MS. Since we do not know the etiology, let alone the pathogenesis, of MS, all clinical measures are "surrogates". There are even differences in the definition of surrogate (Whitaker et al. 1995). I dream of a simple, accurate, precise, responsive and inexpensive urine or saliva test.

Clinical Classification

There is continuous effort to classify patients more accurately into type of course. The Advisory Committee on Clinical Trials of New Agents in MS of the NMSS (USA) surveyed the international clinical research community and has specified consensus definitions of the clinical courses of MS (Lublin and Reingold, 1996).

The recommended course labels are:

1. Relapsing-remitting MS ;
2. Primary progressive MS;
3. Secondary progressive MS;
4. Progressive-relapsing MS.

Because no consensus was reached for relapsing-progressive MS, the category was abandoned. Secondary progressive becomes the preferred term for patients who begin with relapses and whose baseline between attacks progressively worsens.

It is hoped that the new classification will improve patient selection for trials and subsequent generalizability when therapies are applied by practitioners. However, with the exception of a secondary progressive course (Minderhoud et al. 1988), the past type of course is not a very good predictor for future worsening (Ellison et al. 1989, 1994; Goodkin and Rudick 1989; Myers et al. 1993). The EDSS score at entry into the trial appears to be a much more important predictor (Bornstein et al. 1987; Ellison et al. 1992b; Weiner et al. 1989, Weinshenker et al. 1989, 1991).

Clinical Measures (Variables, Outcomes)

Unfortunately, the most widely used clinical rating system, John Kurtzke's Functional Systems Status Scale (FSS) and EDSS scores, have moderate intraobserver, high interobserver variation, and are insensitive to change (unresponsive) (Noseworthy 1994). Nevertheless, when challenged to devise a "better" measure, investigators quickly learn the magnitude of the problem (Whitaker et al. 1995).

At the University of California, Los Angeles, we (B. D. Leake, M. R. Mickey, L. W. Myers, K. Syndulko and W. W. Tourtellotte) have investigated linear, interval, continuous, quantified tests of neurologic function for two decades. Although the analysis of these tests continues, I think that the gains in accuracy and precision within an individual patient are offset by the interpatient differences. The implications of this variability between individuals are: it is likely that standard deviations of raw measures will be high (therefore mandating large sample sizes for therapeutic trials), and some variation on a change score for each person (end minus beginning, slope) will be necessary for a primary outcome measure (Ellison et al. 1994).

There are other difficulties with quantified tests. Although tests administered by a masked (blind to the treatment) examiner are appealing, the instruments and personnel to perform the tests add to the cost. The patients resist lengthy test sessions and dream up many excuses for breaking appointments if they must make a visit in addition to their "regular" one to the trial center. Most importantly, they are severely threatened when they observe worsening in their scores and avoid returning.

I think stratification by the entry EDSS has already markedly improved the situation and may make quantified tests unnecessary.

I agree completely with Noseworthy that the opinions of the patient and the examining neurologist should receive more attention (Noseworthy 1994). Gulick and colleagues reported that the patient and staff will agree (≤1 step) on scores for the EDSS 72% of the time and the FSS 73%–86% of the time (Gulick et al. 1993). The intraclass correlation coefficient (ICC) is 0.84 for the EDSS, but only 0.26 for the FSS sensory score, and up to 0.69 for the pyramidal score (Solari et al. 1993).

Furthermore, anything we can do to simplify the patients' already enormous commitments of time, effort and money will be useful. It may be possible to gather the information for most of the FSS scores and the EDSS score by telephone (Scheinberg et al. 1986). Verdier-Taillefer et al. predicted the neurologists score (±1 point) 73% of the time with a self-administered patient "auto-questionnaire" using linear regression (Verdier-Taillefer et al. 1994).

Are these correlations "good enough?" The correlation coefficients were greater than 0.50 for five of the FSS and the EDSS, but lower for the Brainstem and Mental FSS scores. In aggregate, only the ICC of 0.84 for the EDSS justifies substituting the patient's opinion for the neurologist's (Solari et al. 1993). Therefore, we end up with at least two data sets: the patient's and the neurologist's. Then we encounter the multiple outcomes problem. Goodkin and colleagues may have made a major advance in dealing with multiple outcomes in the methotrexate trial (Goodkin et al. 1995).

A significant advance is the definition of "progression" as a 1.0 step increase in the EDSS, maintained for at least 3 months if the entry EDSS is 5.0 or below, and a 0.5 step if the entry EDSS is 5.5 or greater (Ellison et al. 1994; Goodkin et al. 1995; Jacobs et al. 1994). This definition has made survival analysis a powerful design and analytic technique for full trials.

Trials become more complicated daily. Many investigators are trying to capture changes in cognition since neuropsychologic tests correlate poorly with the EDSS. Now the Food and Drug Administration requires quality of life measures for full (pivotal, Phase III) trials (Devinsky 1995; Vickrey et al. 1995). To cope with these many demands, several task forces have been organized by the NMSS (USA) to develop specific guidelines for clinical scales (including neuropsychologic assessment and health related quality of life questionnaires), imaging and trial design (Whitaker et al. 1995).

If you want to be current in your thinking about the problems of measurement and clinical trial design, in addition to reading Chapters 4–7 of this book, you should consult the compendia edited by Silberberg and by Thompson (Silberberg 1994; Thompson 1995) and the publication by Whitaker et al. (1995).

Laboratory Measures Other than MRI

There are no universally accepted laboratory measures that predict the natural history of an individual or group of patients. There may be laboratory tests that reflect a biologic effect of an intervention (e.g. tumor necrosis factor alpha production by monocytes), but we do not know the relevance of such changes to the disorder called MS.

Nuwer et al. detected a beneficial effect of the combination of methylprednisolone and azathioprine on quantitative visual evoked potentials at the end of the second year of the trial. Although changes in the slopes of standard neurologic examination scores approached statistical significance 1 year later, Kurtzke's Disability Status Scale (DSS) scores never reached statistical significance (Nuwer et al. 1987). The analysis of such evoked potential data must be parametric and with the recognition that there will be many patients who will not exhibit any change for the better or worse (many zeros).

Magnetic Resonance Imaging

Because of marked patient-to-patient variation in the frequency of enhancing lesions, hoped for reductions in sample size may not occur (McFarland et al. 1992). The use of MRI with enhancement reduces the sample size needed for a parallel groups design from 630 without MRI to 90 patients per arm if monthly scans are done for 6 months (50% reduction in lesions/month, a power of 0.8, and alpha = 0.05 (two-tail test)). If an open crossover design is used, the sample size per arm drops from 156 to 12. If patients are selected on a high frequency of MRI lesions 4 months before randomization to a double-masked placebo-controlled trial with 6-monthly MRI, 31 patients per arm are necessary rather than 403. Since more than 400 MRI scans would be necessary, the latter design could be implemented in only a few centers.

Goodkin et al. have pointed out that all unenhanced lesions are not the same when it comes to detecting enlargement. If the baseline lesion is smaller than 0.67 cm^2, then the change must be 45.2% for a reliable value. Larger lesions must change by 24.2% (Goodkin et al. 1992).

Despite the fact that current MRI techniques are useful for detecting subclinical disease "activity", either by enhancing lesions or by lesion load, they correlate poorly with clinical impairment (disability). Magnetization transfer imaging and proton magnetic resonance spectroscopy may eventually be more useful for characterizing demyelination, axonal loss and chemical changes (Arnold et al. 1992; Filippi et al. 1995; Grossman 1994; Miller 1994). Natural history studies may or may not demonstrate relationships between MRI findings and clinical phenomena. In 1992, Thompson et al. were able to separate early relapsing–remitting MS from benign MS by new lesion formation and by enhancement (Thompson et al. 1992). Filippi et al. demonstrated with quantitative measurement of lesion load that monosymptomatic patients with a high MRI "lesion load" at presentation were likely to have a greater load as well as disability 5 years later (Filippi et al. 1994b). They also found subtle changes in T2-weighted supra- and infratentorial lesion load and normal appearing white matter T2 values in secondary progressive patients compared with those showing a benign course (Filippi et al. 1994a). Khoury et al. correlated changes and cumulative changes in EDSS scores, the Ambulation Index, and the number of MRI lesions in 18 patients undergoing frequent MRI, who were followed for 1 year. They concluded that MRI is a valid measure of disease "activity" (Khoury et al. 1994). Filippi et al. performed unenhanced T2-weighted brain MRI scans, separated by an interval of 24–36 months in 281 patients. They correlated changes in EDSS scores with new or enlarging MRI lesions. The correlations were statistically significant ($P = 0.02$ for new lesions and $P = 0.002$ for enlarging lesions), Spearman's rank correlation coefficients were low (0.13 for new lesions, 0.18 for enlarging lesions) (Filippi et al. 1995). On the other hand, MRI activity may increase generally, without any necessary clinical correlation (Capra et al. 1992).

The predictive value of reductions in MRI lesion burden or formation for stabilization of neurologic impairment as measured by the EDSS may not be high. In the interferon beta-1b (Betaseron®) trial there were reductions in brain MRI lesions without improvement in the EDSS change score (McDonald et al. 1994). Unfortunately, as McDonald pointed out, changes in the spinal cord MRI, which are not so easily detected, may be the locus of whatever determines progression.

Might a reduction of MRI lesions give us false hope? In five patients who had failed a variety of treatments, Smith et al. found a decrease in mean monthly contrast enhanced MRI lesions from 8.2 to one within 4 months of starting monthly intravenous pulse cyclophosphamide (Smith et al. 1995). Clinical improvement also occurred. However, full trials of cyclophosphamide have demonstrated marginal to no persisting improvement (Canadian Cooperative Multiple Sclerosis Study Group 1991; Likosky et al. 1991; Weiner et al. 1993.)

It seems a tautology that, if a potential therapeutic agent fails to reduce MRI lesions, it is not promising. If it does stop or reduce them, the agent may be efficacious for some, but not all, of the processes that worsen the clinical state of the patient (progression). This might be so if repair does not occur, or if the processes causing slow progression are unaffected by the agent. We have already discovered that high dose Solumedrol® may stop enhancement for a time but clinical improvement may not follow and new lesions may show up, even though the treatment continues.

The Design Itself

We must still wrestle with the questions, "What are we trying to change – relapses or progression?", and, "How best to measure the change?" I think it might be more useful to rephrase the question to, "Is the patient better, the same or worse, and by how much?"

Preliminary Trials

For preliminary trials, are "historical controls" appropriate if the experimental treatment is less effective than a placebo-treated group from the past 5–10 years? I vote yes.

I was hopeful that enhanced MRI would allow us to use the patient as his or her own control (pre-post design) and gain efficacy information early in the clinical trial pathway, but now I am not so sure (Stone et al. 1995). For example, I have difficulty in reconciling the encouraging report of the effect of mitoxantrone on clinical deterioration and cessation of MRI lesions by Mauch et al. with the very negative studies of Noseworthy et al. and Bastianello and colleagues (Bastianello et al. 1994; Mauch et al. 1992; Noseworthy et al. 1993). Mauch et al. investigated mitoxantrone in ten patients with a rapidly deteriorating course and a total of 169 enhancing lesions. During the 10 months of treatment, only ten lesions appeared in nine patients, and clinical improvement or stabilization occurred.

Noseworthy and colleagues could not confirm this encouraging study (Noseworthy et al. 1993). In 13 patients with chronic progressive MS, eight of 12 had MRI activity on 13 of 29 follow-up evaluations. Comparison with two historical control groups – active and placebo-treated patients with progression of their MS in the Canadian Cooperative Trial of cyclophosphamide and plasma exchange – did not reveal any clinical efficacy.

Bastianello et al. also concluded that low dose mitoxantrone was not a promising therapy for relapsing-remitting MS in a 1-year trial, with only 25 patients (12 placebo, 13 mitoxantrone) and based upon serial gadolinium-DTPA-enhanced MRI. They found no statistically significant differences between the two groups in the average change of the EDSS or in the frequency of new or enlarging enhancing lesions (Bastianello et al. 1994).

Pilot Trials

It has once again been shown that a bias toward the declaration of efficacy is a hazard of "open label" investigations, wherein the examining neurologist is not blinded (masked) (Noseworthy 1994; Noseworthy et al. 1994). Agents for the relapsing-remitting type of MS must be tested against an interferon (active drug control) (Ellison et al. 1994). This will increase the sample sizes dramatically and may slow the development of multiple simultaneous interventions (for example, beta interferon and copolymer 1 and/or azathioprine or methotrexate). Sequential designs, wherein we might wait for "treatment failure" before adding the second agent, will come up, but I think the time to failure based upon clinical measures will be so long that these designs are not feasible. MRI continuing lesions above a threshold value could make this design realistic. Tacitly, we already are moving in this direction in preliminary trials.

Now that we know there are confounding and predictive covariates (EDSS score at entry, age less than or greater than 40 years (Weiner et al. 1992), MRI lesion burden at entry (Filippi et al. 1994b), MRI activity before entry, must we design these into the trial? If we do, I think the distinction between "pilot" and "full" trials will blur. Certainly, if we are to reach the desired power (0.8 or greater) the sample sizes will mushroom enormously. Perhaps it is time to reconsider matched pair designs (Bornstein et al. 1987; Ellison et al. 1980; Sipe et al. 1994).

Full Trials

All the considerations discussed above for pilot trials apply to pivotal or full trials. The inexorable increase in sample size will strike these trials hard. In addition, the variations between clinical sites must be taken into account when sample size calculations are made. Since the Food and Drug Administration now requires health-related quality of life measures for full (pivotal, Phase III) trials, we will face the multiplicity of outcomes problem when we perform the power calculations. For pivotal trials, time to an event (survival analysis) has many advantages, but it may not reduce sample sizes.

Conclusions

Preliminary Trials

1. For preliminary trials of safety, tolerance, and regimen relying on clinical measures for outcome, we can detect interventions that are unlikely to be beneficial by comparison with "historical controls" who have received placebos.
2. If the outcome in the new treatment group is *worse* than in the historical control group, we will not pursue the agent.
3. If the outcome measure is based upon MRI lesion formation (new, enhancing, expanding), we can use the patient as the control if we use a pre-post repeated measures design.
4. If lesions or clinical deterioration continue in the face of the experimental therapy, we conclude the treatment is unlikely to be beneficial.

Pilot (Phase II) Trials

1. These will probably be used less and less.
2. As agents move through preliminary trials, if they appear safe and

tolerable with a well-defined regimen, the agent will be advanced to a full trial immediately if MRI lesions are reduced below a threshold value.

3. A masked (blinded) neurologist evaluator will add to the validity of the trial, but quantified tests by a masked observer may be just as "good".
4. Somehow, if we are going to keep the sample sizes of future trials within reasonable limits, we must find a single primary outcome variable; is it the Kurtzke EDSS?

Full (Pivotal, Phase III) Trials

1. For efficacy trials, we must remember that we are treating human beings rather than MRI lesions.
2. Therefore, there is no substitute for the parallel group, double-masked, placebo or accepted treatment concomitant controlled clinical trial with clinically important outcome measures.
3. Assuming the Kurtzke EDSS is the primary outcome measure, I think stratification of patients into two groups: EDSS score ≤5.5, and EDSS score ≥6.0, has been the single most important clinical advance.
4. On the one hand, because of stratification, Kurtzke's EDSS may be adequate, despite its failings, and "better" measures (continuous, interval) could be unnecessary. If so, we should not devote resources to developing them!
5. On the other hand, some trials will require an "active" or approved treatment group and sample sizes will increase dramatically as the power of the trial is increased to show "equivalence". Continuous, interval measurements or their derivatives are likely to give more precision and help to counter the escalation of the numbers of subjects required.
6. The patient's and the examining (blinded, masked) neurologist's opinions should be investigated as the "gold standard" by which efficacy is finally determined.
7. Let us keep our eyes on the ball: MS is no longer an untreatable condition! We are making incremental gains with increasing frequency and rapidity. You can quote me: I predict Multiple Sclerosis Eradication Day will be 1 January, 2001.

Acknowledgements

Supported by NINDS grant NS08711, the Conrad N. Hilton Foundation, the Nancy Davis Foundation for Multiple Sclerosis, various donors, and the people of the State of California.

References

Albert PS, McFarland HF, Smith ME et al. (1994) Time series for modelling counts from a relapsing-remitting disease: applications to modelling disease activity in multiple sclerosis. Stat Med 13:453–466

Arnold DL, Matthews PM, Francis GS et al. (1992) Proton magnetic resonance spectroscopic imaging for metabolic characterization of demyelinating plaques. Ann Neurol 31(Suppl 3):235–241

Barkhof F, Hommes OR, Scheltens P, Valk J (1991) Quantitative MRI changes in gadolinium-DTPA enhancement after high-dose intravenous methylprednisolose in multiple sclerosis. Neurology 41:1219–1222

Barkhof F, Frequin ST, Hommes OR et al. (1992) A correlative triad of gadolinium-DTPA MRI, EDSS, and CSF-MBP in relapsing multiple sclerosis patients treated with high-dose intravenous methyprednisolone. Neurology 42:63–67

Barkhof F, Tas MW, Frequin ST et al. (1994) Limited duration of the effect of methylprednisolone on changes on MRI in multiple sclerosis. Neuroradiology 36:382–387

Bastianello S, Pozzilli D, D'Andrea F et al. (1994) A controlled trial of mitoxantrone in multiple sclerosis: serial MRI evaluation at one year. Can J Neurol Sci 21:266–270

Bergamaschi R, Citterio A, Filippini G et al. (1993) Clinical trials in multiple sclerosis: a critical review. Acta Neurologica (Napoli) 15:462–474

Bornstein MB, Miller A, Slagle S et al. (1987) A pilot trial of Cop 1 in exacerbating-remitting multiple sclerosis. N Engl J Med 317:408–414

Bornstein MB, Miller A, Slagle S et al. (1991) A placebo-controlled, double-blind, randomized, two-center pilot trial of Cop 1 in chronic progressive multiple sclerosis. Neurology 41:533–539

Broman T (1970) Management of patients with multiple sclerosis. In: Vinken PJ, Bruyn GW (eds) Multiple sclerosis and other demyelinating diseases. North-Holland Publishing Company, Amsterdam, pp 408–425 (Handbook of Clinical Neurology, vol. 9)

Canadian Cooperative Multiple Sclerosis Study Group (1991) The Canadian cooperative trial of cyclophosphamide and plasma exchange in progressive multiple sclerosis. Lancet 337:441–446

Capra R, Marciano N, Vignolo LA et al. (1992) Gadolinium-pentetic acid magnetic resonance imaging in patients with relapsing-remitting multiple sclerosis. Arch Neurol 49:687–689

Devinsky O (1995) Outcome research in neurology: incorporating health-related quality of life. Ann Neurol 37:141–142

Durelli L, Bongioanni MR, Cavallo R et al. (1994) Chronic systemic high-dose recombinant interferon alfa-2a reduces exacerbation rate, MRI signs of disease activity, and lymphocyte interferon gamma production in relapsing-remitting multiple sclerosis. Neurology 44:406–413

Ellison GW, Mickey MR, Myers LW et al. (1980) A pilot study of amantadine treatment of multiple sclerosis. In: Bauer HJ, Poser S, Ritter G (eds) Progress in multiple sclerosis research. Springer; Berlin, pp 407–408

Ellison GW, Myers LW, Mickey MR et al. (1989) The variable course of multiple sclerosis. Neurology 39(Suppl 1):357

Ellison GW, Myers LW, Leake BD et al. (1992a) A preliminary trial of gold sodium thiomalate (gst) for multiple sclerosis. Neurology 42(Suppl 3):209

Ellison GW, Myers LW, Leake BD (1992b) Disability scale influence on rate of worsening of multiple sclerosis patients. Ann Neurol 32:259A

Ellison GW, Myers LW, Leake BD et al. (1994) Design strategies in multiple sclerosis clinical trials. Ann Neurol 36:S108–S112

Filippi M, Barker GJ, Horsfield MA et al. (1994a) Benign and secondary progressive multiple sclerosis: a preliminary quantitative MRI study. J Neurol 241:246–251

Filippi M, Horsfield MA, Morrissey SP et al. (1994b) Quantitative brain MRI lesion load predicts the course of clinically isolated syndromes suggestive of multiple sclerosis. Neurology 44:635–641

Filippi M, Paty DW, Kappos L et al. (1995) Correlations between changes in disability and T2-weighted brain MRI activity in multiple sclerosis: a follow-up study. Neurology 45:255–260

Frank JA, Stone LA, Smith ME et al. (1994) Serial contrast-enhanced magnetic resonance imaging in patients with early relapsing-remitting multiple sclerosis: implications for treatment trials. Ann Neurol 36:S86–S90

Goodkin DE, Rudick RA (1989) Exacerbation rates and adherence to disease type in a prospectively followed MS population: implications for clinical trials. Neurology 39:357

Goodkin DE, Ross JS, Medendorp SV et al. (1992) Magnetic resonance imaging lesion enlargement in multiple sclerosis. Disease-related activity, chance occurrence, or measurement artifact? Arch Neurol 49(Suppl 3):261–263

Goodkin DE, Rudick RA, Medendorp SV et al. (1995) Low-dose (7.5 mg) oral methotrexate reduces the rate of progression in chronic progressive multiple sclerosis. Ann Neurol 37:30–40

Grossman RI (1994) Magnetization transfer in multiple sclerosis. Ann Neurol 36(Suppl):S97–S99

Gulick EE, Cook SD, Troiano R (1993) Comparison of patient and staff assessment of MS patients health status. Acta Neurol Scand 88:87–93

IFNB Multiple Sclerosis Study Group (1993) Interferon beta-1b is effective in relapsing–remitting multiple sclerosis: I. Clinical results of a multicenter, randomized double-blind, placebo-controlled trial. Neurology 43:655–661

IFNB Multiple Sclerosis Study Group, University of British Columbia MS/MRI Analysis Group (1995) Interferon beta-1b in the treatment of multiple sclerosis: final outcome of the randomized controlled trial. Neurology 45:1277–1285

Jacobs LD, Cookfair R, Rudick R et al. (1994) Results of a Phase III trial of intramuscular recombinant beta interferon as treatment for multiple sclerosis [abstract]. Ann Neurol 36:259

Johnson KP, Brooks BR, Cohen JA et al. (1995) Copolymer 1 reduces relapse rate and improves disability in relapsing–remitting multiple sclerosis: results of a Phase III multicenter, double-blind, placebo-controlled trial. Neurology 45:1268–1276

Khoury SJ, Guttmann CR, Orav EJ et al. (1994) Longitudinal MRI in multiple sclerosis: correlation between disability and lesion burden. Neurology 44(Suppl 11):2120–2124

Kidd D, Thompson AJ, Kendall BE et al. (1994) Benign form of multiple sclerosis: MRI evidence for less frequent and less inflammatory disease activity. J Neurol Neurosurg Psychiatry 57(Suppl 9):1070–1072

Kinnunen E, Timonen T, Pirttila T et al. (1993) Effects of recombinant alpha-2b-interferon therapy in patients with progressive MS. Acta Neurol Scand 87:457–460

Likosky WH, Fireman B, Elmore R et al. (1991) Intense immunosuppression in chronic progressive multiple sclerosis: the Kaiser study. J Neurol Neurosurg Psychiatry 54:1055–1060

Lublin FD, Reingold SC (1996) Defining the clinical course of multiple sclerosis: results of an international survey. Neurology: in press

Mauch E, Kornhuber HH, Krapf H et al. (1992) Treatment of multiple sclerosis with mitoxantrone. Eur Arch Psychiatry Clin Neurosci 242:96–102

McDonald WI, Miller DH, Thompson AJ (1994) Are magnetic resonance findings predictive of clinical outcome in therapeutic trials in multiple sclerosis? The dilemma of interferon-beta. Ann Neurol 36:14–18

McFarland HF, Frank JA, Albert PS et al. (1992) Using gadolinium-enhanced magnetic resonance imaging lesions to monitor disease activity in multiple sclerosis. Ann Neurol 32:758–766

Miller DH (1994) Magnetic resonance in monitoring the treatment of multiple sclerosis. Ann Neurol 36:S91–S94

Miller DH, Barkhov F, Berry I et al. (1991) Magnetic resonance imaging in monitoring the treatment of multiple sclerosis: concerted action guidelines. J Neurol Neurosurg Psychiatry 54:683–688

Miller DH, Thompson AJ, Morrissey SP et al. (1992) High dose steroids in acute relapses of multiple sclerosis: MRI evidence for possible mechanism of therapeutic effect. J Neurol Neurosurg Psychiatry 55(Suppl 6):450–453

Minderhoud JM, van der Hoeven JH, Prange AJ (1988) Course and prognosis of chronic progressive multiple sclerosis. Results of an epidemiological study. Acta Neurol Scand 781:10–15

Myers LW, Ellison GW, Leake BD (1993) Progressive phase of multiple sclerosis not a useful entry criterion for therapeutic trials. Ann Neurol 34:312A

Myers LW, Ellison GW, Merrill JE et al. (1995) Pentoxifylline not a promising treatment for multiple sclerosis. Neurology 45(Suppl 4):A419

Nauta JJ, Thompson AJ, Barkhof F et al. (1994) Magnetic resonance imaging in monitoring the treatment of multiple sclerosis patients; statistical power of parallel-groups and crossover designs. J Neurol Sci 122:6–14

Noseworthy JH (1994) Clinical scoring methods for multiple sclerosis. Ann Neurol 36:S80–S85

Noseworthy JH, Hopkins MB, Vandervoort MK et al. (1993) An open-trial evaluation of mitoxantrone in the treatment of progressive MS. Neurology 43:1401–1406

Noseworthy JH, Ebers GC, Vandervoort MK et al. (1994) The impact of blinding on the results of a randomized, placebo-controlled multiple sclerosis clinical trial. Neurology 44:16–20

Nuwer MR, Packwood JW, Myers LW, Ellison GW (1987) Evoked potentials predict the clinical changes in a multiple sclerosis drug study. Neurology 37:1754–1761

Paty DW (1994) The interferon beta-1b clinical trial and its implications for other trials. Ann Neurol 36:S113–S114

Paty DW, Li DR (1993) Interferon beta-1b is effective in relapsing–remitting multiple sclerosis: II. MRI analysis results of a multicenter, randomized, double-blind, placebo-controlled trial.

Neurology 43:662–667
Rudick RA, Goodkin DE (eds) (1992) Treatment of multiple sclerosis: trial design, results, and future perspectives. Springer, London
Scheinberg L, Feldman J, Ratzker P et al. (1986) Self-assessment of neurological impairments in multiple sclerosis. Neurology 36 (Suppl 1):284
Silberberg DH (ed) (1994) Multiple sclerosis: approaches to management. Ann Neurol 36:S1–S162
Sipe JC, Romine JS, Koziol JA et al. (1994) Cladribine in treatment of chronic progressive multiple sclerosis. Lancet 344:9–13
Smith ME, Stone LA, Albert PS et al. (1993) Clinical worsening in multiple sclerosis is associated with increased frequency and area of gadopentetate dimeglumine-enhancing magnetic resonance imaging lesions. Ann Neurol 33:480–489
Smith ME, Albert PS, Stone LA et al. (1995) The use of MRI to evaluate individual heterogeneity in treatment response in multiple sclerosis. Neurology 45:A435
Solari A, Amato MP, Bergamaschi R et al. (1993) Accuracy of self-assessment of the minimal record of disability in patients with multiple sclerosis. Acta Neurol Scand 87:43–46
Stone LA, Frank JA, Albert PS et al. (1995) The effect of interferon-β on blood–brain barrier disruptions demonstrated by contrast-enhanced magnetic resonance imaging in relapsing-remitting multiple sclerosis. Ann Neurol 37:611–619
Thompson AJ (ed) (1995) Measurement in multiple sclerosis. MS Management 2:3–57
Thompson AJ, Miller D, Youl B et al. (1992) Serial gadolinium-enhanced MRI in relapsing/remitting multiple sclerosis of varying disease duration. Neurology 42:60–63
Verdier-Taillefer MH, Roullet E, Cesaro P et al. (1994) Validation of self-reported neurological disability in multiple sclerosis. Int J Epidemiol 23:148–154
Vickrey BG, Hays RD, Harooni R et al. (1995) A health-related quality-of-life measure for multiple sclerosis. Qual Life Res 4:187–206
Weiner HL, Dau P, Khatri B et al. (1989) Double-blind study of true versus sham plasma exchange in patients being treated with immunosuppression for acute attacks of multiple sclerosis. Neurology 39:1143–1149
Weiner HL, Mackin GA, Orav EJ et al. (1992) Effect of age on response of chronic progressive multiple sclerosis patients to cyclophosphamide booster therapy. Neurology 42:465
Weiner HL, Mackin GA, Orav EJ et al. (1993) Intermittent cyclophosphamide plus therapy in progressive multiple sclerosis: final report of the Northeast Cooperative Multiple Sclerosis Treatment Group. Neurology 43:910–918
Weinshenker BG, Bass B, Rice GPA et al. (1989) The natural history of multiple sclerosis: a geographically based study: 2. Predictive value of the early clinical course. Brain 112:1419–1428
Weinshenker BG, Rice GP, Noseworthy JH (1991) The natural history of multiple sclerosis: a geographically based study: 4. Applications to planning and interpretation of clinical therapeutic trials. Brain 114:1057–1067
Whitaker JN, The Advisory Committee on Clinical Trials on New Agents in Multiple Sclerosis of the National Multiple Sclerosis Society (1993) Expanded clinical trials of treatments for multiple sclerosis. Ann Neurol 34:755–756
Whitaker JN, McFarland HF, Rudge P et al. (1995) Outcomes assessment in multiple sclerosis clinical trials: a critical analysis. Multiple Sclerosis 1:37–47
Yudkin PL, Ellison GW, Ghezzi A et al. (1991) Overview of azathioprine treatment in multiple sclerosis. Lancet 338:1051–1055

2 Pathogenesis of Multiple Sclerosis: Relationship to Therapeutic Strategies

Jorge R. Oksenberg and Stephen L. Hauser

Introduction

Among the chronic inflammatory disorders of humans, multiple sclerosis (MS) represents perhaps the most complex puzzle and a frustrating challenge to medical science. Having successfully teased three generations of immunologists and virologists, the underlying biology of MS remains only vaguely understood. The immunology of MS appears complex, in part because there have been so many observations, some conflicting, that do not result in a clear model of pathogenesis. Einstein noted that good science simplified one's understanding of the world, a criterion thus far not met in the MS arena. Certain fundamental questions must be answered before a coherent picture emerges. For example, what is the mechanism of chronic inflammation in MS? What triggers MS? What antigens (if any) are targeted? MS is generally considered to be an autoimmune disease, yet inflammation and selective destruction of central nervous system (CNS) elements may also occur in non-autoimmune conditions, diseases of known etiology including genetic disorders (adrenaleukodystrophy, metachromatic leukodystrophy) or chronic virus infections (HTLV-I or Theiler murine encephalomyelitis virus). The inflammatory changes that occur in MS may ultimately be shown to be secondary rather than primary, and only tentative assumptions of the nature of MS can reasonably be made at this time. This said, recent data from multiple converging sources lend support to the classical concept that MS is mediated by an aberrant immune response directed against one or several myelin proteins of the CNS (Tables 2.1 and 2.2). Such a response will develop only in a genetically susceptible individual, following some as yet undefined environmental exposure. The autoimmune model of the pathogenesis of MS has set the tone for immunotherapy in this disease, first by general immunosuppression using cytotoxic drugs and, more recently, by selectively targeting a specific component of the immune response (Oksenberg 1994).

A primary role for the immune system in the etiology of MS has been debated for more than a century, since the initial suggestion by Pierre Marie in 1884 that lesions of MS might represent a common complication to multiple infectious agents. Spirochaetes were claimed to be the cause of MS in 1917 and during the past 80 years more than 20 infectious agents have been reported, but not confirmed, to cause the disease. Beginning in the 1930s, work by Rivers and others defined the experimental autoimmune disease, experimental allergic encephalomyelitis (EAE), which bore some clinical and pathologic resemblance to human MS. In the cerebrospinal fluid (CSF) of patients, evidence for cellular inflammation and a selective increase in levels of locally synthesized immunoglobulin, was presented in the 1930s and 1940s, respectively. Searches for autoantibodies or other myelinotoxic factors date also from the 1930s. The demonstration in 1961 by Patterson that EAE could be adoptively transferred by specifically sensitized T cells inaugurated the era of T-cell immunology in MS research, an area that in many respects dominates the field to this day.

Table 2.1. MS as an autoimmune disease: evolution of thinking

Date	Development of knowledge
1835	First pathologic description of MS
1884	Relationship to infection is proposed
1932	Encephalitis accompanied by myelin destruction is experimentally produced in monkeys by multiple injections of rabbit cord tissue
1934	CSF inflammatory changes recognized in MS
1947	Elevated immunoglobulin levels in CSF
1960	T-cell mediation of experimental allergic encephalitis (EAE) demonstrated by adoptive transfer
1972	MS genetic susceptibility is associated with the major histocompatibility complex on chromosome 6
1977	The administration of soluble neuroantigens induce tolerance and regulate EAE
1980	IgG of restricted clonality with reactivity to myelin basic protein (MBP) eluted from MS brain
1982	The cellular composition of the inflammatory reaction in the MS plaque is described
1985	Molecular mimicry may operate in MS
1988	Suppression of EAE is achieved by oral administration of MBP
1988	Limited heterogeneity of lymphocytes mediating EAE allows T-cell antigen receptor (TCR)-specific immune intervention
1990	Identification of activated MBP-reactive cells in MS peripheral blood
1993	TCR rearrangements from MS brain lesions encode CDR3 regions identical to those found in T cells recognizing MBP
1993	Superantigens may be implicated in the initiation and/or recurrence of demyelination
1993	MBP-specific TCR transgenic mice develop spontaneous autoimmunity

Table 2.2. Putative autoantigens in MS

Myelin basic protein (MBP)
Proteolipid protein (PLP)
Myelin oligodendrocyte glycoprotein (MOG)
Myelin associated glycoprotein (MAG)
Heat shock proteins
β-arrestin and arrestin
Glial fibrillary acidic protein (GFAP)
Astrocyte-derived calcium-binding protein (S1000β)
Transaldolase

Our present view of the pathogenesis of MS has been markedly enhanced during the past several years by the identification of credible candidate autoantigens, the study of the role of major histocompatibility complex (MHC) gene products, the genetic analysis of the T-cell antigen receptor (TCR), and progress in the understanding of cytokine physiology. In addition, significant advances in the capacity to manipulate, control and understand EAE has led to a true revolution in knowledge of T-cell mediated demyelination. Indeed, sophisticated approaches for treatment of EAE by selective immune intervention are being attempted in MS at the present time (see Chapter 3) (Table 2.3). This review will focus on the immunopathology of the MS plaque, the mechanisms of plaque formation, the analysis of regulatory circuits required to maintain tolerance to CNS antigens, and the genetic basis of susceptibility to MS. We believe that the development of new and more effective therapy is likely to result from the use of new molecular tools to define the immune response in MS and to characterize its genetic basis.

Table 2.3. Experimental strategies for selective immunosuppressive therapy

Monoclonal antibodies to:
T-cell sub populations (CD4)[a]
T cell receptors[b]
Adhesion molecules[a]
Accessory molecules (CD40, CD80)[c]
MHC class II molecules[c]
Cytokine receptors[c]
Activation markers[c]
Macrophages[c]
Cytokines[c]
T-cell vaccination[a]
TCR peptide vaccination[a]
Immunomodulation (COP 1[a], Linomide[a])
Oral induced tolerance[a]
Inhalation induced tolerance[c]
Cytokine receptor analogs and antagonists[a]
Cytokines (IFN-β[a], TGF-β[b], IL-4[c], IL-10[c])
Antigen-induced programmed T-cell death (apoptosis)[c]
Antigen peptides TCR analogs and antagonists[c]
Blocking costimulation pathway (anergy)[c]
Blocking costimulation pathway (Th1/Th2 commitment)[c]
MHC class II–peptides complexes[b]
Anti-IgD peptide conjugates[c]
Superantigen modulation[c]
Metalloprotease inhibitors[c]
Blocking-signal transduction pathways[c]
cAMP-phosphodiesterase inhibitors[c]
Complement inhibitors[c]
Regulation of MHC gene expression[c]
Apoptosis-inducing antigens[c]

[a]Clinical trials
[b]Pre-clinical trial stage
[c]Experimental stage

Immunopathology of the MS Lesion

The pathologic hallmark of MS is the plaque, a well demarcated gray or pink lesion, characterized histologically by complete myelin loss, an absence of oligodendrocytes and relative sparing of axons. MS plaques are multiple, generally asymmetric, and tend to concentrate in deep white matter near the lateral ventricles, corpus callosum, floor of the fourth ventricle, deep periaqueductal region, optic nerves and tracts, corticomedullary junction and cervical spinal cord. The acute MS lesion is characterized by perivascular and parenchymal infiltration of mononuclear cells, both T cells and macrophages, and by myelin breakdown that appears to be mediated by the infiltrating cells. B cells and plasma cells are only rarely present. As lesions evolve, axons traversing the lesion show marked irregular beading; proliferation of astrocytes occurs, and lipid-laden macrophages containing myelin debris are prominent. Progressive fibrillary gliosis ensues and mononuclear cells gradually disappear. In some MS lesions, but not others, proliferation of oligodendrocytes appears to be present initially, but these cells are apparently destroyed as the gliosis progresses. Gliosis is more severe in MS than in most other neuropathologic conditions. In chronic MS lesions, complete, or nearly complete, demyelination, dense gliosis and loss of oligodendroglia are found. In some chronic active MS lesions, gradations in the histologic findings from the center to the lesion edge suggest that lesions expand by concentric outward growth. Axonal preservation is relative rather than absolute. In approximately 10% of lesions there is significant axonal destruction. Rarely, complete destruction of the neuropil and cavitation occur.

Controversy still surrounds the nature of the initial pathologic event in MS. The earliest detectable event in plaque development is an increase in permeability of the blood-brain barrier (BBB), associated with inflammation (McDonald 1994). Following the breach in the BBB, myelin appears to be the primary target of the pathologic immune reaction (Kermode et al. 1990; Raine 1994a). Lassman and colleagues found that oligodendrocytes were preserved in early lesions of relapsing MS but were destroyed in chronic lesions (Ozawa et al. 1994). Oligodendrocytes were also apparently destroyed in early aggressive cases. These findings suggested some variability of oligodendroglial destruction in different clinical forms of MS. Rodriguez et al. (1993) has proposed a different sequence of neuropathologic events. In a study of 11 stereotaxic brain lesion biopsy specimens, uniform widening of inner myelin lamellae (biphasic myelinopathy) and degeneration of inner glial loops ("dying-back" oligodendrogliopathy) were early pathologic abnormalities that preceded complete destruction of myelin sheaths. Because the oligodendrocytes were morphologically preserved in this early stage, the authors proposed that the initial event in MS is the functional interference with the myelinating capacity of these cells. Subsequently, degeneration of both the inner myelin lamellae and the inner oligodendroglial loop occur. As a consequence of this injury, novel or aberrant antigens may be exposed, triggering the infiltration of inflammatory cells (Rodriguez et al. 1993).

As the inflammation proceeds, oligodendrocytes at the periphery of the plaque, as well as astrocytes, proliferate under the influence of factors released into the microenvironment. Such oligodendrocytes, which appear to continue to function as myelinating cells, may be derived from surviving or progenitor cells (Wu and Raine 1992). When inflammation decreases, the edema disappears and conduction is restored, possibly as a result of the expansion of sodium channels into the demyelinated axon (McDonald 1994). Remyelination is not essential to remission.

Upregulation of MHC molecules has been proposed as a marker of plaque activity. Class I MHC antigens have been identified in plaque tissue on endothelial cells, infiltrating lymphocytes and astroglia, while class II determinants are reported to be expressed on endothelial cells, macrophages, microglia and astroglia. On the other hand, a recent study by Bo and colleagues (1994) provides compelling evidence that the only cells in the active lesions expressing class II antigens are macrophages and microglia. In any case, the high expression of MHC class II molecules in MS brains suggests that the local microenvironment may be enriched in MHC-activating factors such as interferon (IFN) -γ, and that antigen is possibly presented to T cells (Traugott et al. 1983). It is important to note, however, that in many silent plaques devoid of T-cell infiltrates, class II MHC may be expressed at high levels on reactive microglia. Upregulation of MHC class II antigens is not unique to MS tissue, as it has also been detected in neurodegenerative diseases and following trauma.

As noted above, the inflammatory reaction in active plaques is dominated by T lymphocytes and macrophages, whereas B lymphocytes and plasma cells are rare. The percentage of plasma cells in the inflammatory infiltrates is significantly higher in late chronic MS compared with acute MS (Lassman et al. 1994). Early studies demonstrated that lymphocytic perivascular cuffs are prominent at the edge of active plaques and are occasionally seen in areas with no evidence of demyelination or macrophage infiltration. T cells in the parenchyma and in the perivascular cuffs consisted of CD8+ (suppressor/cytotoxic) cells and variable numbers of CD4+ (helper/inducer) cells (Hauser et al. 1986b). The selective accumulation and compartmentalization of T cells indicate a specific pattern in the homing of T cells to the lesion, and suggests an immune response to a discrete antigenic complex. Indeed, restricted populations of activated T cells reactive against myelin components are present in the peripheral blood (Allegretta et al. 1990, 1994) and are compartmentalized in the CNS of MS patients (Lee et al. 1991; Oksenberg et al. 1990a; Renno et al. 1994; Usuku et al. 1992).

T Cells and Macrophages

The vast majority of CD4/CD8 T cells in the MS brain bear the common form of the antigen cell receptor (i.e. the α/β heterodimer). The TCR is expressed on the surface of mature T lymphocytes, which subserves T-cell recognition by fragments of antigen associated with MHC molecules. The antigen-binding variable domains of the TCR have a β barrel structure in which a conserved framework of β strands support three hypervariable loops termed complementary determining regions (CDRs). The putative CDR1 and CDR2 loops are encoded within the germline sequences of the variable (V) gene segments, while the CDR3 loops are encoded by the V, diversity (D) and joining (J) genes that rearrange in unique ways in individual developing T-cells, and include the use of non-germline N region nucleotide additions and/or deletions, generating dramatic increases in T-cell diversity (Usuku et al. 1992b). CDR3 regions play a critical role in peptide recognition. Modeling of the trimolecular interaction between the TCR, the MHC antigen-presenting molecules and bound antigenic peptide, suggests that the complementary-determining regions, CDR1 and CDR2 of the TCR, interact primarily with the alpha helical regions of the MHC, and provide the structural framework and topology for the interaction of a particular CDR3 region, (N)Jα and (N)Dβ(N)Jβ, with the peptide bound in the MHC cleft (Chothia et al. 1988; Jorgensen et al. 1992; Katayama et al. 1995). One of the authors (JRO) recently reported the study of TCRAV and TCRBV rearrangements using the polymerase chain reaction and sequence analysis in MS plaques (Oksenberg et al. 1993a). A limited number of TCR-V gene rearrangements were seen in 30 specimens from 16 MS brains. Of eight MS patients who had the MS-associated MHC type human leukocyte antigen (HLA)-DR2 (DRB1*1501, DQA1*0102, DQB1*0602 and either DPB1*0401 or 0402), seven had rearrangements of the TCRBV 5.2 gene in the lesions, compared with only two of seven MS brains from patients who were not DR2-positive. Genetic susceptibility to MS has been shown to be associated with the HLA-DR2 haplotype in caucasoid populations. It is conceivable that the bias in TCRBV gene expression resulted from activation of reactive T cells after encounters with peripheral or local exposed antigens presented by HLA-DR2-associated antigen-presenting molecules, and their subsequent trapping in the brain. In a related observation, Kotzin and colleagues (1991) found that 90% of T-cell lines that could be expanded from peripheral blood of DR2-positive patients and that reacted against the myelin component, myelin basic protein (MBP), expressed TCRBV 5.2 and/or TCRBV 6 genes. We then sequenced BV 5.2 positive cDNA clones from different anatomic regions of the brain of two DR2-positive MS patients. Instead of finding many different CDR3 sequences, as would be expected if no selection by antigen was operating, in the plaques of both patients five predominant amino acid CDR3 motifs were present: BV 5.2(Q)LR or BV 5.2LRGA, BV 5.2LGG, BV 5.2LVAG, BV 5.2LDG, and BV 5.2(Q)PT. None of these sequences was seen in BV 5.2 transcripts from control brain tissue or from the peripheral blood of individuals with the same HLA phenotype. After a search of more than 1500 CDR3 sequences that have been published, a few striking similarities emerged. One of the repeated BV 5.2 motifs found in MS brains contained the basic pattern LRGA at the V–D–J junction, which is identical to that found in a cytotoxic T-cell clone recognizing the MBP sequence 87–106, isolated from the peripheral blood of a DR2-positive MS patient. This CDR3 sequence is also seen in T-cell clones reactive to the MBP peptide 87–99, derived from the spinal cord of Lewis rats with EAE (MBP is the major autoantigen in most rodent models of EAE). Taken together, these results constitute the first evidence for an MBP-specific T-cell response in MS brain tissue. Although both the α and β TCR chains contribute to the peptide and MHC specificity of a T cell, identification of TCRB CDR 3 sequences identical to those found in bona fide T-cell lines known to be reactive against MBP 87–106 strongly suggests that MBP-specific T cells are present in the MS nervous system. The observation that some of the TCR sequences detected in the MS lesions are similar to those expressed by pathogenic encephalitogenic (i.e. disease-inducing) T-cell clones further suggests that these cells may be involved in the disease process. In a recent study, Hara and colleagues (1994) reported that the TCRBV gene sequences expressed by lymphocytes in spinal cord lesions taken from HTLV-I-associated myelopathy/tropical spastic paraparesis (HAM/TSP) autopsy cases, included restricted CDR3 motifs with a striking homology to those reported earlier in MS brains. Because no proviral DNA was amplified in any neuronal cells, including neurons and glial cells, demyelination of the spinal cord as a direct result of viral infection is unlikely. T cells expressing these restricted TCRBV CDR3 motifs may be somehow expanded or activated as a result of infection with HTLV-I. These results raise the possibility that tissue damage in HAM/TSP is mediated by autoreactive T cells, as in MS. An association between HTLV-I infection and MS was suggested in the mid-1980s, but the current weight of evidence argues strongly against a role for this human retrovirus in MS (Hauser et al. 1986a; Reddy et al. 1988; Oksenberg et al. 1990b).

T cells carrying the other form of the TCR, the γ/δ heterodimer, have been also identified in significant numbers in lesions of MS. Using immunocytochemistry, Selmaj and colleagues (1991) showed that γ/δ+ TCR T cells, while absent from control brain tissues, accumulated specifically at the margins of chronic active plaques, in which the acute phase reactant heat shock protein (hsp 65) was coexpressed on immature oligodendrocytes. In addition, clonal expansion of γ/δ T cells was detected in the brain, CSF and peripheral blood of MS patients with acute disease (Shimonkevitz et al. 1993; Wucherpfennig et al. 1992a). Bernard and colleagues reported that the majority of γ/δ cells in chronic plaques expressed the Vγ2 and Vδ2 chains. However, sequence analysis of such transcripts showed no evidence of clonal expansion (Hvas et al. 1993). Striking limited diversity of a Vδ2-Jδ3 TCR rearrangement was detected by Battistini and colleagues (1995) in chronic active lesions. Further studies are needed to ascertain whether γ/δ T cells are involved in the demyelinating process, whether they respond to heat shock and other stress-related proteins, or merely represent a non-specific recruitment of T cells into the CNS. It is noteworthy however, that peripheral blood γ/δ T cells can induce the lysis of fresh human oligodendrocytes in culture (Freedman et al. 1991). Detailed knowledge of the patterns of expression of TCR genes in MS might have implications for the treatment of this disease, given the success of preventing or reversing experimental demyelination with reagents that target specific V-region gene products (Acha-Orbea et al. 1988; Offner et al. 1991). It is important to remember however, that TCR studies on the inflamed brain represent just snapshots, which cover a short chapter in the history of the plaque.

The dynamics of the autoimmune T-cell infiltration into and out of the CNS parenchyma have proved difficult to investigate in humans. A more complete picture is emerging from studies in animal models. EAE can be induced in a variety of animal species, including non-human primates, by injection of myelin proteins or their peptide derivatives, as well as by adoptive transfer of CD4+ activated T cells specific for MBP or proteolipid protein (PLP) (Bernard et al.

1992). EAE is a prototypic experimental model for antigen-specific, T-cell-mediated autoimmunity. Based upon clinical, histologic and genetic similarities to the human disease, EAE is widely considered to be a relevant model for MS. The establishment of inflammatory EAE lesions and clinical disease is a multi-step event. It has been proposed that the first step requires that activated T cells cross the BBB. Activated lymphocytes that bear a memory phenotype (CD44+, Mel 14–), suggesting previous activation by antigen, and also express the adhesion molecule VLA-4 integrin (β1α4), become attached to appropriate receptors on endothelial cells at parajunctional areas, adjacent to the endothelial tight junctions, and then proceed to pass directly into the interstitial matrix. It is of considerable interest that this process occurs without regard to the antigen specificity of a T cell; thus MBP reactive cells cross the BBB with no greater efficiency than do activated cells that do not recognize a CNS antigen (Wekerle et al. 1994). Next, specific CD4+ T cells are reactivated in situ by fragments of myelin antigens presented in the framework of MHC class II molecules on the surface of antigen-presenting cells (macrophages, microglia and perhaps astrocytes). This leads to a second wave of inflammatory recruitment and clinical EAE. Proinflammatory cytokines such as TNF-α and IFN-γ are probably key mediators of the full-blown inflammatory response. Encephalitogenic myelin-specific T cells may not be capable of mediating EAE in the absence of this secondary leukocyte recruitment.

The prototypic EAE susceptible rat strain is Lewis. After injection of an encephalitogenic, MBP-reacting T-cell line into these animals, pathogenic T cells are detectable in the brain within a few hours (Karin et al. 1993). Until day 4, brain lesions are mostly populated by these cells. In contrast, by the time clinical paralysis occurs, the TCR genes rearranged in the CNS are quite diverse, indicating an heterogeneous (polyclonal) T-cell population (Bell et al. 1993; Karin et al. 1993). Following recovery from the acute attack, the TCR repertoire in the lesions is quite restricted again and similar to the early infiltrate. Similarly, in acute MS lesions, TCR gene transcripts are quite heterogeneous, whereas in chronic lesions they are more restricted (Oksenberg et al. 1993a; Wucherpfennig et al. 1992b). What is the likelihood of detecting TCR rearrangements associated with pathogenic T cells in a cellular infiltrate in inflamed brain? Brocke and colleagues recently characterized a murine (SJL/J) encephalitogenic T-cell clone specific for MBP 87–99. This particular clone contains TCRAV and TCRBV sequences homologous to those found in both human T-cell clones reactive to the same epitope and in the MS brain lesions (S. Brocke, personal communication). In addition to sequence homology, these pathogenic cells are of particular interest because they remain anergic in the EAE brain in animals that have recovered from clinical disease after selective immunotherapy with TCR agonist synthetic peptides. By studying chronic MS lesions, the critical signals among the TCRs rearranged in the cellular infiltrate could be deciphered from the noise. This may not have been feasible if more acute lesions had been examined (Oksenberg et al. 1993b).

Recently, the potent proinflammatory and chemoattractant functions of a new superfamily of chemokines were reported (Schall 1991; Schall et al. 1990). These structurally related chemokines share a conserved 4-cysteine motif and are subdivided into two groups, namely C–X–C and C–C, depending on whether or not there is an intervening amino acid between the first two cysteines. The chemokines of the C–X–C class act mainly on neutrophils, whereas the chemokines in the C–C class appear to act on mononuclear cells. RANTES is a member of the C–C class and may have important biologic activities in inflammatory lesions, such as seen in MS. RANTES is a small glycoprotein secreted by activated T cells, monocytes and endothelial cells, and is a chemotactic factor for monocytes and activated CD4+ T cells of the memory phenotype (CD45RO), which is known to accumulate at the site of the MS lesion. Furthermore, RANTES is present in synovial lining cells of patients with rheumatoid arthritis and in delayed-type hypersensitivity reactions. Preliminary data indicate the high expression of mRNA for this cytokine at the edge of active MS plaques (J. Hvas, personal communication).

The waves of cell recruitment into the brain are accompanied by the expression of various cytokines, adhesion molecules, and their receptors (Raine and Canella 1992). In human disease, acute lesions are positive for the adhesion molecule ICAM-1 and its receptor LFA-1, and negative for VCAM-1/VLA-4, whereas chronic lesions are highly positive for both adhesion molecule complexes (Cannella et al. 1991; Raine 1994b). In a more recent study, Cannella and Raine (1995) confirmed the higher expression of VCAM-1 in chronic active plaques compared with acute lesions. VCAM was also present in microglial cells and blood vessels. Strong expression of VLA-4 was detected on cells in perivascular cuffs and in the parenchyma. ICAM-1/LFA-1 was uniformly higher at all stages of lesion formation. The lower expression of VLA-4 in the acute plaque is puzzling because this molecule appears to be required for the entry of CD4+ T cells into the CNS parenchyma (Baron et al. 1993). Furthermore, Yednock and colleagues (1992) showed that the in vivo administration of an antibody against human VLA-4 integrin $\alpha4\beta1$ not only prevented the accumulation of leukocytes in the CNS but also inhibited the development of EAE in Lewis rats. Romanic and Madri (1994) showed that T cells that have transmigrated through endothelial cells in vitro or in vivo exhibit a specific downregulation and decrease in $\alpha4$ expression at the cell surface, providing an explanation to the lower expression of VLA-4 in the acute plaque. Following adhesion, T cells transmigrate through the endothelium and the subendothelial basal lamina into the matrix. Although macrophages are a rich source of enzymes that will disrupt the endothelium and allow traffic into the subendothelial basal lamina, T cells may have their own arsenal of proteases. Leppert and colleagues (1995) recently demonstrated that highly purified normal peripheral blood T lymphocytes express two matrix metalloproteinases, gelatinases A (72 kDa) and B (92 kDa). Both gelatinases are structurally related and share the proteolytic selectivity for basal lamina collagens. Gelatinase B is secreted constitutively, whereas gelatinase A is inducible in vitro on activation. The 72 kDa gelatinase A is also inducible in T cells upon adhesion to endothelial cells after binding to VCAM-1 (Romanic and Madri 1994). Inhibitors of gelatinases may offer new therapeutic avenues for MS and other inflammatory diseases.

T lymphocytes crossing the BBB would encounter perivascular macrophages constitutively expressing MHC class II. This encounter may be sufficient to present myelin antigens to specific T cells (Perry 1994). The resident microglia, lying within the parenchyma, would then become activated as a result of locally released cytokines. Brain parenchymal non-bone-marrow derived cells, such as astrocytes and endothelial cells, may be also capable of functioning as antigen-presenting cells (Fontana et al. 1984; Myers et al. 1993). Conversely, astrocytes may also play a role in limiting the progression of inflammatory lesions by failing to provide appropriate antigen-presenting costimulatory signals to the responding lymphocyte (Weber et al. 1994). A cascade of events that will result in plaque formation and demyelination has been started. Macrophages act not only as antigen-presenting cells to T lymphocytes but also as scavengers that remove debris and serve as a source of growth regulatory molecules and cytokines. Interactions between T cells and macrophages can result in proliferation of each of these cell types through the mediation of such molecules as IL-2 and colony stimulating factors respectively. Furthermore, endothelial and T cells can provide colony stimulating factors to the macrophage to prevent apoptosis and cell death and maintain activation. In addition, activated macrophages can produce an extraordinary number of biologically active molecules with profound effects on lymphocytes and macrophages themselves, as well as on endothelial and CNS cells.

The recruited macrophage is likely to be an additional key mediator of vascular and myelin damage in MS. By depleting the macrophage populations from animals with EAE, either by intraperitoneal injection of silica (Brosnan et al. 1981) or by liposomes containing dichloromethylene diphosphonate (Huitinga et al. 1993), amelioration of disease was achieved. Liposomes, delivered before the onset of clinical signs, will prevent disease, demonstrating that recruited macrophages (liposomes do not actually enter the CNS) also contribute to the effector phase of the disease. Membrane proteins involved in macrophage adherence to the endothelium include the CD11b/CD18 integrin, also known as the type 3 complement receptor (CR3). Intravenous injection of antibodies directed against epitopes in the CR3 molecule suppressed clinical signs of EAE, confirming the role of CR3 in macrophage homing toward inflammatory CNS lesions (Huitinga et al. 1993). Numerous questions remain to be answered in studies of the macrophage in MS. It will be important to determine the time of arrival to the plaque in relation to lymphocytes, and the details of their cell cycle inside the brain. The critical role that the macrophage may play in lesion formation suggests that finding means of controlling macrophage participation at all levels of demyelination could be critical in altering lesion progression.

B Cells and the Humoral Reaction

In most MS patients, an elevated level of intrathecally synthesized immunoglobulins can be detected in the CNS. Although the specificity of these antibodies is mostly unknown, antimyelin specificities have been reported (Bernard et al. 1981; Newcombe et al. 1982; Olsson et al. 1990). The role, if any, of these putative autoantibodies in the pathogenesis of MS is unclear. The antibodies may serve to opsonize the myelin sheath and make it more available for phagocytosis by macrophages. CNS immunoglobulins may also induce in vitro myelinolysis via activation of a Ca^{2+}-dependent myelin-associated protease acting on MBP (Kerlero de Rosbo and Bernard 1989). In the CSF, the presence of membrane attack complexes suggests a possible role for complement-mediated antibody damage in MS (Roddy et al. 1994). Evidence that antibodies may participate in CNS demyelination has been obtained in recent animal experiments. Little or no demyelination is usually observed in EAE induced in Lewis rats by injection of purified MBP or by passive transfer of MBP reactive lymphocytes (Bernard and Kerlero de Rosbo 1992). Extensive demyelination can be induced in these animals by intravenous injection of anti-MOG (myelin oligodendrocyte glycoprotein) monoclonal antibodies when the BBB is breached (Schluesener et al. 1987). It is important to note that polyclonal antibodies against MBP, PLP or myelin associated glycoprotein (MAG) have no such effect. Evidence for an anti-MOG role in the in vitro demyelination effect has also been reported (Kerlero de Rosbo et al. 1990). MOG is a member of the immunoglobulin supergene family and, interestingly, the gene encoding MOG maps within the MHC in human chromosome 6 (Pham-Dinh et al. 1993). It constitutes about 0.05% of CNS myelin proteins, and is located exclusively on oligodendrocyte surfaces and in the outermost lamellae of myelin sheaths, making it readily accessible to the immune attack (Brunner et al. 1989). As suggested by Bernard (Bernard and Kerlero de Rosbo 1992), these studies indicate that antibody-mediated demyelination may not necessarily involve recognition of quantitatively major myelin proteins as previously assumed, but rather of strategically located antigens. In addition, B cells probably participate in the process of antigen presentation to T cells (Parker 1993). The recent availability of B-cell knockout mice (i.e. genetically altered mice lacking immunoglobulin molecules) (Loffert et al. 1994), may allow a better definition of the role of B lymphocytes in autoimmune demyelination.

The Role of Cytokines

During the process of lesion formation, cytokines, growth factors and other small molecules, such as nitric oxide, induce and regulate numerous critical cell functions, including cell recruitment and migration, cell proliferation and cell death. Elucidation of their roles in MS may provide opportunities to use them as potential starting points for therapeutic intervention.

A variety of cytokines regulate the activation, differentiation, and proliferation of T lymphocytes. Under their influence, cells differentiate into two major pathways (Table 2.4). T(helper)h1 cells produce IL-2, IL-3 TNF-β and IFN-γ, and participate in inflammatory responses. Th2 cells produce IL-3, IL-4, IL-5 and IL-10. A third subset of T cells, Th0, with a pattern of cytokine production overlapping both Th1 and Th2, was identified, and may represent a precursor population. In contrast to Th1 cells, Th2 cells depend on IL-4 rather than IL-2 for their autocrine growth, and can proliferate to anti-CD3 antibodies in the absence of accessory cells.

One of the first cytokines to be recognized in MS lesions was IL-2 and its

Table 2.4. CD4+ Th1/Th2 dichotomy

Th1-type response	Th2-type response
Mediators	
IFN-γ	IL-3
IL-2	IL-4
IL-3	IL-5
GM-CSF	IL-6
TNF-β	IL-10
	IL-13
	GM-CSF
Functions	
Inhibition of Th2 (IFN-γ)	Inhibition of Th1 (IL-10)
B cell differentiation (IFN-γ, IL-2) (IgG2a+, IgG2b– and IgG3–)	B cell differentiation (IL-4, IL-5) (IgG1+, IgG4+ and IgGE+)
Promotion of cell-mediated immunity and DTH responses	Promotion of humoral immunity
	Promotion of tolerance
Macrophage Activation (IFN-γ)	Mast cells and eosinophils: differentiation (IL-3, IL-4, IL-5)

At least two different Th cell types arise from a common precursor (Th0 or ThP). IL-2 is the autocrine growth factor for Th1, and IL-4 acts preferentially on Th2 cells. In addition, Th cells are engaged in mutual antagonism. IFN-γ from Th1 and IL-10 from Th2 cells, inhibit the other sub-populations. Preferential activation of one T cell type may explain why the immune response may be predominantly "cellular" in some circumstances, and "humoral" in others.

receptor (Hofman et al. 1986). Since then, a large number of pro-inflammatory (IL-1, IL-6, RANTES, MIP-1α, TNF-α, TNF-β, IFN-γ) and regulatory (IL-10, IL-4, TGF-β) cytokines have been detected in the brain, peripheral blood and CSF of MS patients (Raine 1994a, b). It is probable that, acting in both paracrine and autocrine ways, they constitute a functional network that regulates the cellular interactions that operate in MS.

One of us (SLH) identified the cytokines IL-1 β, TNF-α, and IL-6 by specific radioimmunoassays in the CSF of patients with MS and other neurologic diseases (OND) (Hauser et al. 1990). There was a high incidence of detectable IL-1β in patients with active MS compared with inactive MS or OND patients. TNF-α was also more frequently present in active MS than in OND CSF. By contrast, most MS CSF samples did not contain detectable IL-6. There was no correlation between the degree of CSF pleocytosis and the level of individual cytokines, suggesting that cytokine accumulation may be derived from CNS, and not CSF, cells. Elevated levels of TNF-α in the CSF have been associated in one study with disease progression (Sharief and Hentges 1991), but the reproducibility of the assay system used may have been suboptimal. As IL-1β and TNF-α experimentally induce astrogliosis, demyelination, temperature elevation, lassitude and sleep, these results raise the possibility that these cytokines may contribute to a variety of clinical manifestations in MS.

The role of TNF-α in EAE and MS has been studied extensively. TNF-α, by upregulaton of cytokine production, such as of RANTES for example, enhances lymphocyte–endothelial cell adhesion and is an efficient mediator of cell recruitment in inflammatory infiltrates (Issekutz and Issekutz 1993). Administration of TNF-α augments EAE (Kuroda and Shimamoto 1991), whereas antibodies to TNF-α or TNF-α receptor, and inhibitors of TNF-α synthesis, abrogate the disease (Ruddle et al. 1990). More recently, it has been demonstrated that the modulatory effect of soluble peptide variants of an MBP epitope is through downregulation of TNF-α production (Karin et al. 1994). Finally, injection of TNF-α into the vitreous, a fluid compartment of the CNS, instigates oligodendrocyte disruption and demyelination (Butt and Jenkins 1994). TNF-α is initially expressed as a precursor with a 233 transmembrane amino acid anchor. This precursor is proteolytically processed to yield a mature 157 amino acid cytokine. The sequence in the putative cleavage site reveals homologies with peptide sequences known to be cleaved by metalloproteinase-like enzymes. Two recent papers report that the in vitro and in vivo release of TNF-α is specifically prevented by metalloproteinase inhibitors (Gearing et al. 1994; McGeehan, et al. 1994). Thus, metalloproteinases may act not only as mediators of cell extravasation, but may also increase the inflammatory and homing reactions through TNF processing. From the clinical point of view, synthetic compounds able to block both TNF-α production and matrix degradation may be effective in controlling MS (Gearing et al. 1994; Genain et al. 1995; McGeehan et al. 1994).

Self-Antigens in Multiple Sclerosis

In this paper, we are considering the concept that heightened self-reactivity is in some manner operational in the MS disease process. A critical prerequisite to understanding the molecular basis of an autoimmune disease is knowledge of the autoantigen or autoantigens. Antigen identification will help to define the pathogenesis of the diseases, and may provide new opportunities for novel diagnostic and therapeutic approaches (Table 2.3). The characterization of the autoantigen, in terms of molecular structure and nucleotide or amino acid sequences, can facilitate epitope mapping and accurate definition of antibody binding sites. As already discussed, EAE can be induced in susceptible animals following active immunization with purified MBP or PLP and their derived peptides in a suitable adjuvant, as well as transfer with MBP- or PLP-specific T cells. Because MBP and PLP represent the two predominant myelin proteins (about 30% and 50% of myelin proteins by weight respectively), they have received the most attention as potential autoantigens in MS (Table 2.5) (Friez 1989). Using protein chemistry, electron microscopy and mass spectrometry, Moscarello and colleagues concluded that MBP in MS patients is arrested at the level of the first growth spurt, within the first 6 years of life, and is therefore developmentally immature (Moscarello et al. 1994). The authors postulated that a structural change in MBP is primary and not secondary to the disease process, and that immature myelin is more susceptible to degradation, providing the initial antigenic material to the immune system. This provocative observation has not been confirmed, and it is possible that the observed changes were secondary to MS rather than the inciting event. Nonetheless, the major immune response detected in the laboratory in MS patients is directed against MBP (Olsson et al. 1990; Steinman 1994). MBP reactive T cells appear to concentrate in the CSF, relative to their frequency in peripheral blood (Soderstrom et al. 1993). In addition, Warren and colleagues recently reported that 111 of 116 chronic progressive MS patients had anti-MBP antibody in the CSF (Warren et al. 1994). Most patients who had no anti-MBP antibody in the CSF did

Table 2.5. Incriminating MBP in the pathogenesis of MS

MBP makes up about 30% of central myelin proteins
EAE is inducible in susceptible animals by active immunization with MBP, fragments of MBP, or synthetic peptides from MBP epitopes, when injected in suitable adjuvants
EAE is inducible in susceptible animals by passive transfer of MBP-reactive T-helper cells
Brain derived endothelial cells from guinea pigs are able to present MBP, but not purified protein derivative or ovalbumin, to previously sensitized T cells
It is possible to prevent or even reverse EAE by neutralizing the immune response against MBP
MBP induced lymphoproliferation among MS patients is only slightly higher than in controls, but activated T-cell clones with specificity for MBP are observed in MS patients and not in controls
Extensive molecular homology has been detected between MBP stretches and pathogens such as adenovirus type 2
Antibodies to MBP are regularly found in the CSF of patients with acute optic neuritis and active MS, as well as in CNS tissue of MS patients
Direct cloning and sequencing of TCR rearrangements from MS brain lesions indicated that some of these rearrangements are encoding CDR3 regions identical to those found in T cells recognizing MBP
Immature MBP isoforms may have a higher distribution among MS patients
Linkage was reported between allelic markers located at 5′ of the MBP gene on chromosome 18, and susceptibility to MS in a Finnish population of familial MS patients

have antibodies to PLP. The anti-MBP IgG affinity purified from CNS lesions reacted with the MBP peptide p75–106, a putative dominant T-cell recognition site. Several studies have shown that human MBP-specific T cells predominantly recognize peptides located in the center and in the C-terminal part of the MBP molecule, around residues 84–102 and 143–168 (Kotzin et al. 1991; Martin et al. 1991; Ota, Matsui et al. 1990; Pette et al. 1990; Valli et al. 1993; Wucherpfennig et al. 1994a, b). Although a number of MHC class II determinants can serve as antigen-presenting molecules, the immunodominant epitope 84–102 binds with high affinity to HLA-DR2 molecules (Wucherpfennig et al. 1994a). As detailed above, the analysis of TCR gene rearrangements in the MS brain has also indicated that one of the major immune responses in the lesions of HLA-DR2 patients, is directed to the MBP epitopes 84–102 or 87–106 (Oksenberg et al. 1993b). The importance of MBP reactive cells in autoimmunity was further demonstrated in recent work, where MBP-reactive T-cell clones isolated from the peripheral blood of healthy, unimmunized *Callithrix jacchus* marmosets, efficiently transferred CNS inflammatory disease (Genain et al. 1994). This primate species is characterized by a natural chimerism of bone marrow elements between siblings, that allows the adoptive transfer of cells between individuals across histocompatibility barriers.

EAE mediated by transfer of MBP or PLP reactive T cells is characterized by paralysis and perivascular CNS inflammation, yet, in most models, little demyelination is observed. In contrast, sensitization with CNS tissue homogenates may result in extensive demyelination. This suggests that antigens other than MBP and PLP are involved in demyelination. Highly purified myelin antigens were used by Bernard and colleagues to assess cell-mediated immune responses in MS patients. The greatest incidence of proliferative response by MS peripheral blood lymphocytes was to MOG, as 12 of 24 patients reacted, and of these, eight reacted exclusively to MOG. In contrast, only one control individual of 16 tested reacted positively to this antigen. The incidence of responses to MBP, PLP and MAG did not differ significantly between MS patients and control individuals (Kerlero de Rosbo et al. 1993). Furthermore, they induced demyelinating relapsing EAE disease in rats after a single injection of purified MOG (Johns et al. 1995). As discussed above, reactivity against minor components of myelin, as well as to other antigens including heat shock proteins, β-arrestin and arrestin, glial fibrillary acidic protein and astrocyte-derived calcium-binding protein (S1000β) may play equally important roles in this disease (Selmaj et al. 1991; Ohguro et al. 1993; Kojima et al. 1994; Wekerle et al. 1994) (Table 2.2). Both normal and disease T-cell repertoires against autoantigens may share similar or even identical specificities. Peripheral regulatory mechanisms are then necessary to keep such cells under control in order to prevent their activation and the development of spontaneous autoimmune responses.

Maintenance of Peripheral Self-Tolerance

During T-cell ontogeny in the thymus, lymphoid stem cells undergo maturation and differentiation in consecutive waves of thymic selection (Benoist and Mathis 1992; Marrack and Kappler 1988). Thymocytes that will be useful to the host undergo positive selection, whereas thymocytes with autoreactive potential undergo negative selection by clonal deletion or inactivation. The "affinity/avidity" model may explain the balance between negative and positive selection (Nikolic-Zugic 1994). This hypothesis suggests that only cells bearing receptors with an intermediate affinity/avidity toward self-peptides–MHC complexes would survive selection. Those with lower avidity would fail to be positively selected, whereas the ones with high affinity/avidity would be negatively selected. Thymic regulation is extended to the periphery in the form of clonal anergy, clonal ignorance and exhaustion, idiotype interactions, and suppression (Murphy et al. 1989; Schonrich et al. 1991). It is not completely clear why some of these cells escape this surveillance and later in life participate in autoimmune pathogenic processes, but the multiple events that are required to induce self-reactivity may include tissue damage by trauma or infection and genetically determined susceptibility. Several experimental systems have been used to understand the mechanisms involved in maintenance of peripheral tolerance to myelin antigens. Among others, such studies include myelin immunization (Levine et al. 1968), T-cell vaccination (Ben-Nun et al. 1981), CD8+ T-cell depletion (Jiang et al. 1992), apoptosis induction (Critchfield et al. 1994), CD8 knockout (Koh, et al. 1992) and TCR transgenic mice (Goverman et al. 1993).

A topic of intense recent interest is the possible association of apoptosis with autoimmunity (Carson and Ribeiro 1993; Tan 1994). Apoptosis, or programmed cell death, is a form of cell death characterized by cell shrinkage, nuclear condensation and surface blobbing. In tissues, apoptosis usually affects scattered single cells rather than clusters, and fragments of apoptotic cells are phagocytosed and digested by resident cells. In this way, potentially immunogenic cellular components are exposed, a process that might explain why antibodies in autoimmune diseases, as for example in systemic lupus erythematosus, are directed at multiple antigens. In addition, it appears that apoptosis is one mechanism by which clonal thymic deletion takes place after immature lymphocytes bind autoantigens (Goldstein et al. 1991; Tan 1994). A defect in the deletion of these lymphocytes could predispose to autoimmunity. The MLR/Mp-lpr/lpr mouse, which develops a disease analogous to human lupus, has a molecular abnormality in the APO-1 or *Fas* gene that mediates apoptosis (Watanabe-Fukunaga et al. 1992). Because *lpr* mice do not express the *Fas* receptor, they do not efficiently delete autoaggressive T lymphocytes. It is not clear if apoptotic mechanisms operate in MS.

Oral administration of MBP suppresses EAE by inducing peripheral tolerance. Tolerance can be adoptively transferred by CD8+ T cells, which are generated following oral administration of antigens and release TGF-β after being triggered by the specific antigen. TGF-β suppresses immune responses in the microenvironment, creating a form of bystander suppression that will control the disease (Miller et al. 1992). An alternative mechanism based on the induction of anergy (unresponsiveness) to the autoaggressive T cells by the tolerogen was also proposed (Whitacre et al. 1991). It is possible that a low antigen dose induces suppression whereas a high antigen dose induces clonal anergy (Friedman and Weiner 1994). In a recent study, T-cell clones were isolated from the mesenteric lymph nodes of animals that had been orally tolerized to MBP and had received an intraperitoneal injection of MBP as adjuvant. These mucosal clones were CD4+ and shared TCR usage, MHC restriction, and epitope specificity with encephalitogenic T-cell clones. However, they suppressed EAE that was induced with either MBP or PLP by producing a Th2-like cytokine profile composed of TGF-β, IL-4 and IL-10 (Chen et al. 1994).

It is widely accepted that the lack of second signals or costimulation provided by accessory cells causes mature T lymphocytes to enter a state of tolerance or anergy, in which they fail to proliferate or produce lymphokines, and are refractory to subsequent stimulation by antigen. The B7 costimulatory pathway involves at least two molecules, B7-1 and B7-2, which interact with their count receptors, CD28 and CTL-4, on T cells. Blocking B7-1 interactions during T-cell activation induces functional inactivation in Th1 cells. Consequently, IL-2 and IFN-γ, but not IL-4, production is inhibited, leading to a state of hyporesponsiveness or anergy. Thus, it may be possible to anergize selectively the Th1 cells and enhance the modulatory Th2 response by presentation of antigen without costimulation. For example, Finck and colleagues treated lupus-prone NZB/NZW mice with soluble CTLA4Ig. This protocol resulted in the blocking of autoantibody production and prolonged life, even when treatment was delayed until the most advanced stage of clinical illness (Finck et al. 1994). Conversely, the injection of anti-B7-2 antibody substantially increased disease severity in the EAE model, whereas administration of anti-B7-1 antibody significantly reduced the incidence of EAE, possibly through the generation of Th2 clones (Kuchroo et al. 1995). Since cotreatment with anti-IL 4 antibody prevented disease amelioration, costimulatory molecules may directly affect cytokine secretion.

Infection in Multiple Sclerosis

Infectious agents have been postulated as causes of MS for over a century. Most work has focused on viruses known to be able to induce demyelination in humans and experimental animals (Johnson 1994). The possible role of a virus in MS is supported by data suggesting that some as yet undetermined childhood exposure somehow influences susceptibility to MS. This data is derived from migration studies and from study of apparent point epidemics of MS. Viral infections may also induce exacerbations. Some MS patients have abnormal immune responses to certain viruses. Higher antibody titers against measles, herpex simples, varicella, rubella, Epstein–Barr, influenza C and some parainfluenza strains have been detected in the serum and CSF samples of MS patients compared with controls. The occurrence of viral infections was studied in a group of patients participating in a recent IFN-β clinical trial (Panitch 1994). A strong correlation was found between MS attacks and viral upper respiratory infections. In addition, a number of viruses have been recovered from MS patients' fluids and tissues (Johnson 1994). However, despite data obtained from epidemiologic, serologic and animal studies, no virus has been consistently isolated, or viral material uniquely identified, from MS patients. Nonviral microorganisms or their toxins implicated in demyelination include *Acanthamoeba, Borrelia, Brucella, Campylobacter, Hartmannella,* mycobacterium, trypanosomes, diphtheria toxin and tetanus toxoid (Birnbaum et al. 1993; Brocke et al. 1994). A model even proposing that MS is mediated by prions exists in the literature (Wojtowicz 1993).

The role, if any, of pathogens in MS remains unknown. Mechanisms that may explain a pathogen–MS interaction include polyclonal activation of T and B cells, infection and destruction of regulatory cells, exposure of sequestered or modified antigens, and "molecular mimicry". Molecular mimicry refers to the initiation of an autoimmune response because of sequence or structural homologies between a self-protein and a protein in a viral or bacterial pathogen (Wucherpfennig and Strominger 1995). For example, EAE may be induced by immune sensitization with a peptide sequence from a pathogen with homology to MBP (Fujinami and Oldstone 1985). MBP shares extensive homologies at the amino acid level with measles, influenza and adenovirus. Residues 91–101 of MBP, for example, share stretches of four to six amino acids with adenovirus (Jahnke et al. 1985). Homology may be necessary at only a few amino acids for efficient T-cell recognition to occur. Conservation of the native amino acid sequence at four of ten amino acids of the MBP Ac1–10 epitope is sufficient to induce EAE (Gautam et al. 1992). Tolerance to MBP can be also broken by viral infection of the brain, another "innocent bystander" model. For example, anti-MBP responses are seen in measles encephalitis in humans (Johnson et al. 1984) and HTLV-I infection (Hara et al. 1994). In rats, infection of the brain with the neurotropic coronavirus results in a breakdown in tolerance to MBP, and activation of MBP-reactive T cells capable of transferring EAE (Watanabe et al. 1983). Thus, a neurotrophic virus may infect the nervous system and, by doing so, stimulate an immune response not only to the virus but also to normal nervous system proteins.

An alternative mechanism has recently been proposed, which implicates "exogenous superantigens" in the etiology of autoimmune diseases (Paliard et al. 1991). The term superantigen describes antigens that, at very low concentrations (in the picomolar range), can stimulate subsets of T lymphocytes (Chatila and Geha 1992; Herman et al. 1991; White et al. 1989). Superantigens bind with high affinity to class II MHC molecules outside the antigen binding grove. They interact with the Vβ chain of the TCR in the region of the β-pleated sheet, away from the CDR3 region, the putative antigen binding site. In a non-MHC restricted manner, with no need for antigen processing, the class II superantigen complexes trigger the proliferation of T cells expressing particular TCR-Vβ chains. This stimulation is independent of accessory molecules, and induces the release of cytokines such as IL-2, IFN-γ and TNF-α. A notable feature of superantigenic stimulation is that responding T cells initially mount a vigorous response, but then disappear or display anergy. Two groups of superantigens have been defined: endogenous superantigens (Acha-Orbea and Palmer 1991; Choi et al. 1991), retroviral sequences encoded within the genome, which have been identified in the mouse, but not yet in humans, and exogenous superantigens. This second group includes the toxins of many common bacteria, and possibly components of certain viruses, for example, the nucleocapsid of rabies (Lafon et al. 1992; Misfeldt 1990).

Superantigens are associated with numerous human diseases, such as food poisoning, toxic shock syndrome, scalded skin syndrome, and others (Misfeldt 1990; Zumla 1992). The involvement of exogenous superantigens as etiologic agents in several autoimmune diseases is currently the subject of active investigation (Abe et al. 1993; Conrad et al. 1994; Paliard et al. 1991). Many autoimmune diseases are exacerbated, and perhaps even preceded, by infections. Theoretically, superantigens may reverse the state of anergy on CD4+ T cells tolerant to self-antigens, activating pathogenic pathways. In a recent study, Brocke and colleagues (1993) showed that relapses and exacerbations of EAE could be induced with the superantigen Staphylococcus enterotoxin B (SEB), and, to a lesser extent, with SEA. At least part of the observed effect is due to specific reactivation of autoreactive cells in the periphery and to the production of TNF-α, because administration of anti-TNF antibodies can delay the onset of disease induced by SEB. Interestingly, SEB can prevent disease when given at least 14 days before onset of disease. Burns and colleagues (1992) examined the ability of staphylococcal toxins to stimulate human T cells specific for MBP or PLP, which are putative autoantigens in MS. All myelin antigen-specific T cells responded in proliferation studies to at least one of the nine superantigenic toxins used in this study. In some experiments, the superantigenic toxins were up to 7×10^5-fold more potent in proliferation assays than were the myelin antigens to which the T cells were initially sensitized. The authors suggest that massive superantigen stimulation during infection may be associated with the activation of myelin-specific T cells and disease exacerbation. These results may have important therapeutic implications. MacNeil and colleagues (1992) demonstrated that it is possible to inhibit superantigen recognition with peptides that resemble the site of superantigen interaction on the TCR-β chain.

Activation of T cells by superantigens requires the presence of MHC class II molecules, the cross linking of toxin, or other costimulation. In the absence of these conditions, superantigens such as SEB appear to cause anergy. Trace levels of SEB suppress the pathogenic effect of encephalitogenic BV8-expressing T-cell clones (Ben-Nun and Yossefi 1992). It was recently observed that SEB can form biologically active complexes with soluble TCR molecules in both the absence and presence of class II MHC molecules (Seth et al. 1994). This finding may provide an explanation for the anergic effect of superantigens in vivo in the absence of costimulants or cross linking, and may lead to new approaches for manipulation of the immune response. It is likely that these strategies and methodologies will yield crucial information about environmental factors involved in MS pathogenesis.

Genes Conferring Susceptibility to Multiple Sclerosis

MS is not usually considered a genetic disease in the classic sense. However, the racial and familial clustering of MS, the higher disease incidence in women (roughly 2:1, compared with males), and the high concordance rate in monozygotic twins (25%–30%) compared with dizygotic twins (2%–5%) and non-twin siblings (2%–5%) (Ebers et al. 1986), all suggest genetic influences on susceptibility to MS. A simple model of inheritance for all MS is unlikely and cannot account for the non-linear decrease in disease risk with increasing genetic distance from the MS proband. Although, in some families, a pattern suggestive of autosomal dominant inheritance (parent to child or grandparent to parent to child) is found, more often siblings or first cousins are coaffected, suggesting recessive or oligogenic inheritance. Indeed, concordance estimates in twins and relatives of MS patients differ from predictions based on single-gene inheritance, and suggests a multigenic etiology (Ebers et al. 1986). Although it is likely that genetic heterogeneity exists in MS, a simple mode of inheritance or a single underlying susceptibility gene cannot be ruled out in a subset of pedigrees. Using published data from twin and multiply affected family studies, different genetic models of MS susceptibility were evaluated by Phillips (1993) using mathematical techniques developed by Risch (1990). His analysis favored a model involving multiple interacting susceptibility loci, each with a relatively small contribution to the overall risk. His analysis also indicates that perhaps as many as 15 mutually influenced (epistatic) susceptibility loci are involved in familial MS transmission.

By analyzing backcross experiments in mice and rat strains susceptible to EAE or demyelination caused by Theiler's murine encephalitis virus (TMEV), Blankenhorn and Stranford (1992) concluded that at least six chromosome markers in EAE, and four in TMEV, are associated with susceptibility to immune demyelination. In addition to the MHC and the TCR gene complexes, T-cell suppressor activity and the response to pertussis-induced histamine sensitization, were included as candidate, albeit unconfirmed, genes. The *Bordetella pertussis*-induced histamine sensitization (*Bphs*) locus was mapped telomeric to the TCR-β-chain gene, on the murine chromosome 6 (Sudweeks et al. 1993). It is important to note that pertussis toxin is used as an adjuvant in the induction of

EAE in mice. This region also contains a number of other loci with immunologic relevance.

Early attempts to identify the "MS gene(s)" focused on those polymorphic genes whose products participate in the immune response, such as the genes comprising the MHC on chromosome 6, TCR genes on chromosomes 7 and 14, and immunoglobulin genes. Although suggestive correlations between certain alleles at these loci and the presence of MS have been described, conflicting results are not unusual and critical questions remain unanswered (Oksenberg et al. 1993a).

The Major Histocompatibility Complex

In humans, the MHC, also known as the human leukocyte antigen (HLA) region, consists of linked gene clusters located in the short arm of chromosome 6 at 6p21.3, spanning over 3 million base pairs (Simpson 1988; Trowsdale 1988). An individual's ability to respond to an antigen, whether it be foreign or self, is in part determined by the amino acid sequences of these highly polymorphic molecules (Pullen et al. 1989; Unanue 1992). Not surprisingly, susceptibility to a number of diseases, most of them autoimmune, has been associated with particular class II alleles (Nepom and Erlich 1991; Todd et al. 1988). The association between an MHC determinant and MS was first described in 1972 (Bertrams et al. 1972; Maito et al. 1972). An extensive literature supports this association (Oksenberg and Steinman 1990). The majority of studies have focused on Caucasians of northern European descent, where predisposition to MS has been associated with the HLA-A3, B7, DR2, Dw2 extended haplotype. The class II (HLA-D) region provides the strongest association with MS, and molecular analyses have identified the susceptible DR2 haplotype as HLA-DR2, DRB1*1501, DQA1*0102, DQB1*0602 (Allen et al. 1994; Olerup et al. 1989; Spurkland et al. 1991; Vartdal et al. 1989). Attempts to localize further the susceptibility genes within the DR-DQ region have not provided consensus. The strong linkage disequilibrium across the DR-DQ region and the fact that DRB1*1501 and DQB1*0602 are found exclusively on this DR2 haplotype in northern Europeans (Begovich et al. 1992), has prevented a clear resolution of the relative contribution of each gene. Other as yet undefined genes within this region or specific combinations of particular alleles at the DR and DQ loci may actually confer susceptibility.

Although it is clear from data on multiple ethnic groups that the DR and DQ subregions of the MHC play a role in susceptibility to MS, there is no consensus on the actual gene or genes involved. Because these studies have been performed on various ethnic groups, the apparent contradictions might be reconciled, or at least explained from the geographic and ethnic variation among the different studies. It is possible that different genetic backgrounds may provide different susceptibility patterns for unrelated environmental factors. In addition to the class I and class II genes, the human MHC contains at least 70 additional genes. Other genes mapped in the MHC region include complement proteins C2, factor B and C4, and genes for the steroid 21-hydroxylase, collectively known as class

III genes, as well as genes for tumor necrosis factor (TNF-α and β), genes involved in antigen processing (LMP 1 and LMP 2) and transport (TAP 1 and TAP 2), and possibly genes regulating nonimmune functions and development. The MHC determinants may merely represent markers for other susceptibility genes located in the same chromosomal area. Although there is no direct proof, susceptibility is more likely to be mediated by the class II genes themselves (DR, DQ or both) due to the known functions of these molecules in the normal immune response.

Formal linkage studies of the MHC region in MS sibling pairs have also yielded conflicting results, although pooled data indicate that a small MHC effect may be present. Cumulative data, representing 244 sibling pairs, indicate that 95 pairs (39%) share both haplotypes, 115 pairs (47%) share only one haplotype, and 34 pairs (14%) do not share an HLA haplotype in common. By random segregation of HLA genes, one would expect sharing of 25%, 50% and 25% of genes in common by sibling pairs. Thus a shift towards greater than expected HLA gene sharing by coaffected MS siblings indicates a genetic effect of this region. However, complete HLA discordance in 14% of affected sibling pairs indicates that coinheritance of an HLA gene does not always occur, and suggests that the genetic influence of the HLA region on MS is small (Phillips 1993).

The T-Cell Receptor Complex

T-cell receptor genes were expected to have an impact in the overall genetic susceptibility to MS. Linkage studies have shown a clear influence of the TCR-β-chain gene complex (or genes linked to it) in experimental murine demyelination (Blankenhorn and Stranford 1992). An early approach to identify variations in TCR genes that could affect the development of human disease was based on the detection of polymorphic markers using restriction fragment length polymorphism analysis. Several polymorphisms in human TCR genes have been described and in certain cases were found to correlate with the incidence of MS (Oksenberg and Steinman 1990; Steinman et al. 1992). In contrast, other studies have revealed no association between germline polymorphisms of the TCR and susceptibility to MS (Hillert and Olerlup 1992).

As for MHC genes, a useful approach to test for TCR influences on MS is to test families with multiply-affected siblings using a series of markers located at different regions of the TCR complex (Robinson and Kindt 1992). In a collaborative study, Seboun et al. analyzed the inheritance of TCR-β-chain genes in families, with 40 sibling pairs with relapsing–remitting MS, using both human and murine probes (Seboun et al. 1989). The mean proportion of TCR-β haplotypes identical by descent inherited by MS sibling pairs was significantly increased compared with expected values, whereas the distribution of haplotype sharing was random when MS patients were compared with their unaffected siblings. Additional support for an effect of TCR-β inheritance in MS sibling pairs was presented in preliminary form for an English data set. The association between MS and the sharing of TCR-β haplotypes in families is not absolute (Lynch et al. 1991) and its actual contribution to susceptibility largely remains to be defined.

Other Candidate Markers

A multiallelic tetranucleotide repeat polymorphism identified 5′ to the MBP gene on chromosome 18 may be associated with MS (Boylan et al. 1990a, b). More recently, this genetic marker was studied in a homogeneous pool of 21 Finnish MS families (Tienari et al. 1992). A significant association was found between MS patients and the MBP marker, mostly attributable to the higher frequency of an 1.27 kb allele among patients in comparison to controls. The same Finnish group have since reported a highly significant two-locus linkage in MS, when MBP was analyzed in conjunction with the HLA locus (Tienari et al. 1994). Subsequent reports in other populations have failed to confirm linkage or association between MS and this genomic segment (Graham et al. 1993; Rose et al. 1993; Wood et al. 1994). Most of these studies, however, used a short stretch of the repeat and potentially informative polymorphisms may therefore have been missed.

In the past 5 years, genes that participate in antigen processing have been mapped to the MHC class II region (Monaco 1992; Trowsdale 1993). Two of these genes, which map between HLA-DNA and HLA-DOB genes, belong to the ATP-binding cassette transporter superfamily. They have been named TAP1 and TAP2, for transporters associated with antigen processing, and it was proposed that their products form a complex that transports peptides into the lumen of the endoplasmic reticulum for interaction with MHC class I molecules. Two additional genes, LMP2 and LMP7, which map close to TAP1 and TAP2, encode products that are related to subunits of a large cytoplasmic complex called the proteasome, thought to be involved in degradation of proteins in the cytoplasm. Limited polymorphism has been detected in both sets of genes. Powis and colleagues (1992) demonstrated that, in the rat system, allelic variation within TAP2 determines the peptides assembled in MHC class I RT1.Aa molecules, and their subsequent recognition by allogeneic T cells. Due to their location in the MHC class II cluster and their possible involvement in antigen processing of endogenous class I restricted proteins, it is tempting to postulate that polymorphism in the TAP and LMP genes may be involved in antigen peptide selection that might lead to autoimmunity. However, no association was detected between LMP or TAP polymorphisms and MS susceptibility (Liblau et al. 1993; Szafer et al. 1994). Further studies will be required to discover the extent of polymorphism in these genes, and to test whether different alleles contribute to autoimmune susceptibility.

A recent study employing transgenic methodology may shed light on some functional aspects of genetically determined susceptibility to autoimmunity (Scott et al. 1994). In this experimental model, transgenic expression of an influenza hemagglutinin (HA) on islet β cells, was combined with a diabetogenic BV8.3 TCR transgene specific for a class II-restricted HA peptide. Double transgenic mice displayed either resistance or susceptibility to spontaneous autoimmune diabetes, depending on genetic contributions from either of two common inbred strains, BALB/c or B10.D2. Functional studies of autoreactive CD4+ T cells from resistant mice showed, contrary to expectations, no clonal anergy, clonal deletion or receptor desensitization; rather, there was a non-

MHC-encoded predisposition toward differentiation to a non-pathogenic effector phenotype (regulatory Th2 cells versus proinflammatory Th1 cells). T cells from resistant double negative transgenic mice also showed evidence of prior activation by antigen, suggesting that disease may be under genetically controlled active regulation by autoreactive Th2 cells.

With the advent of genomic screening, a comprehensive and ambitious approach is now possible for the genetic dissection of complex traits such as MS susceptibility (Lander and Schork 1994). The goal in genomic screening is to scan the entire human genome for chromosomal regions that may harbor susceptibility genes. Regions linked to the disease can then be studied by positional cloning methods. This strategy takes advantage of two rapidly developing sets of tools: a large number of highly polymorphic microsatellite markers, and modern statistical techniques (Dawson et al. 1990; Pericak-Vance et al. 1991). Microsatellites are tandem DNA repeats (2–4 bases) characterized by the high degree of polymorphism in the number of repeated units. These markers were first identified about 5 years ago, and have since become the polymorphism markers of choice for genetic studies (Weber 1990; Weber and May 1989). Recent work has now generated microsatellite maps of every chromosome, and more refined maps are in progress as part of the human genome initiative. Genomic screening with anonymous markers followed by detailed analysis of candidate regions using positional cloning methods, represent a powerful tool to identify susceptibility genes. By collecting appropriate pedigrees, it will be possible to perform an efficient screen of the entire human genome to identify the genetic components of MS. Their characterization will help to define the basic etiology of the disease, improve diagnostic ability and risk assessment, and influence therapy.

References

Abe J, Kotzin BL, Meissner C et al. (1993) Characterization of T cell repertorie changes in acute Kawasaki disease. J Exp Med 177:791–796

Acha-Orbea H, Palmer E (1991) Mls – a retrovirus exploits the immune system. Immunol Today 12:356–361

Acha-Orbea H, Mitchell DJ, Timmermann L et al. (1988) Limited heterogeneity of T cell receptors from lymphocytes mediating autoimmune encephalomyelitis allows specific immune intervention. Cell 54:263–273

Allegretta M, Nicklas JA, Sriram S, Albertini RJ (1990) T cells responsive to myelin basic protein in patients with multiple sclerosis. Science 247:718–721

Allegretta M, Albertini RJ, Howell MD et al. (1994) Homologies between T cell receptor junctional sequences unique to multiple sclerosis and T cells mediating experimental allergic encephalomyelitis. J Clin Invest 94:105–109

Allen M, Sandberg-Wollheim M, Sjogren K et al. (1994) Association of susceptibility to multiple sclerosis in Sweden with HLA class II DRB1 and DQB1 alleles. Hum Immunol 39:41–48

Baron JL, Madri JA, Ruddle NH, Hashim G, Janeway CA (1993) Surface expression of α4 integrin by CD4 T cells is required for their entry into brain parenchyma. J Exp Med 177:57–68

Battistini L, Selmaj K, Kowal C et al. (1995) Multiple sclerosis: limited diversity of the Vδ2-Jδ3 T cell receptor in chronic active lesions. Ann Neurol 37:198–203

Begovich AB, McKlure GR, Suraj V et al. (1992) Polymorphism, recombination and linkage disequilibrium within the HLA class II region. J Immunol 148:249–258

Bell RB, Lindsey JW, Sobel RA, Hodgkinson S, Steinman L (1993) Diverse T cell receptor V beta usage in the central nervous system in experimental allergic encephalomyelitis. J Immunol

150:4085–4092

Ben-Nun A, Yossefi S (1992) Staphylococcal enterotoxin B as a potent suppressant of T lymphocytes: trace levels suppress T lymphocyte proliferative responses. Eur J Immunol 22:1495–1503

Ben-Nun A, Wekerle H, Cohen IR (1981) Vaccination against autoimmune encephalomyelitis using attenuated cells of a T-lymphocyte line reactive against myelin basic protein. Nature 292:60–61

Benoist C, Mathis D (1992) Generation of the alpha/beta repertoire. Curr Opin Immunol 4:156–161

Bernard CCA, Kerlero de Rosbo N (1992) Multiple sclerosis: an autoimmune disease of multifactorial etiology. Curr Opin Immunol 4:760–765

Bernard CCA, Randell VB, Horvath L, Carnegie PR, Mackay IR (1981) Antibody to myelin basic protein in extracts of multiple sclerosis brain. Immunol 43:447–457

Bernard CCA, Mandel TE, Mackay IR (1992) Experimental models of human autoimmune disease: overview and prototypes. In: Rose NR, Mackay IR (eds) The autoimmune diseases, vol. II. Academic Press, San Diego, pp 47–106

Bertrams J, Kuwert E, Liedtke U (1972) HLA antigens and multiple sclerosis. Tissue Antigens 2:405–408

Birnbaum G, Kotilinek L, Albrecht BS (1993) Spinal fluid lymphocytes from a subgroup of multiple sclerosis patients respond to mycobacterial antigens. Ann Neurol 34:18–24

Blankenhorn EP, Stranford SA (1992) Genetic factors in demyelinating diseases: genes that control demyelination due to experimental allergic encephalomyelitis and Theiler's murine encephalitis virus. Reg Immunol 4:331–343

Bo L, Mark S, Kong P, Nyland H, Pardo CA, Trapp BD (1994) Detection of MHC class II antigens on macrophages and microglia, but not astrocytes and endothelia, in active MS lesions. J Neuroimmunol 51:135–146

Boylan KB, Ayers TM, Popko B et al. (1990a) Repetitive DNA (TGGA)n 5′ to the human myelin basic protein gene: a new oligonucleotide repetitive sequence showing length polymorphism. Genomics 6:16–22

Boylan KB, Takahashi N, Paty DW et al. (1990b) DNA length polymorphism 5′ to the myelin basic protein gene is associated with multiple sclerosis. Ann Neurol 27:291–297

Brocke S, Gaur A, Piercy C et al. (1993) Induction of relapsing paralysis in experimental allergic encephalomyelitis by bacterial superantigen. Nature 365:642–645

Brocke S, Veromaa T, Weissman IL, Gijbels K, Steinman L (1994) Infection and multiple sclerosis: a possible role for superantigens? Trends Microbiol 2:250–254

Brosnan CF, Bornstein MB, Bloom BR (1981) The effect of macrophage depletion on the clinical and pathologic expression of experimental allergic encephalomyelitis. J Immunol 126:614–620

Brunner C, Lassmann H, Waehneldet TV, Matthieu J-M, Linington C (1989) Differential ultrastructural localization of myelin basic protein, myelin oligodendroglia glycoprotein, and 2′,3′-cyclic nucleotide 3′-phosphodiesterase in the CNS of adult rats. J Neurochem 52:296–304

Burns J, Littlefield K, Gill J, Trotter JL (1992) Bacterial toxin superantigens activate human T lymphocytes reactive with myelin autoantigens. Eur J Immunol 32:352–357

Butt AM, Jenkins HG (1994) Morphological changes in oligodendrocytes in the intact mouse optic nerve following intravitreal injection of tumor necrosis factor. J Neuroimmunol 51:27–33

Cannella B, Raine CS (1995) The adhesion molecule and cytokine profile of multiple sclerosis lesions. Ann Neurol 37:424–435

Cannella B, Cross AH, Raine CS (1991) Relapsing autoimmune demyelination: a role for vascular addressins. J Neuroimmunol 35:295–300

Carson DA, Ribeiro JM (1993) Apoptosis and disease. Lancet 341:1251–1254

Chatila T, Geha RS (1992) Superantigens. Curr Opin Immunol 4:74–78

Chen Y, Kuchroo VK, Inobe J-I, Hafler DA, Weiner HL (1994) Regulatory T cell clones induced by oral tolerance: suppression of autoimmune encephalomyelitis. Science 265:1237–1240

Choi Y, Kappler JW, Marrack P (1991) A superantigen encoded in the open reading frame of the 3′ long terminal repeat of mouse mammary tumor virus. Nature 350:203–207

Chothia C, Boswell D, Lesk AM (1988) The outline structure of the T cell alpha-beta receptor. EMBO J 7:3745–3755

Conrad B, Weidmann E, Trucco G et al. (1994) Evidence for superantigen in insulin-dependent diabetes mellitus aetiology. Nature 371:351–355

Critchfield JM, Racke M, Zuniga-Pflucker JC et al. (1994) T cell deletion in high antigen dose therapy of autoimmune encephalomyelitis. Science 263:1139–1143

Dawson DV, Kaplan EB, Elston RC (1990) Extensions to sib-pair linkage test applicable to disorders characterized by delayed onset. Genet Epidemiol 7:453–456

Ebers GC, Bulman DE, Sadovnick AD et al. (1986) A population-based study of multiple sclerosis in twins. N Engl J Med 315:1638–1642

Finck BK, Linsley PS, Wofsy D (1994) Treatment of murine lupus with CTLA4Ig. Science 265:1225–1227

Fontana A, Fierz W, Bodmer S et al. (1984) Astrocytes present myelin basic protein to encephalitogenic T cell lines. Nature 307:273–276

Freedman MS, Ruifs TC, Selin LK, Antel JP (1991) Peripheral blood gamma/delta T cells lyse fresh human brain-derived oligodendrocytes. Ann Neurol 30:253–257

Friedman R, Weiner HL (1994) Induction of anergy or active suppression following oral tolerance is determined by antigen dosage. Proc Natl Acad Sci USA 91:6688–6692

Friez W (1989) Multiple sclerosis as autoimmune disease: myelin antigens. Res Immunol 140:181–185

Fujinami RS, Oldstone MBA (1985) Amino acid homology between the encephalitogenic site of myelin basic protein and virus: mechanism for autoimmunity. Science 230:1043–1045

Gautam A, Pearson C, Smilek D, Steinman L, McDevitt HO (1992) A polyalanine peptide containing only five native basic protein residues induces autoimmune encephalomyelitis. J Exp Med 176:605–609

Gearing AJH, Beckett P, Christodoulou M (1994) Processing of tumor necrosis factor-alpha precursor by metalloproteinases. Nature 370:555–557

Genain CP, Lee-Parritz D, Nguyen M-H et al. (1994) In healthy primates, circulating autoreactive T cells mediate autoimmune disease. J Clin Invest 94:1339–1345

Genain CP, Roberts T, Davis RL et al. (1995) Prevention of autoimmune demyelination in non-human primates by a cAMP-specific phosphodiesterase inhibitor. Proc Natl Acad Sci USA 92:3601–3605

Goldstein P, Ojcius DM, Young CD (1991) Cell death mechanisms and the immune system. Immunol Rev 10:267–293

Goverman J, Woods A, Larson L et al. (1993) Transgenic mice that express a myelin basic protein-specific T cell receptor develop spontaneous autoimmunity. Cell 72:551–560

Graham CA, Kirk CW, Nevin NC et al. (1993) Lack of association between myelin basic protein gene microsatellite and multiple sclerosis. Lancet 341:1596

Hara H, Morita M, Iwaki T et al. (1994) Detection of HTLV-I proviral DNA and analysis of TCR V beta CDR3 sequences in spinal cord of HAM/TSP. J Exp Med 180:831–839

Hauser SL, Aubert C, Burks JS et al. (1986a) Analysis of human T lymphotropic virus sequences in multiple sclerosis. Nature 322:176–177

Hauser SL, Bhan AK, Gilles F et al. (1986b) Immunocytochemical analysis of the cellular infiltrates in multiple sclerosis lesions. Ann Neurol 19:578–587

Hauser SL, Doolittle TH, Linclon R, Brown RH, Dinarello CA (1990) Cytokine accumulation in CSF of multiple sclerosis patients: frequent detection of interleukin-1 and tumor necrosis factor but not interleukin-6. Neurology 40:1735–1739

Herman A, Kappler JW, Marrack P, Pullen AM (1991) Superantigens: mechanism of T-cell stimulation and role in immune responses. Annu Rev Immunol 9:745–772

Hillert J, Olerlup O (1992) Germ-line polymorphism of TCR genes and disease susceptibility – fact or hypothesis? Immunol Today 13:47–49

Hofman FM, von Hanwehr RI, Dinarello CA et al. (1986) Immunoregulatory molecules and IL-2 receptors identified in multiple sclerosis brain. J Immunol 136:3239–3245

Huitinga I, Damoiseaux JG, Dopp EA, Dijkstra CD (1993) Treatment with anti-CR3 antibodies ED7 and ED8 suppresses experimental allergic encephalomyelitis in Lewis rat. Eur J Immunol 23:709–715

Hvas J, Oksenberg JR, Fernando R, Steinman L, Bernard CCA (1993) Gamma/delta T-cell receptor repertoire in brain lesions of patients with multiple sclerosis. J Neuroimmunol 46:225–234

Issekutz AC, Issekutz TB (1993) Quantitation and kinetics of blood monocyte migration to acute inflammatory reactions, and IL-1α, tumor necrosis factor-α, and IFN-γ. J Immunol 151:2105–2115

Jahnke U, Fischer E, Alvord EA (1985) Sequence homology between certain viral proteins and proteins related to encephalomyelitis and neuritis. Science 229:282–284

Jiang H, Zhang S-L, Pernis B (1992) Role of CD8+ T cells in murine experimental allergic encephalomyelitis. Science 256:1213–1215

Johns TG, Kerlero de Rosbo N, Menon KK, Abo S, Gonzalez MF, Bernard CCA (1995) Myelin oligodendrocyte glycoprotein induces a demyelinating encephalomyelitis resembling multiple sclerosis. J Immunol 154:5536–5541

Johnson RT (1994) The virology of demyelinating diseases. Ann Neurol 36:S54–S60

Johnson RT, Griffin RE, Hirsch RL et al. (1984) Measles encephalomyelitis: clinical and immunological studies. N Engl J Med 310:137–141

Jorgensen JL, Esser U, Fazekas de St Groth B, Reay P, Davis MM (1992) Mapping TCR-peptide contacts by variant peptide immunization of single-chain transgenics. Nature 355:224–230

Karin N, Szafer F, Mitchell DJ, Gold DP, Steinman L (1993) Selective and nonselective stages in homing of T lymphocytes to the central nervous system during experimental allergic encephalomyelitis. J Immunol 150:4116–4124

Karin N, Mitchel DJ, Ling N, Brocke S, Steinman L (1994) Reversal of experimental autoimmune encephalomyelitis by a soluble peptide variant of a myelin basic protein epitope: T cell receptor antagonism and reduction of IFN-γ and TNF-α production. J Exp Med 180:2227–2237

Katayama CD, Eidelman FJ, Duncan A, Hooshmand F, Hedrick SM (1995) Predicted complementarity determining regions of the T cell antigen receptor determine antigen specificity. EMBO J 14:927–938

Kerlero de Rosbo N, Bernard CCA (1989) Multiple sclerosis brain immunoglobulins stimulate myelin basic protein degradation in human myelin: a new cause of demyelination. J Neurochem 53:513–518

Kerlero de Rosbo N, Honegger P, Lassmann H, Matthieu J (1990) Demyelination induced in aggregating brain cell cultures by a monoclonal antibody against MOG. J Neurochem 55:583–587

Kerlero de Rosbo N, Milo R, Lees MB et al. (1993) Reactivity to myelin antigens in multiple sclerosis. J Clin Invest 92:2602–2608

Kermode AG, Thompson AJ, Tufts P et al. (1990) Breakdown of the blood–brain barrier precedes symptoms and other MRI signs of new lesions in multiple sclerosis. Brain 113:1477–1489

Koh D-R, Fung-Leung W-P, Ho A et al. (1992) Less mortality but more relapses in experimental allergic encephalomyelitis in CD8–/– mice. Science 256:1210–1213

Kojima K, Berger T, Lassmann H et al. (1994) Experimental autoimmune panencephalitis and uveoretinitis transferred to Lewis rat by T lymphocytes specific for the S100β molecule, a calcium binding protein of astroglia. J Exp Med 180:817–829

Kotzin B, Karaturi S, Chou Y et al. (1991) Preferential T cell receptor Vβ usage in myelin basic protein reactive to T cell clones from patients with multiple sclerosis. Proc Natl Acad Sci USA 88:9161–9165

Kuchroo VK, Prabhu Das M, Brown JA et al. (1995) B7-1 and B7-2 costimulatory molecules activate differentially the Thl/Th2 developmental pathways: application to autoimmune disease therapy. Cell 80:707–718

Kuroda Y, Shimamoto Y (1991) Human tumor necrosis factor-alpha augments experimental allergic encephalomyelitis in rats. J Neuroimmunol 34:159–164

Lafon M, Mireille L, Martinez-Arends A et al. (1992) Evidence for a viral superantigen in humans. Nature 358:507–510

Lander ES, Schork NJ (1994) Genetic dissection of complex traits. Science 265:2037–2048

Lassman H, Suchanek G., Ozawa K (1994) Histopathology and the blood–cerebrospinal fluid barrier in multiple sclerosis. Ann Neurol 36:S42–S46

Lee SJ, Wucherpfennig KW, Brod SA, Benjamin D (1991) Common T cell receptor V beta usage in oligoclonal T lymphocytes derived from cerebrospinal fluid and blood of patients with multiple sclerosis. Ann Neurol 29:33–40

Leppert D, Waubant E, Galardy R, Bunnett NW, Hauser SL (1995) T-cell gelatinases mediate basement membrane transmigration in vitro. J Immunol 154:4379–4389

Levine S, Hoenig EM, Kies MW (1968) Allergic encephalomyelitis: passive transfer prevented by encephalitogen. Science 161:1155–1157

Liblau R, van Endert PM, Sandberg-Wollheim M et al. (1993) Antigen processing gene polymorphisms in HLA-DR2 multiple sclerosis. Neurology 43:1192–1197

Loffert D, Schaal S, Ehlich A et al. (1994) Early B-cell development in the mouse: insights from mutations introduced by gene targeting. Immunol Rev 137:135–153

Lynch SG, Rose JW, Petajan JH et al. (1991) Discordance of T-cell receptor beta-chain genes in familial multiple sclerosis. Ann Neurol 30:229–241

MacNeil D, Fraga E, Singh B (1992) Inhibition of superantigen recognition by peptides of the variable region of the T cell receptor beta chain. Eur J Immunol 22:937–941

Maito S, Manerow N, Mickey MR, Terasaki PI (1972) Multiple sclerosis: association with HL-A3. Tissue Antigens 2:1–4

Marrack P, Kappler J (1988) The T cell repertoire for antigen and MHC. Immunol Today 9:308–315

McDonald WI (1994) The pathological and clinical dynamics of multiple sclerosis. J Neuropathol Exp Neurol 53:338–343

McGeehan GM, Becherer JD, Bast RC et al. (1994) Regulation of tumor necrosis factor-alpha processing by a metalloproteinase inhibitor. Nature 370:558–561

Martin R, Howell MD, Jaraquemada D et al. (1991) A myelin basic protein peptide is recognized in the context of four HLA-DR types associated with multiple sclerosis. J Exp Med 173:19–24

Miller A, Lider O, Roberts B, Sporn B, Weiner HL (1992) Suppressor T cells generated by oral tolerization to myelin basic protein suppress both in vitro and in vivo immune responses by the release of TGF beta after antigen-specific triggering. Proc Natl Acad Sci USA 89:421–425

Misfeldt ML (1990) Microbial superantigens. Infect Immun 58:2409–2413

Monaco JJ (1992) Genes in the MHC that may affect antigen processing. Curr Opin Immunol 4:70–73

Moscarello MA, Wood DD, Ackerley C, Boulias C (1994) Myelin in multiple sclerosis is developmentally immature. J Clin Invest 94:146–154

Murphy KW, Weaver CT, Elish M (1989) Peripheral tolerance to allogeneic class II histocompatibility antigens expressed in transgenic mice: evidence against a clonal deletion mechanism. Proc Natl Acad Sci USA 86:10034–10038

Myers KJ, Dougherty JP, Ron Y (1993) In vivo antigen presentation by both brain parenchymal cells and hematopoietically derived cells during the induction of experimental autoimmune encephalomyelitis. J Immunol 15:2252–2260

Nepom G, Erlich HA (1991) MHC-class II molecules and autoimmunity. Ann Rev Immunol 9:493–525

Newcombe J, Glynn P, Cuzner ML (1982) Analysis by transfer electrophoresis of reactivity of IgG with brain proteins in multiple sclerosis. J Neurochem 39:1192–1194

Nikolic-Zugic J (1994) A relationship between positive and negative selection. In: Nikolic-Zugic J (ed) Intrathymic T-cell development. Molecular Biology Intelligence Unit, RG Landes Company, Austin, pp 115–126

Offner H, Hashim G, Vandenbark A (1991) T cell receptor peptide therapy triggers autoregulation of experimental encephalomyelitis. Science 251:430–432

Ohguro H, Chiba S, Igarashi Y et al. (1993) Beta-arrestin and arrestin are recognized by autoantibodies in sera from multiple sclerosis patients. Proc Natl Acad Sci USA 90:3241–3245

Oksenberg JR (1994) Selective targeting of the immune response in autoimmune demyelination. West J Med 161:255–259

Oksenberg JR, Steinman L (1990) The role of the MHC and T cell receptor in susceptibility to multiple sclerosis. Curr Opin Immunol 2:619–621

Oksenberg JR, Stuart S, Begovich AB et al. (1990a) Limited heterogeneity of rearranged T-cell receptor V alpha transcripts in brains of multiple sclerosis patients. Nature 345:344–346

Oksenberg JR, Mantegazza R, Sakai K, Bernard CCA, Steinman L (1990b) HTLV-1 sequences are not detected in peripheral blood genomic DNA or in brain cDNA of multiple sclerosis patients. Ann Neurol 28:574–577

Oksenberg JR, Panzara MA, Begovich AB et al. (1993a) Selection for T-cell receptor Vβ-Dβ-Jβ gene rearrangements with specificity for a myelin basic protein peptide in brain lesions of multiple sclerosis. Nature 362:68–70

Oksenberg JR, Begovich AB, Erlich E, Steinman L (1993b) Genetic factors in multiple sclerosis. JAMA 270:2362–2369

Olerup O, Hillert J, Fredrikson S et al. (1989) Primarily chronic progressive and relapsing/remitting MS: two immunogenetically distinct disease entities. Proc Natl Acad Sci USA 86:7113–7117

Olsson T, Baig S, Hojeberg B, Link H (1990) Antimyelin basic protein and antimyelin antibody-producing cells in MS. Ann Neurol 27:132–136

Ota K, Matsui M, Milford E et al. (1990) T cell recognition of an immunodominant myelin basic protein epitope in multiple sclerosis. Nature 346:183–187

Ozawa K, Suchanek G, Breitschopf H et al. (1994) Patterns of oligodendroglia pathology in multiple sclerosis. Brain 117:1311–1322

Paliard X, West S, Lafferty J et al. (1991) Evidence for the effects of a superantigen in rheumatoid arthritis. Science 253:325–329

Panitch HS (1994) Influence of infection on exacerbations of multiple sclerosis. Ann Neurol 36:S25–S28

Parker DC (1993) The function of antigen recognition in T cell-dependent B cell activation. Semin Immunol 5:413–420

Pericak-Vance MA, Bebout JL, Gaskell PCJ et al. (1991) Linkage studies in familial Alzheimer disease: evidence for chromosome linkage. Am J Hum Genet 48:1034–1050

Perry VH (1994) Macrophages and the nervous system. Neuroscience Intelligence Unit, RG Landes Company, Austin

Pette M, Fujita K, Kitze B et al. (1990) Myelin basic protein specific T cell lines from MS patients and healthy individuals. Neurology 40:1770–1776

Pham-Dinh D, Mattei M, Nussbaumm JC et al. (1993) Myelin/oligodendrocyte glycoprotein is a member of a subset of the immunoglobulin superfamily encoded within the major histo-

compatibility complex. Proc Natl Acad Sci USA 90:7990–7994
Phillips JT (1993) Genetic susceptibility models in multiple sclerosis. In: Rosenberg RN, Prusiner SB, DiMauro S, Barchi RL, Kunkel LM (eds) The molecular and genetic basis of neurological disease. Butterworth-Heinemann, Boston, pp 41–46
Powis SJ, Deverson EV, Coadwell WJ et al. (1992) Effect of polymorphism of an MHC linked transporter on the peptides assembled in a class I molecule. Nature 357:211–215
Pullen AM, Kappler JW, Marrack P (1989) Tolerance to self antigens shapes the T-cell repertoire. Immunol Rev 107:125–139
Raine CS (1994a) The Dale E. McFarlin memorial lecture. The immunology of the multiple sclerosis lesion. Ann Neurol 36:S61–S72
Raine CS (1994b) Multiple sclerosis: immune system molecule expression in the central nervous system. J Neuropathol Exp Neurol 53:328–337
Raine CS, Canella B (1992) Adhesion molecules and central nervous system inflammation. Semin Neurosci 4:201–211
Reddy EP, Sandberg-Wollheim M, Mettus RC et al. (1988) Amplification and molecular cloning of HTLV-I sequences from DNA of multiple sclerosis patients. Science 243:529–533
Renno T, Zeine R, Girard JM et al. (1994) Selective enrichment of Th1 CD45RB low CD4+ T cells in autoimmune infiltrates in experimental allergic encephalomyelitis. Int Immunol 6:347–354
Risch N (1990) Linkage strategies for genetically complex traits: I. Multilocus models. Am J Hum Genet 46:222–228
Robinson MA, Kindt JT (1992) Linkage between T cell receptor genes and susceptibility to multiple sclerosis: a complex issue. Reg Immunol 4:274–283
Roddy J, Clark I, Hazelman BC, Compston DA, Scolding NJ (1994) Cerebrospinal fluid concentrations of the complement MAC inhibitor CD59 in multiple sclerosis patients and in patients with other neurological disorders. J Neurol 241:557–560
Rodriguez M, Scheithauer BW, Forbes G, Kelly PJ (1993) Oligodendrocyte injury is an early event in lesions of multiple sclerosis. Mayo Clin Proc 68:627–636
Romanic AM, Madri JA (1994) The induction of 72-kD gelatinase in T cells upon adhesion to endothelial cells is VCAM-1 dependent. J Cell Biol 125:1165–1178
Rose J, Gerken S, Lynch S et al. (1993) Genetic susceptibility in familial multiple sclerosis not linked to the myelin basic protein gene. Lancet 342:1179–1181
Ruddle NH, Bergman CM, McGrath KM et al. (1990) An antibody to lymphotoxin and tumor necrosis factor prevents transfer of experimental allergic encephalomyelitis. J Exp Med 172:1193–2000
Schall TJ (1991) Biology of the RANTES/sis cytokine family. Cytokine 3:165–183
Schall TJ, Bacon K, Toy KJ, Goeddel DV (1990) Selective attraction of monocytes and T lymphocytes of the memory phenotype by cytokine RANTES. Nature 347:669–671
Schluesener HJ, Sobel RA, Linington C, Weiner HL (1987) Monoclonal antibodies against a myelin oligodendrocyte glycoprotein induces relapses and demyelination in central nervous system autoimmune disease. J Immunol 139:4016–4021
Schonrich G, Kalinke U, Momburg F et al. (1991) Down-regulation of T cell receptors on self reactive T cells as a novel mechanism for extrathymic tolerance induction. Cell 65:293–304
Scott B, Liblau R, Degermann S et al. (1994) A role for non-MHC genetic polymorphism in susceptibility to spontaneous autoimmunity. Immunity 1:73–82
Seboun E, Robinson MA, Doolittle TH et al. (1989) A susceptibility locus for multiple sclerosis is linked to the T cell receptor beta chain complex. Cell 57:1095–1100
Selmaj K, Brosnan CF, Raine CS (1991) Colocalization of TCR γδ lymphocytes and hsp65+ oligodendrocytes in multiple sclerosis. Proc Natl Acad Sci USA 88:6452–6456
Seth A, Stern LJ, Ottenhoff THM et al. (1994) Binary and ternary complexes between T-cell receptor, class II MHC and superantigen in vitro. Nature 369:324–327
Sharief MK, Hentges R (1991) Association between TNF alpha and disease progression in patients with multiple sclerosis. N Engl J Med 325:467–472
Shimonkevitz R, Colburn C, Burnham JA, Murray RS, Kotzin BL (1993) Clonal expansion of activated γ/δ T cells in recent-onset multiple sclerosis. Proc Natl Acad Sci USA 90:923–927
Simpson E (1988) Function of the MHC. Immunol Suppl 1:27–30
Soderstrom M, Link H, Sim JB et al. (1993) T cells recognizing multiple peptides of myelin basic protein are found in the blood and enriched in the cerebrospinal fluid in optic neuritis and multiple sclerosis. Scand J Immunol 37:355–368
Spurkland A, Ronningen K, Vandvik B, Thorsby E, Vartdal F (1991) HLA-DQA1 and HLA-DQB1 genes may jointly determine susceptibility to develop multiple sclerosis. Hum Immunol 30:69–75
Steinman L (1994) Specific motifs in T cell receptor VβDβJβ gene sequences in multiple sclerosis

lesions in brain. Behring Inst Mitt 94:148–157
Steinman L, Oksenberg JR, Bernard CCA (1992) Association of susceptibility to multiple sclerosis with TCR genes. Immunol Today 13:49–51
Sudweeks JD, Todd JH, Blankenhorn EP et al. (1993) Locus controlling *Bordetella pertussis*-induced histamine sensitization (Bphs), an autoimmune disease-susceptibility gene, maps distal to T-cell receptor beta chain gene on mouse chromosome 6. Proc Natl Acad Sci USA 90:3700–3704
Szafer F, Oksenberg JR, Steinman L (1994) New allelic polymorphisms in TAP genes. Immunogenetics 39:374
Tan EM (1994) Autoimmunity and apoptosis. J Exp Med 179:1083–1086
Tienari PJ, Wikstrom J, Sajantila A, Palo J, Peltonen L (1992) Genetic susceptibility to multiple sclerosis linked to myelin basic protein gene. Lancet 340:987–991
Tienari PJ, Terwilliger JD, Ott J, Palo J, Peltonen L (1994) Two-locus linkage analysis in multiple sclerosis. Genomics 19:320–325
Todd JA, Acha-Orbea H, Bell JI et al. (1988) A molecular basis for MHC class II-associated autoimmunity. Science 240:1003–1009
Traugott U, Reinherz E, Raine CS (1983) Multiple sclerosis: distribution of T cell subsets within active lesions. Science 219:308–310
Trowsdale J (1988) Molecular genetics of the MHC. Immunol Suppl 1:21–23
Trowsdale J (1993) Genomic structure and function in the MHC. Trends Genet 9:117–122
Unanue ER (1992) Cellular studies on antigen presentation by class II MHC molecules. Curr Opin Immunol 4:63–69
Usuku K, Joshi N, Hatem CJ et al. (1992a) T-cell receptor expression by cerebro-spinal fluid cells in multiple sclerosis. Neurology 42(Suppl 3):187a
Usuku K, Joshi N, Hauser SL (1992b) T-cell receptors: Germline polymorphism and patterns of usage in demyelinating diseases. Crit Rev Immunol 11:381–393
Valli A, Sette A, Kappos L et al. (1993) Binding of myelin basic protein peptides to human histocompatibility leukocyte antigen class II molecules and their recognition by T cells from multiple sclerosis patients. J Clin Invest 91:616–628
Vartdal F, Sollid L, Vandvik B, Markussen G, Thorsby E (1989) Patients with multiple sclerosis carry DQb1 genes which encode shared polymorphic amino acid sequences. Hum Immunol 25:103–110
Warren KG, Catz I, Johnson E, Mielke B (1994) Anti-myelin basic protein and anti-proteolipid protein specific forms of multiple sclerosis. Ann Neurol 35:280–289
Watanabe R, Wege H, ter Meujlen V (1983) Adoptive transfer of EAE-like lesions from rats with corona virus-induced demyelination and encephalomyelitis. Nature 305:50–53
Watanabe-Fukunaga R, Brannon CI, Copeland NG, Jenkins NA, Netaga S (1992) Lymphoproliferation disorder in mice explained by defects in *Fas* antigen that mediates apopotosis. Nature 356:314–317
Weber F, Meinl E, Aloisi F et al. (1994) Human astrocytes are only partially competent antigen presenting cells. Brain 117:59–69
Weber JL (1990) Informativeness of human (dC-dA)n (dG-dT)n polymorphisms. Genomics 7:524–530
Weber JL, May PE (1989) Abundant class of human DNA polymorphisms which can be typed using the polymerase chain reaction. Am J Hum Genet 44:388–396
Wekerle H, Kojima K, Lannes-Vieira J, Lassmann H, Linington C (1994) Animal models. Ann Neurol 36:S47–S53
Whitacre CC, Gienapp IE, Orosz C, Bitar DM (1991) Oral tolerance in experimental autoimmune encephalomyelitis: III. Evidence for clonal anergy. J Immunol 147:2155–2163
White J, Herman A, Pullen AM et al. (1989) The V beta-specific superantigen staphylococcal enterotoxin B: stimulation of mature T cells and clonal deletion in neonatal mice. Cell 56:2409–2413
Wojtowicz S (1993) Multiple sclerosis and prions. Med Hypoth 40:48–54
Wood NW, Holmans P, Clayton D, Robertson N, Compston DAS (1994) No linkage or association between multiple sclerosis and the myelin basic protein gene in affected sibling pairs. J Neurol Neurosurg Psychiatry 57:1191–1194
Wu E, Raine CS (1992) Multiple sclerosis: interactions between oligodendrocytes and hypertrophic astrocytes and their occurrence in other, non-demyelinating conditions. Lab Invest 67:88–99
Wucherpfennig KW, Strominger JL (1995) Molecular mimicry in T cell-mediated autoimmunity: viral peptides activate human T cell clones specific for myelin basic protein. Cell 80:695–705
Wucherpfennig KW, Newcombe J, Li H et al. (1992a) Gamma/delta T cell repertoire in acute multiple sclerosis lesions. Proc Natl Acad Sci USA 89:4588–4592
Wucherpfennig K, Newcombe J, Li H et al. (1992b) Polyclonal TCR Vα-Vβ repertoire in active

multiple sclerosis lesions. J Exp Med 175:993–1002
Wucherpfennig KW, Sette A, Southwood S et al. (1994a) Structural requirements for binding of an immunodominant myelin basic protein peptide to DR 2 isotypes and for its recognition by human T cell clones. J Exp Med 179:279–290
Wucherpfennig KW, Zhang J, Witek C et al. (1994b) Clonal expansion and persistance of human T cells specific for an immunodominant myelin basic protein peptide. J Immunol 152:5581–5592
Yednock TA, Cannon C, Fritz L et al. (1992) Prevention of experimental autoimmune encephalo myelitis by antibodies against α4b1 integrin. Nature 356:63–66
Zumla A (1992) Superantigens, T cells, and microbes. Clin Infect Dis 15:313–320

Additional Bibliography

Challoner PB, Smith KT, Parker JD et al. (1995) Plaque associated expression of human herpes virus 6 in multiple sclerosis. Proc Natl Acad Sci USA 92:7440–7444
Cook SD, Pohowsky-Cochan C, Bansil S, Dowling PC (1995) Evidence for MS as an infectious disease. Acta Neurol Scand Suppl 161:34–42
Ebers GC, Sadovnick AD, Risch NJ (1995) A genetic basis for familial aggregation in MS, Canadian Collaborative Study Group. Nature 377:150–151
Kellar-Wood HF, Wood NW, Holmans P, Clayton D, Robertson N, Compston DA (1995) MS and the HLA-D region: linkage and association studies. J Neuroimmunol 58:183–190
Li F, Linan MJ, Stein MC, Faustman DL (1995) Reduced expression of peptide-loaded HLA class I molecules on multiple sclerosis lymphocytes. Ann Neurol 38:147–154
Medaer R, Stinissen P, Troyen L, Raus J, Zhang J (1995) Depletion of MBP autoreactive T cells by T-cell vaccination: pilot trial in multiple sclerosis. Lancet 346:807–808
van Noort JM, van Sechel AC, Bajramovic JJ et al. (1995) The small heat-shock protein alpha B-cristallin as candidate autoantigen in multiple sclerosis. Nature 375:798–801
Wei S, Charmley P, Birchfield RI, Concannon P (1995) Human T-cell receptor Vβ gene polymorphism and multiple sclerosis. Am J Hum Genet 56:963–969

3 Future of Multiple Sclerosis Therapeutics: Rational Approaches Targeting Putative Pathogenic Mechanisms

Subramaniam Sriram

History of Therapy of Multiple Sclerosis

Since the initial description of multiple sclerosis (MS) as a distinct nosological entity 100 years ago, the etiology of the disease has remained an enigma. The lack of clear clinical criteria for the diagnosis of MS, marked variability in the natural history and lack of good markers of disease progression, have contributed to the frustration in designing and conducting successful therapeutic trials in MS (McKhann 1990). Today, the development of consortiums that plan and execute multicenter clinical trials, and also the use of MRI scans, raise the possibility of developing more sensitive surrogate markers for determining clinical response to therapy (IFNB Multiple Sclerosis Study Group 1993). A review of our present understanding of the etiology of MS is reviewed in the preceding chapter. In this chapter, we will review therapeutic strategies that have been implemented or are currently being designed in the context of our present understanding of the pathogenesis of MS.

Since the etiology of MS is unknown, understanding the pathology has helped us better to "hypothesize" the cause of MS and help to design strategies for its treatment (Raine 1994; Whitaker 1994). Acute MS lesions show marked perivenous inflammation, with a preponderance of T lymphocytes (Hauser et al. 1986). These lesions resemble, at least in part, postinfectious or postvaccination syndromes, seen either as a consequence of rabies vaccination or following viral exanthems (Lampert 1978). This observation has led to treatment strategies targeting lymphocyte surface antigens either to delete them or to render them inactive (Steinman 1991). Also, a reliable experimental model of central nervous system (CNS) inflammation became available when Rivers et al. showed the development of an acute inflammatory demyelinating disease in monkeys after immunization with crude brain extract in adjuvant (Rivers and Schwentker 1935). In 1936, Putnam, writing about MS, referred it as, "An acute process in many cases that may represent an allergic response to the partial administration (or response) to toxins or organ extracts" (Putnam 1936). These observations set the stage for MS to be viewed as an "autoallergic or autoimmune" process. To reconcile the environmental factors that may play a role in the pathogenesis of MS, it is now generally believed that an external agent, such as a virus, may act as a trigger to initiate an autoallergic response that proceeds to develop into an inflammatory demyelinating disease (McFarlin and McFarland 1982). The concept that MS is an autoimmune disease has powerfully influenced treatment strategies over the last decade.

Basis for Multiple Sclerosis as an Autoimmune Disease

The evidence that MS is an autoimmune disease is circumstantial (Dhib-Jalbut and McFarlin 1990). The association between MS and certain genes of the major histocompatibility complex (MHC) provides the strongest argument to link MS as an autoimmune disease (Olerup and Hillert 1990; Tiwari and Terasaki 1985). In addition, many similarities between MS and the experimental counterpart, experimental allergic encephalitis (EAE) have furthered this association. EAE shares many of the clinical and pathologic features seen in MS, but it does not necessarily follow that the autoantigens that induce EAE are identical or closely related to those in MS (McFarlin and McFarland 1982). Attempts to discover the autoantigen in MS have been inconclusive perhaps because technology available today is not sufficiently sensitive to detect relevant reactivity to autoantigen. If Koch's postulates for defining the causative agent of an infectious disease were to be applied to MS, only successful therapy aimed at eliminating that clonal population of T cells that react to the antigen is likely conclusively to demonstrate a causal association between an antigen and MS (Owens and Sriram 1995; Zamvil and Steinman 1989).

Paradigm for Central Nervous System Inflammation and Demyelination

Since therapy should start a priori with certain assumptions, two murine models (Theiler's murine encephalomyelitis and EAE) have been used to design and test therapies in MS (Alvord et al. 1984; Dal-Canto and Rabinowitz 1982). Over the last two decades, EAE has become the principal model system used to understand the pathophysiologic processes underlying inflammatory, autoimmune demyelination in the CNS, and to test the efficacy of immunotherapeutic agents (Martenson 1984). Unlike other experimental autoimmune diseases, a chronic relapsing form of EAE (CR-EAE) can be induced in mice and guinea pigs (Fritz et al. 1983; Lassman and Wisniewski 1979; Lublin et al. 1981). The ability to follow the incidence and severity of relapses makes CR-EAE an important model, since success or failure of a compound can be ascertained in an established disease, which is a clinically more relevant setting. Unfortunately, many immunotherapeutic studies in EAE have been conducted in the acute monophasic form of EAE, and therefore the efficacy of these therapies in established CR-EAE remains to be seen. It should also be emphasized that the EAE model is no acid test for the success or failure of subsequent therapies in MS. Gamma interferon has been shown to prevent EAE in mice, while its administration to MS patients worsens the disease (Voorthuis et al. 1990; Weinstock-Guttmann et al. 1995). Thus, treatment results in EAE are not necessarily the same in MS patients. Beta interferon was used in MS prior to its study in EAE, and is just now being studied in EAE to clarify its mechanisms of action. As a corollary, the lack of evidence of a particular compound in EAE does not necessarily exclude its therapeutic role in MS.

An ideal form of immunotherapy for autoimmune disease is one that would exclusively delete or render unresponsive a large portion of the autoreactive repertoire while leaving the rest of the immune system intact. The application of such a principle has been successful in EAE, in which the autoantigens (peptides) are known and the relevant T-cell and MHC genes that control the immune responses have limited heterogeneity. The extension of these very principles to the treatment of human disease such as MS has been hampered by the failure to demonstrate immune reactivity to a particular antigen exclusively in patients with autoimmune disease or the presence of T cells with a restricted repertoire to autoantigens. Another assumption in the approach of antigen-specific therapies in autoimmune disease is that the autoantigen, and hence the autoreactive T-cell repertoire, is fixed over time. However, results from studies in EAE suggest otherwise. Nine days after immunization of PLJ mice with MBP a T-cell response restricted to peptide 1-11 of Myelin basic protein (MBP) is seen. However, 21–180 days later, reactivity to several new determinants of MBP (p35–47, p81–100 and p121–140) occurs. This phenomena, termed determinant spreading, suggests that the autoreactive repertoire changes and hence becomes a "moving target" for successful application of antigen-specific therapies. This not withstanding, a number of studies to delete "putative autoantigen reactive cells" are scheduled to go into trials over the next few years.

For the next decade, while the search for a better test to demonstrate the presence of key autoantigens will continue, immunotherapy of MS will focus on means to limit inflammation, prevent demyelination and promote remyelination. The development of the immune response after the expansion of the autoreactive T-cell repertoire is complex. Nonetheless, it is possible to contain the extent of the inflammation without knowledge of the autoantigen. This limitation of the inflammatory process is likely to occur at multiple levels, as illustrated in Figure 3.1, and is likely to be the focus of the immunotherapies listed in Table 3.1 over the ensuing years.

Target 1. The "Initial Hit": Role of Agents that Prevent the Migration of Cells Across the Blood–Brain Barrier

Lymphocyte migration across the blood-brain barrier is a key event in the development of inflammatory lesions and, as such, represents an opportunity for potential therapeutic intervention. MRI scans show a breakdown in the blood–

brain barrier, presumably indicating areas of extravasation of lymphocytes into the brain parenchyma, in patients undergoing clinical relapses. High dose methylprednisolone restores the integrity of the blood–brain barrier and thereby alleviates the symptoms of MS.

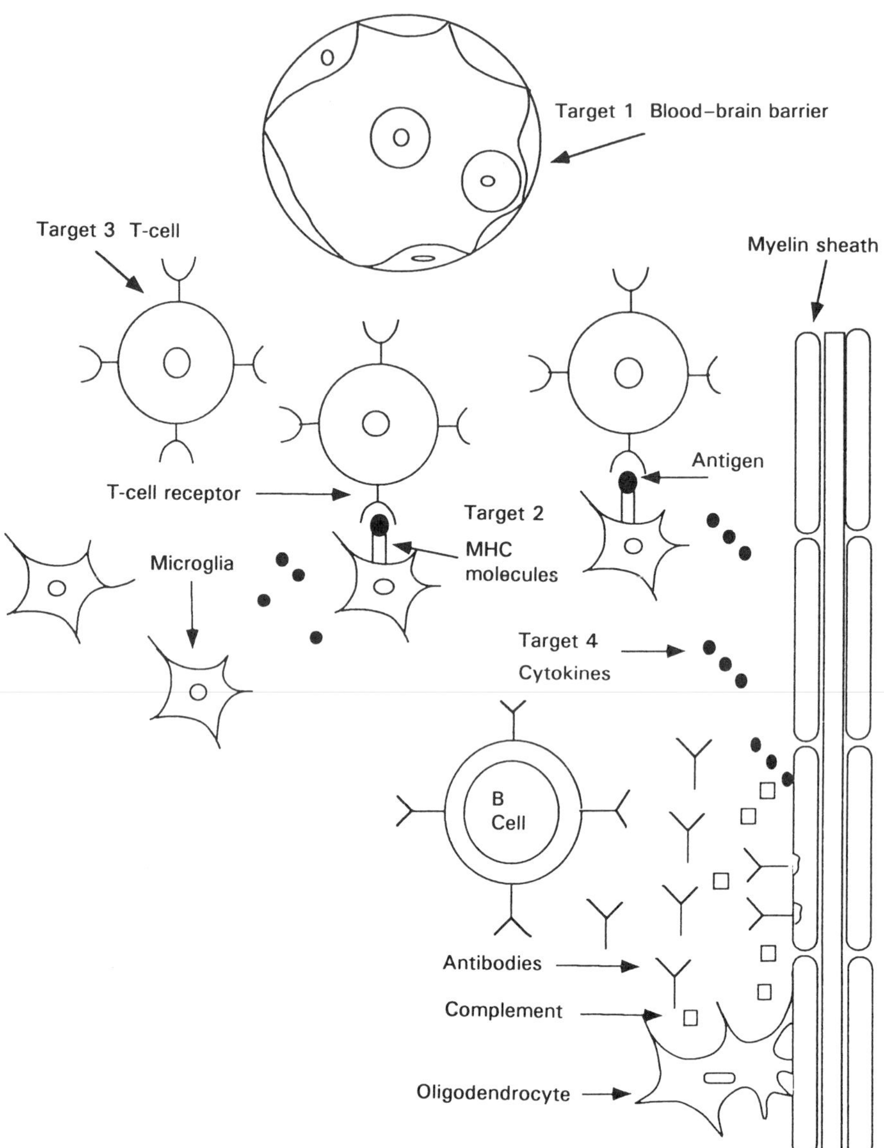

Figure 3.1. Immunotherapy of MS. Representation of the cascade of events that lead from breakdown of the blood–brain barrier to demyelination. Also represented are points in the inflammatory cascade where immune intervention is likely to result in reversal of inflammation and demyelination.

Table 3.1. Strategies for immunotherapy of multiple sclerosis

Target	Strategy	Pharmacologic agents
Blood–brain barrier	Reduces extravasation of lymphocytes into brain	Glucocorticoids[a] Antibodies to adhesion molecules, VLA-4[c], ICAM[c], L-Selectin[c] TGF-β[b], IFN-β
MHC class II antigens	Inhibits T-cell–MHC interaction	Antibodies to MHC class II antigens[c] Vaccination with MHC beta chain peptides[c]
	Decreases expression of MHC class II molecules	IL-10[c], TGF-β[b], IFN-β[a]
Alternate leukocyte antigens	Decreases costimultion of T cells	Antibodies to B7[c], CD52[b]
Antigenic peptide	Altered peptide ligand	Altered self-peptides[c]
	Decoy peptide	Copolymer 1[d]
	Anergy	High dose peptide[b], oral tolerance[b], soluble class II MHC peptide complexes[a]
Non-polymorphic molecules on T cells	Delete helper T cells	Antibodies to CD4[b], CD3[b], CD52[b]
Signaling molecules in T cells	Impede T-cell signaling responsible for T-cell expansion	Cyclosporine[b], FK 506[c], anti-IL-2 receptor antibodies[c] Antibodies to T cell receptor[c]
T-cell receptor	Inactivation of autoreactive T cells	T-cell receptor peptide vaccination[b]
Cytokines	Decrease action of proinflammatory cytokines	Antibodies to TNF-α[c], IL-1[c] and IL-12[c]; antibodies to IL-2[c] receptor, IL-1R antagonist[c]
	Enhance action of immuno-suppressive cytokines	Alpha and beta interferon[a], IL-10[c], TGF-β[b]
	Soluble receptors to cytokines	Soluble TNF receptor[c]
	Switch from Th1 to Th2 type cytokines	Pentoxyfylline[b], mercuric chloride[c], oral tolerance[b]
Oligodendrocytes	Remyelination	Oligodendrocyte-specific growth factors[c]
Broad spectrum immunosuppressants	Prevent expansion of T cells	2-Chlorodeoxyadenosine[b]

[a]Accepted treatment modality.
[b]Phase I/Phase II clinical trial.
[c]Preclinical trial.
[d]Phase III clinical trial.

Extravasation is a carefully regulated process in the CNS, controlled by cell surface adhesion molecules, cytokines and chemokines. Studies in EAE have revealed that, normally, only activated lymphocytes can cross the blood–brain barrier. If activated lymphocytes are not specific for CNS proteins, inflammation does not develop (Wekerle et al. 1986). Cells that do encounter antigen within the CNS are stimulated to secrete cytokines, which increase the expression of adhesion molecules on endothelial cells. This permits entry of non-activated lymphocytes and macrophages, forming a breach in the blood–brain barrier and development of inflammation.

Immunohistochemical staining has documented the increased expression of important adhesion molecules on endothelium in inflamed areas of the CNS in both EAE and MS (Cannella et al. 1991, Washington et al. 1994). The relative importance of these cell surface receptors is not clear but the contribution of very late antigen 4 (VLA-4) and its ligand, vascular cell adhesion molecule 1 (VCAM-1), has been the subject of several recent studies. VLA-4 belongs to the integrin family of receptors and is expressed on activated T cells. VCAM-1 is absent on normal endothelial cells but expression is induced by cytokines. Because expression of both of these molecules is restricted to activation and inflammation, they are logical targets for blockade of extravasation. Administration of antibodies to VLA-4 prevented EAE in Lewis rats (Yednock et al. 1992). Subsequently, a T-cell clone, which expressed high levels of VLA-4, was shown to be encephalitogenic, whereas variants of the same clone expressing lower levels of VLA-4 were unable to transfer disease. In this study, administration of antibodies to either VLA-4 or VCAM delayed the onset of paralysis (Baron et al. 1993). In contrast to both of these studies, blocking of a distinct pair of adhesion molecules, intercellular adhesion molecule 1 (ICAM-1) and lymphocyte function associated antigen 1 (LFA-1) did not affect the onset or severity of paralysis in EAE (Cannella et al. 1993). In fact, worsening of disease was observed in some mice that received anti-LFA-1 antibodies. This highlights the fact that, while adhesion molecules do play a role in lymphocyte accumulation in the CNS, blocking interactions between these molecules may not always have the desired effect. Since multiple molecules are involved in the process, interfering with only one interaction may not significantly influence extravasation. Even with repeated administration of antibody, only delays in the onset of paralysis were observed. A cocktail of antibodies to the critical receptors or ligands might have a more profound effect on inflammation, but treatment with monoclonal antibodies may ultimately be limited by the development of antibodies that neutralize the monoclonal.

Cytokines also influence lymphocyte migration by regulating expression of adhesion molecules or acting as chemotactic factors. Administration of anti-inflammatory cytokines and therapies designed to block the action of pro-inflammatory cytokines exert effects on multiple levels, including lymphocyte migration. For example, transforming growth factor beta (TGF-β2) has been shown to prevent and treat EAE. While TGF β affects T-cell proliferation, it also decreases the migration of lymphocytes through endothelial cells in vitro; administration of TGF-β to mice inhibits the migration of lymphocytes into the CNS in vivo. Tumor necrosis factor (TNF) induces expression of many adhesion molecules. Therefore, antibodies to TNF may affect T-cell trafficking in addition to blocking the cytotoxicity of TNF. Both TGF-β and anti-TNF strategies have been shown to ameliorate EAE and are being evaluated in clinical trials.

Other agents that alter blood–brain barrier permeability, such as prazosin, may also be useful in limiting CNS inflammation. Unfortunately, all of these approaches may have little effect beyond influencing the extent of damage unless given continuously. It seems likely that inhibitors of lymphocyte migration would be more useful for acute exacerbations of MS than for halting chronic disease progression.

Target 2. Major Histocompatibility Complex Antigens: Immune Response Molecules

Although there is a strong association between the susceptibility to develop MS and MHC class II molecules, the nature of this association is not clear (Olerup and Hillert 1990). It is presumed (given the function of the MHC molecules) that the link between MHC antigens and MS relates to a particular peptide that is presented by the MHC molecule to T cells. In order for T-cell responses to occur, protein antigens must be processed into 15–20 amino acid length peptides by antigen-presenting cells, bind non-covalently to MHC class II molecules and be presented to T cells. Any process that competes or displaces autopeptides is likely to prevent the generation of a T-cell response. Two strategies have arisen from the knowledge that autoreactive T cells recognize specific autopeptides presented by MHC class II molecules. In EAE, wherein the autopeptides are known, it is possible to treat and prevent EAE by displacing the autopeptides with non-encephalitogenic peptides that have a higher affinity to self-MHC class II molecules (Oksenberg et al. 1993a). This form of "decoy or designer peptides" therapy is feasible if the autopeptide in MS is known. Other limitations of peptide-based therapy are the short half-life of the peptides in vivo, the unlikely presumptions that autoimmune disease is dictated by a single or a limited number of self-peptides and that the autoimmune response to the peptides is fixed for the length of the disease. So far, designer peptides have not been tested in CR-EAE (Smilek et al. 1991). It is thought that copolymer 1, a drug currently in trials for the treatment of MS, acts in a manner similar to "decoy" peptides (Chapter 13).

An alternate strategy is to target the MHC molecule. The association between MS and a limited number of HLA-D molecules is high. The majority of MS patients have either HLA-DR2 or the DR4 allele (Olerup and Hillert 1990). This association is across almost all major ethnic groups. Studies in EAE have shown that therapy with antibodies to the MHC molecule is successful in the prevention and in the treatment of acute and CR-EAE in mice, as well as in monkeys treated with HLA-DR antibodies that cross-reacted with MHC class II molecules of monkeys (Jonkers et al. 1988; Sriram et al. 1987). The attractiveness of targeting MHC molecules is that, since most individuals are heterozygous at the MHC locus, inhibition of function of one of the alleles is unlikely to lead to global immunosuppression. This approach is referred to as allele-specific therapy. We have extended this approach by using MHC class II beta chain proteins as vaccines to generate auto-anti-MHC class II antibodies. In so doing, animals vaccinated with self-MHC peptides of the MHC antigens that are associated with disease susceptibility generate auto-MHC class II antibodies. Animals vaccinated in this manner are resistant to the development of EAE; furthermore, if animals are vaccinated after the development of the acute attack, there is a reduction in the severity and the number of clinical relapses (Topham et al. 1994). Vaccination with MHC antigens does not depend upon knowledge of the autoantigen or the T-cell receptor. A Phase I clinical trial of DR4 beta chain hypervariable region peptides has begun in patients with rheumatoid arthritis (RA) in view of the high frequency of the DR4 allele in patients with RA.

Target 3. T Cells: Deletion of the Autoreactive T-Cell Repertoire

The excitement that followed the knowledge that there is a restricted use of T-cell receptor genes in EAE, and the relative ease of deleting these autoreactive T cells to prevent and treat EAE, have been difficult to duplicate in MS (Acha-Orbea et al. 1988; Ben-Nun et al. 1981; Vandenbark et al. 1989; Zamvil et al. 1988). As might have been expected, attempts to isolate T-cell clones of relevance in human autoimmune disease have been complicated by a number of factors, the most difficult being the ability to establish their pathogenicity (Allegretta et al. 1990; Hafler et al. 1988; Ota et al. 1990; Pette et al. 1990). In the absence of a clearly defined reactivity to autopeptide(s) in disease-affected individuals, investigators have attempted to clone relevant T-cell receptor (TCR) genes from brains of individuals with MS. Oksenberg et al. have found a sequence motif within the CDR3 of TCR Vβ of certain human and rodent T-cell clones that recognize peptides of MBP (Oksenberg et al. 1990; Oksenberg et al. 1993b). Since the rodent T cells bearing this TCR sequence were pathogenic, the authors inferred that the human T-cell clones may also be responsible for disease. However, the TCR profile is but a snapshot in time of a disease that proceeds over decades. It is not known if the same TCR motifs are present or are pathogenic at all times. Certain restricted V gene usage in T cells has also been seen in mice during recovery from EAE. These TCR genes are thought to play a role in recovery; deleting this TCR made EAE worse (Kumar and Sercarz 1993). These limitations have dampened the initial enthusiasm that MS and other autoimmune diseases may be treated by a set of precision tools that only target the autoreactive T-cell repertoire.

Oral Tolerance

The oral administration of tissue specific antigens has been shown to lead to amelioration of disease in several autoimmune models of disease, including EAE. The mechanism by which oral administration of antigen induces suppression of autoimmune disease is not clear. Both induction of T-cell anergy and induction of suppressor cells have been proposed as means by which reduction of disease activity is seen to occur (Khoury et al. 1992; Weiner et al. 1994). The latter process has been termed "antigen driven bystander suppression". This mechanism is mediated by CD8+ suppressor T cells and involves the secretion of TGF-β or other suppressive cytokines (Weiner et al. 1994). Because of the bystander effect, the necessity to know the exact antigen is no longer relevant.

The first therapeutic trial of oral tolerance in patients with MS was found to be safe, but efficacy was not rigorously assessed (Weiner et al. 1993). The results of an ongoing Phase III, placebo-controlled clinical trial on oral bovine myelin in patients with MS will help to determine the future role of this therapeutic approach. In a similar trial in orally administered solubilized type II collagen to patients with RA produced a small, but statistically significant, clinical benefit

(Trentham et al. 1993). These results should be interpreted cautiously because of differences in the baseline characteristics of patients, and the lack of a wash-out period for patients who were previously treated with immunosuppressive drugs.

CD4 Molecules

The CD4 molecule is an important coreceptor, which is involved in establishing a better contact between T cells and MHC class II antigens on antigen-presenting cells. Deletion of CD4+ T cells is successful in the prevention and treatment of virtually every known animal model of autoimmune disease (Sriram et al. 1988). In addition, animals immunized with antigens under the umbrella of anti-CD4 antibody therapy are rendered tolerant. This may have deleterious consequences when given to individuals with a chronic disease, such as toxoplasmosis (Vollmer et al. 1987). The potential toxicity notwithstanding, there have been two published reports of the effect of monoclonal antibodies on CD4 in MS (Lindsey et al. 1994). This most recent study also showed no statistical difference in the number of enhancing lesions on sequential MRI scans at a time when all patients had a greater than 75% decrease in circulating CD4 cells. At least six open label trials of anti-CD4 antibodies have been completed in RA (Elliott and Maini 1994). While the safety of the study, at least for the short term, has been good, there has been no consistent improvement in clinical scores. The major reservation with this therapy is the marked depression of CD4 counts that persists for 18 months. It is now known that the ability of the thymus to repopulate fresh, naive CD4 cells decreases significantly with age (Mackall et al. 1995). Any benefit from therapy for a chronic disease that might necessitate reduction of CD4 counts for extended periods may be offset by the risks of intercurrent infections.

Alternate Leukocyte Antigens

T-cell activation and expansion requires not only the interaction between the T-cell receptor, antigenic peptide and the MHC class II antigen, but also other associated signals. These include the interaction between the CD28 molecule on T cells with that of B7 molecule on antigen-presenting cells. The fusion product of CTLA-4 and immunoglobulin interferes with this interaction and is successful in the prevention of a number of autoimmune diseases, including EAE (Perrin et al. 1995).

CD52 is a pan-lymphocyte glycoprotein with no clearly defined function. CAMPATH-1 is a humanized antibody to CD52, administration of which induces profound lymphopenia. Preliminary studies on the efficacy of CD52 antibody in RA and MS have been completed. Seven MS patients who received CAMPATH-1 have shown a decrease in the number of MRI lesions during the period of lymphopenia when compared with MRI scans carried out prior to being on the protocol (Moreau et al. 1994). A therapeutic benefit was also seen in RA patients treated with CAMPATH-1 (Isaacs et al. 1992).

IL-2 and IL-2 Receptor

Since T cells are thought to play a major role in disease pathogenesis, a rational approach has been to limit their growth and expansion. T-cell growth is mediated by IL-2 and its receptor, IL-2R. Agents that block the proliferation of T cells by interfering with subcellular signaling pathways established following interaction of antigen with TCR, or through blocking of the IL-2R have been successful in the management of transplantation rejection. Cyclosporine and FK506 interfere with the pathways that determine cell cycle progression. The multicenter trial of cyclosporine in MS showed a modest success in delaying clinical progression (Multiple Sclerosis Study Group 1990). Trials with other drugs that interfere with signaling through the TCR or the IL-2 receptor are being planned (Waldmann 1993). It is expected that the decreased toxicity of these agents will offer advantages over cyclosporine.

Target 4. Cytokines

While the term cytokines is used to connote molecules that regulate the growth and proliferation of cells, the term signaling molecules is perhaps more appropriate, since cytokines alter the function and expression of many molecules, including those that determine cell growth and differentiation (Heremans et al. 1989). Cytokines made by T cells at the inflammatory site are thought to be important mediators of demyelination in EAE and MS. CD4+ T cells are divided by their cytokine profile into Th1 and Th2 subtypes. CD4+ Th1 cells are high producers of IL-2, TNF and IFN-γ, while Th2 T cells produce IL-4 and IL-10. Functionally, Th1-type cells are responsible for delayed type hypersensitivity response, while Th2 cells promote B-cell growth and antibody formation. Several factors including the route of administration of antigen, MHC antigens and circulating cytokines dictate whether the T-cell response is likely to be Th1 or Th2 following immunization with antigen (Liblau et al. 1995). IL-12 and IFN-γ administered at the time of immunization are likely to lead to a Th1 response while IL-4 and IL-10 strongly direct the development of the Th2-type immune response. Recent data has indicated that Th1 cells are pathogenic in EAE and that recovery from EAE is regulated by T cells of the Th2 phenotype (Karpus et al. 1992). Stable MS patients exhibit a Th2 cytokine pattern in circulatory mononuclear cells, while active MS patients exhibit a Th1 pattern (Rieckmann 1994).

Pathologic studies in MS have established the inflammatory nature of the lesions in the brain and the increase in the levels of certain cytokine molecules in the CSF (Beck et al. 1988; Hauser et al. 1990). While it may be simplistic to deduce the functions of cytokines when studied in vitro from those that are present in vivo at sites of inflammation, certain assumptions about their functions are nonetheless becoming clear. Thus, IFN-γ, perhaps due to its proinflammatory properties, worsens MS (Panitch and Bever 1993). Another proinflammatory cytokine, TNF, is secreted by macrophages and T cells and is myelinotoxic in organ cultures (Selmaj and Raine 1988; Selmaj et al. 1991). Increased levels of TNF are seen in the CSF of patients with MS, which appears to correlate with disease severity (Sharief and Hentges 1991). TGF-β, a molecule that is secreted by T cells, macrophages and platelets, has been seen in the CSF of patients recovering from clinical relapses, suggesting that it might play a role in promoting recovery. TGF-β is a potent cytokine that arrests growth of T cells at the G_1 to S phase transition. The attractiveness of cytokines as therapeutic agents is in part due to the fact that the molecules occur during inflammation and play a role in the natural recovery from EAE (Johns et al. 1991; Johns and Sriram 1993; Racke et al. 1993; Racke et al. 1991; Sharief and Hentges 1991).

Approaches to Cytokine-Based Therapies

Antibodies to Proinflammatory Cytokines

The traditional approach to counter the effect of naturally occurring proinflammatory cytokines has been the use of monoclonal antibodies to soluble proinflammatory cytokines such as TNF-α. In EAE, severity of the disease correlates with the quantity of TNF made by T cells, and anti-TNF antibody reverses acute EAE (Ruddle et al. 1990). Preliminary trials with anti-TNF antibody have been completed in patients with RA and extension of these trials into MS patients is currently under way. The studies of anti-TNF antibody in RA have shown significant decreases in levels of C-reactive protein and sedimentation rate, along with reduction of pain and swelling. IL-12 has potent proinflammatory properties and in vitro has been shown to induce the secretion of IFN-γ, IL-1 and TNF by T cells. It is believed to play a key role in regulating the T-cell cytokine profile toward proinflammatory responses. Antibodies to IL-12 are protective in EAE and, furthermore, anti-IL-12 antibodies are able to switch the immune response from Th1 to a Th2 subtype (see below). Use of IL-12 or IFN-γ antagonists would be attractive therapeutic strategies.

Naturally Occurring Antagonists to Proinflammatory Cytokines: IFN-α, IFN-β, IL-1Ra, TGF-β

Interferons alpha and beta have demonstrated efficacy in placebo-controlled clinical trials (Chapter 11) (Durelli et al. 1994; IFNB Multiple Sclerosis Study Group 1993). Although the mechanisms of action of IFN-β and IFN-α are not known, there is indirect evidence to suggest that each counteracts the effects of IFN-γ. IFN-α and IFN-β also appear to induce the production of TGF-β (see below), thereby further suppressing the immune response of macrophages.

IL-1 consists of two structurally related polypeptides, IL-1α and IL-1β, each of which has a broad spectrum of activities. A third related molecule is IL-1Ra, (receptor antagonist), which inhibits the activity of IL-1. IL-1 is produced mostly by macrophages and T cells and, with TNF, is responsible for the systemic symptoms that accompany sepsis. No clear role for IL-1 in MS has been proposed (Carrieri 1994). However, the known anti-inflammatory effects of IL-1Ra in EAE may warrant a study in MS (Mannie et al. 1987).

TGF-β is a homodimeric protein that has diverse effects on cell growth and on the secretion of various growth factors. Importantly TGF-β counteracts the proinflammatory effects of both TNF-α and IFN-γ, and prevents the expansion of T cells, B cells and NK cells. In addition, it controls CNS inflammation by reducing the migration of lymphocytes across the blood–brain barrier. In view of these properties, TGF-β is now in Phase I clinical trials.

Cytokine Switching Agents

If MS is considered to be disease-mediated by Th1-type cells, then factors that switch the immune response from Th1 to Th2 are likely to promote recovery. Attempts to dictate the cytokine profile of the immune response to Th2 have been made in vitro and in vivo. These have included the administration of anti-IL-12 antibodies or concomitant administration of IL-4 or IL-10 during immunization with antigen. Non-specific agents, such as mercuric chloride or pentoxyphylline (an inhibitor of cAMP), have also been shown to act in a similar manner to switch the immune response from Th1 to Th-2 (Rott et al. 1993; Saoudi et al. 1993). Whether similar strategies will be successful in an established immune response is of interest.

Proinflammatory Cytokine Receptors

In a manner analogous to the use of MHC peptide-binding antagonists, soluble receptors can be used to bind circulating cytokines and prevent their effects at the end organ. The receptors for TNF have been cloned and studies are being planned to determine if administration of excess soluble receptors can prevent the effects of the cytokines at the end organs.

Target 5. Broad Spectrum Antilymphocytic Agents

Cyclophosphamide, azathioprine and high dose corticosteroids have all been used with limited benefit in the management of MS. Limited efficacy, requirement of long term administration, short term and long term adverse events have limited their more general acceptance in clinical practice (Ebers 1993). In spite of these limitations, certain antilymphocytic agents are currently being evaluated in patients with MS. A highly specific antilymphocytic agent, 2-chlorodeoxyadenosine, which kills both resting and dividing lymphocytes, has been shown to be of benefit in patients with chronic progressive MS (Sipe et al. 1994) (Chapter 14). The results of ongoing studies with this agent are awaited with interest.

Target 6. Agents that Induce Remyelination

Since the mechanism of demyelination is not known, it may appear premature to determine if any remyelinating agents may be on the horizon. The explosion in knowledge of growth factors that affect neurons and glia are currently being explored in many degenerative diseases. In vitro cell culture experiments have suggested that fibroblast-derived growth factor and platelet-derived growth factor can potentiate oligodendrocyte growth, and other factors, such as ciliary neurotrophic growth factor, can prevent oligodendrocyte death (Louis 1993).

Conclusions

Given the inherent difficulties in performing double-blinded clinical trials in MS and the number of candidate autoantigens that are potentially available for investigation, antigen-specific therapy aimed at eliminating a clone of antigen reactive cells in MS appears, for the moment, a difficult task. Oral tolerance, if proven to be successful in the treatment of MS, may obviate the need to identify the antigen. Clinical trials, even if unsuccessful in proving benefit, are likely to provide clues to the underlying disease processes. The lack of clinical benefit seen in patients with MS and RA, whose peripheral CD4+ cells become depleted following treatment with monoclonal anti-CD4 antibodies, is causing a paradigm shift in understanding the pathogenesis of the disease. We may become less "CD4 centric" in viewing therapies for MS and may be forced to re-examine some of the basic assumptions underlying this disease.

For the next decade, while the search for a better test to demonstrate the presence of key autoantigens will continue, immunotherapy of MS will focus on the means to limit inflammation. Attempts to influence the natural course of the disease have been successful with cytokines at least for the short term. If the mechanism by which certain cytokines act is known, then drugs may be designed that interfere with either the binding or the signaling of these molecules. Synthesis of organic compounds that perform these functions, that have minimal side effects and can be administered orally and monitored easily, will form an important area of research over the next 10 years. It is quite likely that the understanding of the cause of MS may ultimately be achieved by reasoning prompted by the successes and failures of therapeutic agents.

References

Acha-Orbea H, Mitchell DJ, Timmerman L et al. (1988) Limited heterogeneity of T cell receptors from lymphocytes mediating EAE allows specific immune intervention. Cell 54:263–273

Allegretta M, Nicklas JA, Sriram S et al. (1990) T cells responsive to myelin basic protein in patients with multiple sclerosis. Science 247:718–721

Alvord E, Kies M, Suckling A (1984) Experimental allergic encephalomyelitis: a good model for multiple sclerosis. Liss, New York

Baron JL, Madri JA, Ruddle NH et al. (1993) Surface expression of alpha 4 integrin by CD4 T cells is required for their entry into brain parenchyma. J Exp Med 177:57–68

Beck J, Rondot P, Catinot L (1988) Increased production of interferon gamma and TNF in MS: do cytokines trigger relapses? Acta Neurol Scand 78:318–326
Ben-Nun A, Wekerle H, Cohen IR (1981) Vaccination against autoimmune encephalomyelitis with T lymphocyte line cells reactive against myelin basic protein. Nature 292:60–61
Cannella B, Cross AH, Raine CS (1991) Adhesion related molecules in the central nervous system. Upregulation correlates with inflammatory cell influx during relapsing EAE. Lab Invest 65:23–33
Cannella B, Cross AH, Raine CS (1993) Anti-adhesion molecule therapy in experimental autoimmune encephalomyelitis. J Neuroimmunol 46:43–55
Carrieri PB (1994) The role of cytokines in multiple sclerosis. Int. M S J 1:53–59
Dal-Canto MC, Rabinowitz SG (1982) Experimental models of virus induced demyelination. Ann Neurol 11:109–121
Dhib-Jalbut S, McFarlin DE (1990) Immunology of MS. Ann Allergy 64:433–434
Durelli L, Bongioanni MR, Cavallo R et al. (1994) Chronic systemic high dose recombinant interferon alpha 2a reduces exacerbation rate, MRI signs of disease activity and lymphocyte interferon gamma production in relapsing remitting MS. Neurology 44:406–413
Ebers GC (1993) Treatment of multiple sclerosis. Lancet 343:275–279
Elliott MJ, Maini RN (1994) New directions for biological therapy in rheumatoid arthritis. Int Arch Allergy Immunol 104:112–125
Fritz RB, Chou C-H, McFarlin DE (1983) Relapsing murine experimental allergic encephalomyelitis induced by myelin basic protein. J Immunol 130:1024–1211
Hafler DA, Duby AD, Lee SJ et al. (1988) Oligoclonal T cells in the CSF of patients with MS. J Exp Med 167:1313–1322
Hauser SL, Bhan AK, Gilles F et al. (1986) Immunocytochemical analysis of the cellular infiltrates in MS lesions. Ann Neurol 19:578–587
Hauser SL, Doolittle TH, Lincoln R (1990) Cytokine accumulation in CSF of MS patients: frequent detection of IL1 and TNF but not IL6. Neurology 40:1735–1739
Heremans H, Dillen C, Dijkmans R et al. (1989) The role of cytokines in various animal models of inflammation. Lymphokine Res 8:329–333
IFNβ Multiple Sclerosis Study Group (1993) Interferon beta-1b is effective in relapsing-remitting multiple sclerosis: I. Clinical results of a multicenter, randomized, double blind, placebo-controlled trial. Neurology 43:655–661
Isaacs JD, Watts RA, Hazelman BL et al. (1992) Humanized antibody therapy for rheumatoid arthritis. Lancet 340:748–752
Johns LD, Sriram S (1993) Experimental allergic encephalomyelitis: neutralizing antibody to TGF-β1 enhances the clinical severity of the disease. J Immunol 47:1–9
Johns LD, Flanders KC, Ranges GE et al. (1991) Successful treatment of experimental allergic encephalomyelitis with transforming growth factor-beta 1. J Immunol 147:1792–1803
Jonkers MR, Lambalgen DV, Mitchell SK et al. (1988) Successful treatment of EAE in rhesus monkeys with MHC class II specific monoclonal antibodies. J Autoimmun 1:399–414
Karpus WJ, Gould KE, Swanborg RH (1992) CD4+ suppressor cells of autoimmune encephalomyelitis respond to T cell receptor associated determinants on effector cells by IL4 secretion. Eur J Immunol 22:1757–1763
Khoury SJ, Hancock WW, Weiner HL (1992) Oral tolerance to MBP and natural recovery from EAE are associated with down regulation of inflammatory cytokines and differential upregulation of TGFβ, IL4 and prostaglandin E expression in brain. J Exp Med 176:1355–1372
Kumar V, Sercarz E (1993) The involvement of T cell receptor peptide-specific regulatory CD4+ T cells in recovery from antigen-induced autoimmune disease. J Exp Med 178:909–916
Lampert PW (1978) Autoimmune and virus induced demyelinating diseases. Am J Pathol 91:195–208
Lassman H, Wisniewski HM (1979) Chronic relapsing EAE; clinopathological comparison with multiple sclerosis. Arch Neurol 36:490–495
Liblau RS, Singer SM, McDevitt HO (1995) Th1 and Th2 CD4+ T cells in the pathogenesis of autoimmune disease. Immunol Today 16:34–39
Lindsey JW, Hodgkinson S, Mehta R et al. (1994) Repeated treatment with chimeric anti CD4 antibody in MS. Ann Neurol 36:183–188
Louis JC (1993) CNTF protects oligodendrocytes against natural and TNF induced cell death. Science 259:689–692
Lublin FD, Maurer PH, Berry RG et al. (1981) Delayed relapsing experimental allergic encephalomyelitis in mice. J Immunol 126:819–824
Mackall CL, Fleischer TA, Brown MR et al. (1995) Age, thymopoeisis, and CD4+ T lympocyte regeneration after intense chemotherapy. N Engl J Med 332:143–149

Mannie MD, Dinarello CA, Paterson PY (1987) Interleukin 1 and myelin basic protein synergistically augment adoptive transfer activity of lymphocytes mediating experimental autoimmune encephalomyelitis in Lewis rats. J Immunol 138:4229–4235

Martenson RE (1984) EAE: a good model for multiple sclerosis. Prog Clin Biol Res 146:165–172

McFarlin DE, McFarland HF (1982) Multiple sclerosis. N Engl J Med 307:1183–1188

McKhann GM (1990) Therapeutic trials for MS. Ann Neurol 27:589–590

Moreau T, Thorpe J, Miller D et al. (1994) Preliminary evidence from MRI for reduction in disease activity after lymphocyte depletion in MS. Lancet 344:298–302

Multiple Sclerosis Study Group (1990) Efficacy and toxicity of cyclosporine in chronic progressive MS: a randomized, double blind, placebo controlled clinical trial. Ann Neurol 27:592–605

Oksenberg JR, Stuart S, Begovich AB et al. (1990) Limited heterogeneity of rearranged T cell receptor Vα transcripts in brains of MS patients. Nature 345:344–349

Oksenberg JR, Panzarra MA, Steinman L (1993a) Multiple sclerosis: from immunogentics to immunotherapy. J Neurol Sci 115(Suppl):S29–S37

Oksenberg JR, Panzarra MA, Begovich AB et al. (1993b) Selection for T cell receptor V β-D β-J gene rearrangements with specificity for a myelin basic protein peptide in brain lesions of multiple sclerosis. Nature 362:68–70

Olerup O, Hillert J (1990) HLA associated genetic susceptibility in MS. Tissue Antigens 38:1–15

Ota K, Matsui M, Milford EL et al. (1990) T cell recognition of an immunodominant myelin basic protein epitope in multiple sclerosis. Nature 346:183–187

Owens T, Sriram S (1995) The immunology of MS and its animal model, experimental allergic encephalomyelitis. Neurol Clin North Am 13:51–73

Panitch HS, Bever CT (1993) Clinical trials of interferons in MS. What have we learned? J Neuroimmunol 46:155–164

Perrin PJ, Scott D, Quigley L et al. (1995) Role of B7:CD28/CTLA-4 in the induction of chronic relapsing experimental allergic encephalomyelitis. J Immunol 154:1481–1490

Pette M, Fujita K, Wilkinson D et al. (1990) Myelin auto-reactivity in MS: recognition of MBP in the context of HLA-DR2 products by T cells of MS patients and healthy donors. Proc Natl Acad Sci USA 87:7968–7972

Putnam TJ (1936) Studies in MS: similarities between some forms of encephalomyelitis and MS. Arch Neurol 35:1289–1308

Racke MK, Dhib-Jalbut S, Cannella B et al. (1991) Prevention and treatment of chronic relapsing experimental allergic encephalomyelitis by transforming growth factor-β1. J Immunol 146:3012–3017

Racke M, Sriram S, Carlino J et al. (1993) Long-term treatment of chronic relapsing experimental allergic encephalomyelitis by transforming growth factor-β2. Neuroimmunol 46:175–184

Raine CS (1994) Multiple sclerosis: immune system molecule expression in the central nervous system. J Neuropathol Exp Neurol 53:328–337

Rieckmann P, Albrecht M, Kitze B et al. (1994) Cytokine mRNA levels in mononuclear blood cells from patients with multiple sclerosis. Neurology 44:1523–1526

Rivers TM, Schwentker FF (1935) Encephalomyelitis accompanied by myelin destruction experimentally produced in monkeys. J Exp Med 61:689–702

Rott O, Cash E, Fleischer B (1993) Phosphodiesterase inhibitor pentoxyphylline a selective suppressor of T helper type 1, but not type 2-associated lymphokine production, prevents induction of experimental autoimmune encephalomyelitis in Lewis rats. Eur J Immunol 23:1745–1751

Ruddle NH, Bergman CM, McGrath ML et al. (1990) An antibody to lymphotoxin prevents EAE. J Exp Med 172:1193–1200

Saoudi A, Kuhn J, Hyugen K et al. (1993) Th2 activated cells prevent experimental autoimmune uveoretinitis, a Th1-dependent autoimmune disease. Eur J Immunol 23:3096–3103

Selmaj K, Raine CS (1988) Tumor necrosis factor mediates myelin and oligodendrocyte damage in vivo. Ann Neurol 23:339–346

Selmaj K, Raine CS, Cannella B et al. (1991) Identification of lymphotoxin and tumor necrosis factor in multiple sclerosis. 87:949–954

Sharief MK, Hentges R (1991) Association between TNF alpha and disease progression in patients with MS. N Engl J Med 325:467–472

Sipe JC, Romine JS, Koziol JA et al. (1994) Cladarabine in the treatment of chronic progressive MS. Lancet 344:9–14

Smilek DE, Wraith DC, Hodgkinson S et al. (1991) A single amino acid change in a MBP protein confers the capacity to prevent rather than cause EAE. Proc Natl Acad Sci USA 88:9633–9637

Sriram S, Topham DJ, Carroll L (1987) Haplotype-specific suppression of experimental allergic encephalomyelitis with anti-IA antibodies. J Immunol 139:1485–1489

Sriram S, Carroll L, Fortin S et al. (1988) In vivo immunomodulation by monoclonal anti-CD4 antibody: II. Effect on T cell response to myelin basic protein and experimental allergic encephalomyelitis. J Immunol 141:464–468

Steinman L (1991) The development of rational strategies for the selective immunotherapy against autoimmune disease. Adv Immunol 49:357–369

Tiwari JL, Terasaki PI (1985) HLA and disease association. Springer, New York, pp 182–185

Topham DJ, Arimilli S, Nag B et al. (1994) A synthetic peptide from the third hypervariable region of major histocompatibility complex class II β chain as a vaccine for treatment of experimental autoimmune encephalomyelitis. Proc Natl Acad Sci USA 91:8005–8009

Trentham DE, Dyenesius-Trentham RA, Orav EJ et al. (1993) Effect of oral administration of type II collagen on rheumatoid arthritis. Science 261:1727–1331

Vandenbark AA, Hashim G, Offner H (1989) Immunization with synthetic T-cell receptor V-region peptide protects against experimental autoimmune encephalomyelitis. Nature 341:544–547

Vollmer T, Vollmer MK, Steinman L et al. (1987) Depletion of CD4 lymphocytes reactivates toxoplasmosis in the CNS. J Immunol 138:3731–3741

Voorthuis JAC, Uitdehaag BMJ, DeGroot CJA et al. (1990) Suppression of EAE by intraventricular administration of IFN gamma in Lewis rats. Clin Exp Immunol 81:183–188

Waldmann TA (1993) The IL2/IL2R receptor system: a target for rational immune intervention. Immunol Today 14:264–270

Washington R, Burton J, Todd RF, Newman W, Bragovic L, Dore-Duffy P (1994) Expression of immunologically relevant endothelial cell activation antigens on isolated central nervous system microvessels from patients with multiple sclerosis. Ann Neurol 35:89–97

Weiner HL, Mackin GA, Matsui M et al. (1993) Double blind pilot trial of oral tolerization with myelin antigens in MS. Science 259:1321–1324

Weiner HL, Friedman A, Miller A et al. (1994) Oral tolerance: immunologic mechanisms and treatment of animal and human organ-specific autoimmune diseases by oral administration of autoantigens. Ann Rev Immunol 12:809–837

Weinstock-Guttmann B, Ransohoff RM, Kinkel P et al. (1995) The interferons: biological effects, mechanism of action and use in MS. Ann Neurol 37:7–15

Wekerle H, Linnington C, Lassman H et al. (1986) Cellular immune reactivity within the CNS. Trends Neurosci 9:271–276

Whitaker JN (1994) Rationale for immunotherapy in multiple sclerosis. Ann Neurol 36 Suppl:S103–S107

Yednock TA, Cannon C, Fritz LC et al. (1992) Prevention of EAE by antibodies against alpha beta integrin. Nature 356:63–66

Zamvil SS, Steinman LS (1990) The T lymphocyte in EAE. Ann Rev Immunol 8:579–621

Zamvil SS, Mitchell DJ, Lee NE et al. (1988) Predominant expression of a T cell receptor Vβ gene subfamily in autoimmune encephalomyelitis. J Exp Med 167:1586–1596

4 Statistical and Design Considerations for Multiple Sclerosis Clinical Trials

John Petkau

Introduction

Several statistical issues of current relevance to the design of clinical trials of therapies in multiple sclerosis (MS) and to the analysis of the resulting data will be discussed in this chapter. Weiss and Stadlan (1992) provide a comprehensive discussion of the major elements to be considered in the design of MS clinical trials, which continues to be relevant. The objective here is to focus on emerging issues, which have become more relevant because of recent therapeutic advances in MS and increasing recognition of the possibilities for application of alternative statistical methodology in MS clinical trials.

The focus throughout the chapter will be on statistical aspects of the conduct of pivotal (Phase III) clinical trials. In some instances, the discussion will concern statistical methodology that has long been available but may not have been used to full advantage in MS clinical trials. In others, it will concern possibilities for the application of more recently developed statistical methodology. The discussion throughout the chapter will be within the frequentist statistical framework where control of the probabilities of Type 1 and Type 2 errors for tests of hypotheses and the coverage probabilities of confidence intervals in repeated sampling are the basic requirements.

The realistic expectation that a clinical trial will demonstrate the efficacy of an agent has direct implications for its design. Of primary importance among these is the ethical requirement that the accumulating efficacy data be monitored on a regular basis so that the trial can be terminated early if convincing evidence of efficacy becomes available. In the past, MS clinical trials have usually been designed with a primary endpoint of a clinical response at a specified time following entry to the trial. In such trials, efficacy evidence on the primary endpoint becomes available only after the first patients entered into the trial reach the specified time target, and the scope for early termination is limited unless patient entry takes place over an extended period of time. The current trend to more frequent use of time-to-event responses as primary endpoints opens new possibilities to consider early termination of MS clinical trials following interim analyses. These interim analyses should be carried out in such a way that they do not adversely affect the statistical properties of the design; to accomplish this, a plan for these interim analyses must be explicitly incorporated into the design. However, in some trials, events either internal or external to the trial may prompt an interim analysis at a time when none was planned, thereby forcing a change in this plan. A large body of statistical methodology has been developed to facilitate both planned and unplanned interim analyses. A survey of this methodology for two-armed clinical trials with a single primary endpoint will be the first major topic of this chapter.

The question of how to measure the efficacy of a therapy is a fundamental issue for any clinical trial and has long been a source of concern for MS clinical trials. The most widely accepted outcome measure, the Kurtzke Expanded Disability Status Scale (EDSS) (Kurtzke 1983) does not provide a comprehensive clinical assessment due to its heavy reliance on ambulation, its insensitivity to cognitive decline and its poor assessment of upper extremity function (Whitaker et al. 1995). Given the multidimensional nature of MS, it may be unrealistic to expect that any single measure could adequately describe the effects of an experimental therapy. Thus, there is considerable interest in the development of a revised multidimensional clinical assessment system to measure reliably the most relevant clinical dimensions of the disease: perhaps ambulation, upper extremity function, cognitive function and vision. The second major topic addressed in this chapter concerns approaches for the design of clinical trials where the efficacy of a therapy is to be measured by such a multidimensional outcome measure.

Beyond these two major topics, several others will be discussed very briefly. These include issues arising in MS clinical trials involving more than two arms, the design of active control clinical trials, the varied uses of covariance analysis in the context of clinical trials, and the need for longitudinal analysis of data collected in MS clinical trials.

A Two-Armed Clinical Trial with a Single Primary Endpoint

In this section, we consider a very simple clinical trial with a single primary endpoint, which provides the context for concrete illustrations in our discussion of several issues in this chapter and allows us to make some conceptual points, which are of importance in what follows. The trial will be placebo-controlled and randomized, with n_1 patients assigned to arm 1 (placebo) and n_2 patients to arm 2 (experimental therapy), so the total number of patients randomized will be $n = n_1 + n_2$. The single outcome measure is a continuous response variable and it is known that the variability of the response is the same in both arms in the population of patients under investigation. A beneficial effect of the therapy corresponds to a lowering of the mean response on this primary endpoint from that in the placebo group. If μ_1 and μ_2 are the underlying mean responses on the two arms, then the *parameter of interest* is $\mu_1 - \mu_2$, the difference in these underlying population means.

How large a clinical trial should be planned? In the usual approach to designing clinical trials, this decision is based on the power of a test of the null hypothesis of no difference in the underlying population means, H_0: $\mu_1 - \mu_2 = 0$ Suppose an equal number of patients will be randomized to each arm so that $n_1 = n_2 = n/2$. Table 4.1 illustrates (approximate) sample sizes required for a level $\alpha = 0.05$ two-sided test to achieve a power of $1 - \beta$, or a probability of Type 2 error of β, when the magnitude of treatment effect to be detected is given by

$$\Delta = (\mu_1 - \mu_2)/\sigma,$$

the difference in the underlying population means standardized by the common underlying population standard deviation σ.

The values in Table 4.1 can be obtained from the general formula for the (approximate) sample size required per arm for this very simple context, namely,

$$n/2 = 2(z_\beta + z_{\alpha/2})^2/\Delta^2.$$

With $\alpha = 0.05$ and $1 - \beta = 0.80$, for example, the formula yields

$$n/2 = 2(0.84 + 1.96)^2/\Delta^2 = 15.7/\Delta^2,$$

which leads directly to the entries in the first column of Table 4.1. This general formula will be required several times in the discussion that follows.

At the end of the trial, the difference in the underlying mean responses can be estimated by the difference in the corresponding sample means, $\overline{X}_1 - \overline{X}_2$. Dividing by the standard error (SE) yields the usual Z-statistic for testing the null hypothesis of no difference in the underlying population means, H_0: $\mu_1 - \mu_2 = 0$, which allows the calculation of a P-value to summarize the strength of evidence the data provide in support of a treatment effect. Of considerably greater utility is a confidence interval for the difference in the underlying population means, which provides a range of plausible values for $\mu_1 - \mu_2$, thereby indicating the possible magnitude of the treatment effect. Provided the sample sizes, n_1 and n_2, are reasonably large, these techniques can be used even if the continuous response data are not normally distributed. Further details are provided in Appendix A.

Table 4.1. Required sample sizes for a two-armed clinical trial with a single primary endpoint (two-sided level $\alpha = 0.05$ test)

	$1 - \beta$ = power		
Δ^a = treatment effect	0.80	0.90	0.95
0.10	1570	2102	2599
0.25	252	337	416
0.50	63	85	104
0.75	28	38	47
1.00	16	22	26

$\Delta^a = (\mu_1 - \mu_2)/\sigma$, the standardized difference in the underlying population means on the two arms

It is important to recognize that these techniques can be applied to a great variety of problems arising in the context of clinical trials where the objective is comparison of two arms. In general, there is a parameter of interest, θ, which forms the basis of the comparison of the two arms. With binary response data, for example, the parameter of interest might be the difference in the two underlying proportions, or perhaps the log odds ratio. Similarly, with time-to-event response data, the parameter of interest might be the difference in the two underlying median response times, or perhaps the hazard ratio. Based on the data collected in the clinical trial, an estimate $\hat{\theta}$ of the parameter of interest would be available and the above techniques would again apply (see Appendix A). Thus, this very simple example captures the essence of most problems arising in the context of clinical trials where the objective is a comparison of two arms. It follows that conclusions based on investigation of this simple example are relevant in a much broader context.

Interim Analysis for Two-Armed Clinical Trials

Most clinical trials in MS involve staggered patient entry with patient responses accumulated over an extended period, usually several years. Monitoring of such trials for regular review of the logistics, adherence to protocol, accrual rates and other issues relating to the quality of the trial is desirable because early attention to these issues may allow corrective measures to be taken by the study investigators. Of course, the safety data must be regularly reviewed. A data monitoring committee would typically be responsible for recommendations concerning actions to be taken as a result of these reviews.

In this context, it is natural also to consider regular reviews of the efficacy data, ideally shortly in advance of some of the planned meetings of the data monitoring committee. If a convincing difference between the two arms emerged prior to the planned end of the trial, it might then be desirable to terminate the trial early. If this occurred prior to completion of patient entry, termination of patient entry onto the apparently inferior treatment would be ethically required. If treatment of some patients was continuing, there would be an ethical requirement to terminate the treatment of patients on the apparently inferior treatment. Even if only planned follow-up was continuing, there would be an ethical imperative to announce the results as quickly as possible so that patients outside the trial could benefit from this information.

When interim analyses are not explicitly incorporated into the design, considerable care is required in assessing whether a difference that emerges prior to the planned end of the clinical trial can be considered convincing. A cautious perspective on such unplanned interim analyses is that any difference that emerges during the course of the trial should be viewed as a result of continuously monitoring the data, but undertaking a more formal analysis only when the data appear interesting (Pocock and Hughes 1989). From this point of view, such unplanned interim analyses are equivalent to testing repeatedly the null hypothesis on the accumulating data. However, such repeated testing results in considerable inflation of α, the overall probability of Type 1 error, above the fixed nominal level of the individual tests. The magnitude of this inflation was first systematically studied by Armitage et al. (1969) and is illustrated in Table 4.2 for the special case where patient responses are normally distributed with known variances and equal numbers of responses are collected between each successive repeated two-sided test.

Considerable inflation of the overall Type 1 error is possible even with a modest number of tests, so repeated tests at the usual nominal levels are not adequate as guidelines for considering possible early termination of a trial. As pointed out by Armitage et al. (1969), adjustment of the nominal level of the individual tests to a smaller level would allow control of the overall Type 1 error at any desired level; the appropriate adjusted nominal level would depend upon the number and timing of the tests to be carried out. Such repeated significance testing designs for the continuous monitoring of accumulating data are discussed by Armitage (1975), who details the application of the techniques of sequential analysis to clinical trials.

It is often argued that the continuous assessment of the accumulating data required by such fully sequential designs is simply too difficult to organize, particularly for long term and large clinical trials involving multiple centers. These difficulties may have been overstated in the past and the continual improvement of the capability for electronic data transfer means that continuous monitoring can be a practical possibility. In the context of a trial with a data monitoring committee with primary responsibility for making recommendations concerning early termination, such continuous monitoring may be irrelevant because the committee will only be in a position to make recommendations at its regularly scheduled meetings. What is required is a planned schedule of interim analyses, which is synchronized with the meetings of the data monitoring committee and a corresponding stopping rule with well understood properties to provide guidance to the data monitoring committee with respect to early termination of the clinical trial.

A considerable amount of literature focused on meeting this need has been published since the late 1970s; Jennison and Turnbull (1990) provide a fairly

Table 4.2. Overall Type 1 error α produced by repeated significance tests at a fixed nominal level α' on accumulating normal data[a]

	α' = nominal level	
No. repeated tests	0.05	0.01
1	0.05	0.01
2	0.08	0.02
5	0.14	0.03
10	0.19	0.05
20	0.25	0.06
50	0.32	0.09
100	0.37	0.11
200	0.42	0.13
500	0.49	0.15

[a]Extracted from Armitage et al. (1969, Table 2)

recent review intended for a statistical audience. The early work was directed at the development of classes of *group sequential designs*, which allow repeated assessment of the accumulating data after groups of predetermined numbers of patients have responded. A variety of more flexible procedures for such interim analyses were developed subsequently to overcome some of the limitations imposed by these group sequential designs. This body of methodology will be briefly surveyed in the remainder of this section.

The discussion here will be limited to symmetric designs for two-sided testing of the null hypothesis of no difference between the two arms. Although not commonly employed in the clinical trials context, a one-sided test may sometimes be more appropriate. Alternatively, an asymmetric two-sided design may occasionally be desired. Adaptation of this methodology to these circumstances is straightforward.

Three Classes of Group Sequential Designs

Suppose the number of interim analyses to be carried out is K, where the Kth interim analysis corresponds to the final analysis to be carried out at the planned end of the trial. Our initial description of these designs will be for the idealized case of normally distributed responses with known variance and with successive interim analyses carried out after equal-sized groups of responses where, within each group, an equal number of responses are obtained on both arms. These designs can then be described in terms of the K cut-off values for the Z-statistics at the successive interim analyses, denoted $z_1, z_2, \ldots, z_K$; if the Z-statistic at the kth interim analysis is larger than z_k in magnitude, then the design would call for termination of the trial at the kth interim analysis with the rejection of the null hypothesis of no difference between the two arms. For example, although not recommended for use due to the resulting inflation of the overall Type 1 error, the naive repeated significance testing designs of Table 4.2 correspond to the choices $z_1 = z_2 = \ldots = z_K = 1.960$ for the nominal level of $\alpha' = 0.05$ and $z_1 = z_2 = \ldots = z_K = 2.576$ for the nominal level of $\alpha' = 0.01$. Equivalently, these designs can be described in terms of the nominal levels of the tests carried out at the successive interim analyses, denoted $\alpha_1, \alpha_2, \ldots, \alpha_K$; the design would call for termination of the trial at the kth interim analysis if the *P*-value of the test carried out at the kth interim analysis is smaller than α_k. For example, the naive repeated significance testing designs of Table 4.2 correspond to the choice $\alpha_1 = \alpha_2 = \ldots = \alpha_K = \alpha'$, the fixed nominal level of the individual tests.

Pocock Designs

Pocock (1977) was the first to carry out a detailed investigation of a class of group sequential designs. He proposed application of the repeated significance tests discussed by Armitage (1975) in a group sequential fashion. For this class, each of the K interim analyses is carried out at the same nominal level

Table 4.3. Three classes of two-sided group sequential designs for overall Type 1 error $\alpha = 0.05$

		Pocock		O'Brien/Fleming		Peto/Haybittle	
K = number of interim analyses	Interim analysis	Z	*P*	Z	*P*	Z	*P*
2	1	2.178	0.029	2.798	0.005	3.291	0.001
	2	2.178	0.029	1.977	0.048	1.960	0.050
5	1	2.413	0.016	4.562	0.00001	3.291	0.001
	2	2.413	0.016	3.226	0.0013	3.291	0.001
	3	2.413	0.016	2.634	0.008	3.291	0.001
	4	2.413	0.016	2.281	0.023	3.291	0.001
	5	2.413	0.016	2.040	0.041	1.960	0.050

($\alpha_1 = \alpha_2 = \ldots = \alpha_K$), chosen so that the resulting probability of Type 1 error of the design is equal to the desired level of α. Equivalently, these designs are based on constant cut-off values for the Z-statistics; that is, $z_1 = z_2 = \ldots = z_K$. Pocock tabulated these cut-off values as well as the number of observations required per group in order to achieve specified power, thereby facilitating implementation of this class of designs. For two-sided tests with overall level $\alpha = 0.05$, these cut-off values and corresponding nominal levels for $K = 2$ and $K = 5$ interim analyses appear in Table 4.3 (above). For $K = 5$, for example, the nominal level for each interim analysis is $\alpha_k = 0.016$, with a corresponding Z-statistic cut-off of $z_k = 2.413$. Note that if the trial proceeds to its planned conclusion without early stopping, the cut-off of $z_K = 2.413$ for the final analysis (the Kth interim analysis) is substantially larger than 1.960, the cut-off value for the corresponding fixed sample size procedure. With this design, if the trial proceeds to its planned conclusion without early stopping, a *P*-value of less than $\alpha_K = 0.016$ would have to be achieved at the final analysis in order to be able to claim a significant difference between the two arms at the overall level of $\alpha = 0.05$.

Pocock (1977) also evaluated the average number of groups before termination of the trial under the alternative hypothesis, thereby providing a broader description of the properties of this class of designs. As should be expected, these designs require a somewhat larger planned number of patients than the corresponding fixed sample size design and this number increases with K, the number of planned interim analyses. However, the primary objective of such a sequential design is to allow for early termination of the trial if an important difference emerges between the two arms. Pocock showed that, with this class of design, substantial gains in this aspect are achieved by carrying out two or three interim analyses and little further is gained beyond $K = 5$ interim analyses.

O'Brien/Fleming Designs

A second class of group sequential designs, having the general form of the classical Wald sequential probability ratio test, was proposed by O'Brien and Fleming (1979) in the context of using a χ^2 test to compare two proportions. For interim analyses planned after successive groups of equal numbers of observations, the cut-off values are

$$z_k = z_K\sqrt{K/k}$$

where z_K, the cut-off for the final analysis (the Kth interim analysis), is determined so the overall level of the design is equal to α, the desired probability of Type 1 error. O'Brien and Fleming approximated these cut-off values by simulation, but exact values are provided by Jennison and Turnbull (1989).

Compared with the Pocock designs, the O'Brien/Fleming designs are based on much more stringent tests in the early stages of a clinical trial but less stringent tests in the later stages (see Table 4.3). For $K = 5$ and an overall two-sided level of $\alpha = 0.05$, for example, the cut-off for the final analysis is $z_K = 2.040$; this leads to cut-offs of $z_1 = 4.562$, $z_2 = 3.226$, $z_3 = 2.634$ and $z_4 = 2.281$. Thus, with the O'Brien/Fleming class of designs, early termination occurs only if rather extreme differences emerge at the earlier stages of the trial. This conservatism has the consequence that the cut-off for the Z-statistic in the final analysis needs to be only slightly larger than 1.960, the value for the corresponding fixed sample size procedure. It follows that, with this class of designs, the power is only slightly smaller, and hence the required sample size is only slightly larger, than with the corresponding fixed sample size procedures. For practical purposes, the clinical trial can be designed as a fixed sample size trial and this may be viewed as a very attractive feature.

Peto/Haybittle Designs

A third class of group sequential designs that is very conservative with respect to early stopping at all stages prior to the final analysis was suggested by Peto et al. (1976). Their suggestion was simply to carry out all interim analyses prior to the final analysis at a very low nominal level, say 0.001 (that is, $\alpha_1 = \alpha_2 = \ldots = \alpha_{K-1} = 0.001$, or equivalently, $z_1 = z_2 = \ldots = z_{K-1} = 3.291$). In the event that no early termination takes place, their suggestion was to carry out the final analysis at the desired overall level of α (see Table 4.3). Haybittle (1971) had earlier carried out simulation experiments to examine the properties of effectively this same stopping rule in the context of monitoring long-term clinical trials with survival data. Of course, if the desired overall level of α is used as the nominal level for the final analysis, then the actual overall level is inflated, but, with such a low nominal level at all the earlier interim analyses, the inflation is negligible and can be ignored for practical purposes. Due to their very conservative nature, the properties of this class of designs are very similar to the corresponding fixed sample size procedure; early stopping occurs only if very strong differences emerge.

Properties of Group Sequential Designs

Various authors have investigated the extent to which the properties of these classes of group sequential designs depend upon the special context of equal sized groups of normally distributed responses with known variances within which they were developed. As long as the group sizes are not too small, the distributions of many different types of test statistics corresponding to successive interim analyses can be approximated by the normal distribution, although there are often technical issues concerned with how best to make such an approximation. In such cases, one should expect approximately the same properties and Pocock (1977) provides the results of simulations illustrating this to be the case for test statistics based on binary, exponential and ranked data. The requirement of equal sized groups will usually be difficult to satisfy in practice, but Pocock (1977) and O'Brien and Fleming (1979) provide simulation results indicating that modest deviations from this pattern have essentially no effect on the properties of these designs. Of course, if it is known in advance that there will be substantial deviation from this pattern, the appropriate cut-off values z_1, z_2,..., z_K for the anticipated pattern of interim analyses should be computed and incorporated into the design. Except for the Peto/Haybittle class of designs, these computations are somewhat intricate, so the advice of a statistician should be sought in such circumstances.

Pocock (1982) provides a detailed comparison of these three classes of group sequential designs for the case of $K = 2$ and $K = 5$ interim analyses. Not surprisingly, with respect to early termination properties, the Peto/Haybittle class is dominated by the other two classes. His overall finding is that the Pocock class has the advantage over the O'Brien/Fleming class for alternatives that can be detected with larger power, but the differences between these two classes of designs are substantial only for alternatives that can be detected with large power where termination would typically occur at the very early stages; treatment effects of this magnitude are rare in the context of clinical trials. Further, as already noted, the Pocock class suffers from the disadvantage of a larger maximum sample size and the difficulty of interpretation for a trial that does not reach the stopping boundary but still achieves a *P*-value considerably less than the overall level of α on the final analysis. Combined with a general preference on the part of many investigators for more stringent tests at early stages of a clinical trial, a preference that can also be justified on Bayesian theoretical grounds, these features have led to considerable popularity of the O'Brien/Fleming class of group sequential designs.

The use of these designs in clinical trials where the response is time to an event such as sustained treatment failure, for example, and some patients will be lost to follow-up, or censored, has attracted a great deal of attention. The time-to-event experience on the two arms would typically be compared with a non-parametric test statistic, usually the log-rank statistic or a modification of the Wilcoxon statistic, which takes into account the censoring. Gail et al. (1982) present simulations that illustrate that the properties of these group sequential designs for equal sized groups hold to a very good approximation for the log-rank test, provided the interim analyses are carried out after equally spaced numbers of events. By investigating the properties of a general class of nonparametric test statistics for censored survival data, Tsiatis (1982) was able to provide the theoretical justification underlying this result. Both Tsiatis (1982) and Slud and Wei (1982) showed that this result does not hold for the usual form of the modified Wilcoxon statistic due to Gehan. The latter authors showed how group sequential designs for this test statistic could nevertheless be constructed; their technique applies very generally and is described together with other more flexible approaches below.

The work of these and other authors led to an increased appreciation of the importance of the *information fraction* or *information time* in such sequential trials. A definition of this concept and a simple example is provided in Appendix B. The importance of this concept is that cut-off values for the case of equal sized groups of normally distributed responses with known variances, such as those in Table 4.3, will be approximately correct for a wide variety of test statistics that might be used to compare the efficacy of two treatments, provided the interim analyses are carried out at equally spaced information fractions. More generally, provided a suitable normal approximation is available for the distribution of the successive test statistics based on the accumulating data, appropriate cut-off values for any sequence of information fractions corresponding to the times of anticipated interim analyses can be evaluated in the context of a clinical trial with normally distributed responses having known variances (see Lan and Zucker (1993) for a more detailed discussion).

Thus, for any particular type of clinical trial, it is essential to be able to determine the information fraction. This is usually reasonably straightforward. For the case of comparing the mean levels of a continuous response on two arms, it is shown in Appendix B that the information fraction will typically be very close to the fraction of the total planned responses currently available, so that equally spaced information fractions correspond closely to equal sized groups of responses. For the case of comparing the time-to-event experience on two arms with the log-rank test, the information fraction can be estimated by the current number of events divided by the number expected at the termination of the trial. Thus, the cut-off values for equal sized groups are approximately correct, provided the interim analyses for the log-rank test are carried out at equally spaced numbers of events. With staggered patient entry, this would mean that a considerable time would elapse between the start of the trial and the first interim analysis, but the time intervals between interim analyses would then shorten as more patients entered and events occurred more frequently. This has the advantage of avoiding a premature survival analysis based on very few events. If the schedule of interim analyses is instead at fixed calendar times, then the number of events between successive interim analyses could vary considerably. Fortunately, the simulation results of DeMets and Gail (1985) suggest that using the cut-offs appropriate for equally spaced numbers of events at fixed calendar times typically has only a modest impact on the properties of the log-rank test, particularly with the O'Brien/Fleming class of designs. Nevertheless, rather than relying on these limited empirical results, a better approach would be to estimate the information fractions corresponding to the desired timing of interim analyses (based on knowledge of time-to-event patterns from previous studies) and to compute the corresponding appropriate cut-offs for use in the design. As already mentioned, these computations are somewhat intricate, so the advice of a statistician should be sought in such circumstances.

More Flexible Approaches

The Pocock and O'Brien/Fleming classes of group sequential designs require advance specification of the number of interim analyses (K) as well as the schedule of information fractions at which these will occur. It should be possible to specify an anticipated schedule in advance, and the trial would be designed on that basis, but a clinical trial is a complex undertaking and circumstances could emerge during the trial that would require a change to this planned schedule. Various authors have attempted to address this difficulty by developing more flexible approaches that require less advance specification; these are now described briefly.

Slud and Wei Approach

Slud and Wei (1982) pointed out that one can think of these group sequential designs as "spending" the Type 1 error α over the K interim analyses to be carried out. They suggested specifying positive constants $\pi_1, \pi_2, \ldots, \pi_K$ with $\Sigma\pi_k = \alpha$, where π_k is the portion of the Type 1 error to be "spent" at the kth interim analysis; that is, the cut-offs to determine the stopping boundary are evaluated so that, under the null hypothesis, the probability of stopping at the kth interim analysis, but not earlier is equal to π_k. They recommended an increasing sequence for the constants $\{\pi_k\}$. The cut-off for the kth interim analysis depends only on $\pi_1, \pi_2, \ldots, \pi_k$ and the joint distribution of the successive test statistics at the corresponding times, so the cut-off for the kth interim analysis can be evaluated after the time for the kth interim analysis is selected. Thus, there is no need to specify the schedule of the interim analyses in advance, although the schedule should not depend upon the accumulated data. On the other hand, K must be specified in advance to avoid the possibility of spending the entire Type 1 error before the termination of the trial. The Slud and Wei method is quite generally applicable, although, depending on the form of the joint distribution of the successive test statistics, evaluating the cut-off corresponding to the amount of Type 1 error to be spent at a particular interim analysis may be more difficult than in the simple problem of normally distributed responses with known variances.

Spending Functions

Lan and DeMets (1983) proposed a related approach based on specifying an increasing function of the information fraction to characterize the rate at which the Type 1 error is spent. The cut-off for the kth interim analysis when the information fraction is f_k, is evaluated so that the probability of stopping at this interim analysis is equal to the increase in this spending function from the time of the previous interim analysis (when the information fraction was f_{k-1}). The cut-off for the kth interim analysis depends only on $f_1, f_2, \ldots, f_k$ and the particular Type 1 error spending function selected at the outset, so the cut-off for the kth interim analysis can be evaluated after the information fraction at which the kth interim analysis is to be carried out is selected. The choice of the successive information fractions should not depend upon the accumulated data, but there is no need to specify either the schedule of the interim analyses or their number in advance.

Lan and DeMets (1983) explore the properties of several spending functions and provide versions that closely approximate the Pocock and O'Brien/Fleming boundaries when interim analyses occur at equally spaced information fractions. Thus, investigators who find those classes of designs attractive can use this approach to gain the additional flexibility of not having to specify the number or schedule of the interim analyses in advance. This accommodates the situation, for example, where interim analyses were planned at regular times but patient recruitment is slower than expected, leading to an extension of the trial and the need to carry out additional interim analyses, with the result that both the number and schedule (in terms of information fractions) of the interim analyses could be quite different to what was originally anticipated. The specification of a spending function adjusts to this situation and provides a monitoring boundary without affecting the desired overall level. Kim and DeMets (1987, 1992) discuss the design aspects of this approach.

The flexibility the spending function approach provides for the scheduling of future interim analyses might be perceived as a potential danger. If a rather large value of the test statistic is observed at an interim analysis, but this value does not reach the stopping boundary, a natural inclination would be to increase the frequency of the interim monitoring. Such data-dependent scheduling of future interim analyses will inflate the overall Type 1 error, but to what extent? Lan and DeMets (1989) provide simulation results for two different scenarios, which involve doubling the frequency of future interim analyses as soon as a large test statistic is observed at an interim analysis. For a small number of planned interim analyses, the results for both the Pocock-type and the O'Brien/Fleming-type spending functions indicate the effect on the overall Type 1 and 2 errors is exceedingly small. In a detailed investigation of the effects of violations on the Type 1 errors of plans for interim analyses, Proschan et al. (1992) investigate much more aggressive behavior with these same spending functions. In the cases they consider, even with extraordinary efforts, the Type 1 error is inflated by less than 6% and 11% for the O'Brien/Fleming-type and Pocock-type spending functions respectively. Thus, this approach provides a considerable degree of built-in protection against inflation of the Type 1 error due to the scheduling of more frequent interim analyses based on data trends.

Stochastic Curtailment or Conditional Power

Halperin et al. (1982) describe an extension of *curtailed sampling*, where a trial is terminated as soon as the accumulated data make the final conclusion inevitable, which can be useful to assist with data monitoring deliberations for unplanned interim analyses. Suppose a trial has been designed as a fixed sample size procedure to test a null hypothesis H_0, using a statistic $S(n)$ based on the responses of n patients. The design has $P(\text{Type 1 error}) = \alpha$ and $P(\text{Type 2 error}) = \beta$; that is, when H_0 is true,

$$P\{S(n) \text{ will reject } H_0\} = \alpha,$$

and when H_1, a particular alternative hypothesis of interest, is true,

$$P\{S(n) \text{ will reject } H_0\} = 1 - \beta.$$

Curtailed sampling merely notes that if, at some time prior to the planned termination of the trial when the responses of m patients are available, we can be *certain* that $S(n)$ will reject H_0 or that $S(n)$ will not reject H_0, then we might as well terminate the experiment. This curtailment has no impact on the final decision and therefore it also has no impact on the Type 1 and Type 2 errors. That such curtailment is sometimes possible before the planned end of an experiment is easiest to appreciate in the case of binary responses, but the idea also applies with test statistics based on ranks such as the Wilcoxon statistic (Alling 1963; Halperin and Ware 1974). Nevertheless, circumstances in which the idea can be applied are rather specialized, and opportunities for such curtailment will occur only rarely in large clinical trials, unless the trial is already rather close to its planned end where early termination offers little advantage.

Stochastic curtailment is much more broadly applicable. Rather than insisting the final decision be inevitable before terminating, the idea is to require only that the final decision be determined with high probability. That is, after m responses, when the statistic $S(m)$ is available, we might be willing to terminate the trial with the rejection of H_0 if, even when H_0 is true,

$$P\{S(n) \text{ will reject } H_0 \mid S(m)\} \geq \gamma,$$

or to terminate the trial with the acceptance of H_0 if, even when H_1 is true,

$$P\{S(n) \text{ will reject } H_0 \mid S(m)\} \leq 1-\gamma',$$

where γ and γ' are some suitably large constants, perhaps 0.8 or 0.9.

To provide a more comprehensive description, the probability that $S(n)$ will reject H_0 could be calculated not only under H_0 and H_1 but for the entire range of values of the underlying parameter of interest that describes the relative efficacy of the two arms. Halperin et al. (1982) illustrate such conditional (on the data observed up to the current point in time) power calculations. This *conditional power function* provides a convenient way to describe the likelihood of different possible outcomes at the planned termination, and hence can assist in deliberations of whether to terminate the trial at the current time. Of course, the Type 1 and Type 2 errors will be inflated above their nominal values due to multiple looks at the accumulating data. If the number and scheduled times of the looks at the data are specified in advance, then the actual inflation due to such a design can be evaluated (see Lan and Wittes 1994, for example). However, Lan et al. (1982) showed that, irrespective of the number of looks at the accumulating data, the stochastic curtailment scheme described above yields

$$P(\text{Type 1 error}) < \alpha/\gamma$$

and

$$P(\text{Type 2 error}) < \beta/\gamma'.$$

Thus, if $\gamma = \gamma' = 0.80$, the errors are inflated at most by 25%, whereas if $\gamma = \gamma' = 0.90$, the errors are inflated at most by about 11%.

Under the cautious view that any unplanned interim analyses should be viewed as a result of continuously monitoring the data, but undertaking a more formal analysis only when the data appears interesting, these inequalities insure that stochastic curtailment offers protection against excessive inflation of errors when used for unplanned interim analyses. A stochastic curtailment scheme could be adopted as a formal stopping rule with the test based on $S(n)$ upon planned termination designed to have level $\alpha\gamma$ and power $1-\beta\gamma'$ so that the resulting bounds on the errors are equal to the desired nominal levels of α and β, but such designs are quite conservative with respect to early stopping. This conservatism results in considerable flexibility, allowing one to carry out unplanned interim analyses at arbitrary and even data-dependent times, but the desirability of such a design would very much depend upon the value of this extreme flexibility in the context under consideration. For further discussion of this approach, see Jennison and Turnbull (1990), Davis and Hardy (1994) and Lan and Wittes (1994).

Repeated Confidence Intervals

A major limitation of these group sequential designs is their focus on hypothesis testing and *P*-values. Formally, the only information provided at an interim analysis would be the value of the current Z-statistic and the corresponding nominal *P*-value; comparison with the stopping rule would indicate whether early termination was appropriate. A confidence interval that provides an estimate of the treatment effect and clearly reflects the precision with which this effect is determined would be of greater use to the data monitoring committee considering the termination of the trial, but the usual fixed sample size confidence intervals evaluated at each interim analysis would lead to an overall coverage probability considerably lower than the nominal.

Jennison and Turnbull (1984, 1989) have shown how, corresponding to any design for the interim analyses, a confidence interval for the treatment effect can be generated at each interim analysis so that the collection of repeated confidence intervals corresponding to successive interim analyses has a specified probability that *all* contain the true value of the parameter of interest. If used as a stopping rule, these repeated confidence intervals are equivalent to the underlying designs from which they are derived, but they also provide data summaries, which can be used at interim analyses without danger of overinterpretation. As a price of the very strong guarantee of coverage these repeated confidence intervals provide, the individual intervals can be rather wide, but they are valid regardless of the stopping rule utilized for termination of the trial. They remain valid, for example, when it is decided to continue the trial despite the planned stopping boundary having been reached. So, beyond providing data summaries at interim analyses, the primary use for repeated confidence intervals may be in contexts where the stopping rule is not clearly defined. Jennison and Turnbull (1989) provide a detailed discussion of many potential applications of this methodology.

Discussion

It is important to note that there remain open questions concerning how inference should be carried out following the termination of a sequential study. These tend to be of most importance when a study is terminated in its early stages. For example, studies that stop early tend to overestimate the true treatment effect; the magnitude of this phenomenon for group sequential designs has been illustrated by Hughes and Pocock (1988) and Pocock and Hughes (1989). This raises the question of what adjustments to account for this phenomenon, if any, should be made to estimates and confidence intervals for the treatment effect. A closely related question is what *P*-value should be ascribed to a particular outcome upon termination. These questions have generated a large body of statistical literature. For the purpose of this chapter it is most relevant to appreciate that this difficulty is greatest with those designs that permit early stopping more readily.

There are additional reasons for caution with respect to very early stopping. Early patients may not be representative and, if a reasonable fraction of the patients remain to be entered, the randomization scheme may not yet have achieved balance. Trials that stop early are necessarily based on a relatively small number of responses and even a large estimated treatment effect may not be convincing; a very wide confidence interval will necessarily result. It seems now generally accepted that, for major trials, early interim analysis based on limited data should be based on fairly stringent nominal significance levels.

Clinical trials are complex undertakings, so the decision whether or not to terminate a trial will depend upon much more than simply crossing a specified stopping boundary. Trials may be stopped prior to reaching the stopping boundary due to safety considerations, difficulties of patient accrual, or information external to the trial. The primary endpoint may have reached the stopping boundary but a secondary endpoint might be indicating a negative effect; in some instances, this might be an adequate reason for continuing the study. Of course, early stopping will result in less information than anticipated on primary and secondary endpoints, side effects, the effect of prognostic factors, subgroups, and so on. All these factors will have to be weighed by the data monitoring committee when considering the termination of a study. Nevertheless, formalized plans for the interim analyses, specified in advance but with adequate flexibility to accommodate complications that might arise, provide a valuable objective guideline to assist the deliberations of a data monitoring committee.

Multiple Outcome Measures

Well designed and carefully executed clinical trials are an expensive and time-consuming undertaking, which require a substantial commitment on the part of investigators. There is a natural tendency, therefore, to wish to study as many different aspects of treatment efficacy as possible during the course of any proposed clinical trial. As a consequence, most clinical trials involve multiple outcome measures. For MS clinical trials, the consensus seems to be that several outcome measures are essential adequately to describe the effects of a therapy on the most relevant clinical dimensions of this complex disease. Suitable component measures may not be available currently for some of these dimensions. The question of how to construct the component measures, or how to choose among several candidates, is a challenging problem (LaRocca 1989). The focus here is on thc issuc that arises subsequently: what approaches are available for the design of clinical trials where the efficacy of a therapy is to be assessed by such a multidimensional outcome measure?

A naive approach to the analysis and reporting of the results of the trial would consist of carrying out a detailed analysis on each of the outcome measures separately, and then attempting to provide an overall summary. An obvious danger is that, due to pressures on journal space or for other reasons, only the results for outcome measures demonstrating a treatment effect will be reported, or, at the very least, these results will be emphasized. If done carefully and completely, such a detailed report would provide readers with a comprehensive description, thereby allowing them to draw their own conclusions. Unfortunately, the readers may not appreciate that such multiple testing greatly increases the chances of false positive findings and may interpret such a published report as providing much more evidence of efficacy than is warranted.

This difficulty is reasonably well understood and one of two approaches has typically been used to deal with this problem. The most common approach is to designate one of the outcome measures as the primary endpoint at the design stage of the trial, with all other important outcome measures designated as secondary endpoints. The primary endpoint becomes the basis for designing the study and the assessment of the relative efficacy of the two arms on this endpoint is highlighted in the published report of the trial. The assessment on the secondary endpoints is viewed as more exploratory than definitive.

When investigators find it difficult to select a single outcome measure as the primary endpoint, a second approach sometimes employed consists of combining the most important outcome measures into a single composite outcome measure, which is specified in advance of the trial and designated as the primary endpoint. This approach is most common with binary responses where the composite outcome is usually defined to be a positive response if the patient provides a positive response on any of the original outcome measures. For example, in their approach to the design and analysis of the low dose oral methotrexate clinical trial in chronic progressive MS, Goodkin et al. (1992, 1995) first designated changes they viewed as clinically significant on each of four outcome measures (Expanded Disability Status Scale (EDSS), Ambulation Index, the Box and Block Test, and the 9-Hole Peg Test), thereby effectively converting responses on these four outcome measures into binary responses. The composite outcome measure employed as the single primary endpoint was "treatment failure", defined as worsening of the designated amount sustained for a minimum of 2 months on any of the four components. Such a binary composite outcome measure is quite easy to understand and Goodkin et al. (1992) discuss some potential advantages of this approach. They also point out that such a composite measure will be most useful when the individual components are unrelated in terms of detecting clinically meaningful change, are relatively sensitive and each highly specific.

The use of prespecified composite outcome measures is not limited to the case of component outcome measures based on binary responses. Indeed, the EDSS is exactly such a prespecified composite, where the method of combining assessments on several dimensions into an overall classification of the patient's state of disability was carefully developed on the basis of subject matter knowledge and subsequently refined in the light of experience (Kurtzke 1983). Of course, the interpretation of a treatment effect on any composite outcome measure can become quite obscure due to the inevitable blurring of the role of the components once combined, but, as noted by Goodkin et al. (1992), the main difficulty with this general approach is that, even if the most important component outcome measures for the particular context under consideration can be agreed upon, how the composite outcome measure should be constructed will usually not be clear. A lengthy process of empirical assessment and validation is likely to be required before newly developed prespecified composite outcome measures find general acceptance.

More empirical work is urgently needed, both to validate outcome measures currently in use in MS clinical trials and to provide a better understanding of the relationships between these outcome measures; these relationships are likely to differ according to the stage of the disease as well as other factors. Developing a single prespecified composite outcome measure that could gain general acceptance as a primary endpoint in the wide variety of circumstances of interest in clinical trials in MS seems too ambitious a goal. A more realistic goal would be to obtain general agreement on the most relevant clinical dimensions of MS and to develop valid, reliable and sensitive outcome measures, possibly composite, focused on each of these clinical dimensions. A task force to address this problem has been organized with the support of the National Multiple Sclerosis Society.

Suppose we accept the view that several outcome measures, intended to address different clinical dimensions of MS (ambulation, upper extremity function, cognitive function and vision, for example) but possibly interrelated, are essential adequately to describe the effects of a therapy. In some MS trials, depending on the stage of the disease under study or the nature of the treatment effect anticipated, it may be possible to restrict attention to one of these component outcome measures, which could then be designated as the primary endpoint. However, typically more than one component, and often perhaps all components, would need to be included as primary endpoints. When a number (J) of different outcome measures are to be considered and there is no agreement on how these should be combined into a prespecified composite, methods to overcome the inflation of Type 1 error due to multiple testing on these different endpoints are required. In the remainder of this section, we describe three possible approaches to this problem and compare their performance.

Three Approaches to Multiple Outcome Measures

The approaches to be described deal with a specified collection of J outcome measures, which are to be considered simultaneously as primary endpoints. In the first approach (Bonferroni adjustment), separate tests to assess treatment efficacy are carried out on each of the J components. In the latter two approaches (based on Hotelling's T^2 statistic and linear combinations of Z-statistics), a single global statistic based on all J components is used to assess treatment efficacy. These global statistics can be viewed as composite outcome measures, where the method of combining the components is determined on a statistical basis from the data in the current clinical trial.

Bonferroni Adjustment

A common approach to multiple comparisons of two treatment arms on different outcome measures consists of carrying out the individual comparisons separately, but with Type 1 error levels adjusted in such a way that the overall probability of one or more Type 1 error is no larger than the desired value of α. If the outcome measures are statistically independent, so that patients' responses on any outcome measure are uncorrelated with those on any other outcome measure, then a simple exact adjustment is available. Each comparison should be carried out at level $\alpha^* = 1 - (1 - \alpha)^{1/J}$ (Miller 1981). For the usual values of α, this leads to adjusted levels only slightly larger than α/J. With $\alpha = 0.05$, for example, $\alpha^* = 0.0102$ when $J = 5$, and $\alpha^* = 0.0051$ when $J = 10$.

Typically, the outcome measures would not be statistically independent. To deal with multiple testing of correlated outcomes, an adjustment based on the Bonferroni inequality (Miller 1981) can be employed. This inequality establishes that, if separate tests, each with Type 1 error level of α' are carried out on each of the J different outcomes, then the probability of incorrectly declaring one or more significant difference is no greater than $J\alpha'$. Carrying out the individual comparisons at the level $\alpha' = \alpha/J$ results in an overall Type 1 error no greater than α, thereby yielding a conservative method. Pocock et al. (1987) demonstrate that, for the case of normally distributed and equally correlated outcomes, the extent of this conservatism is slight provided the pairwise correlation among the outcomes is no more than 0.5. The great advantage of this approach is its simplicity.

For this method, the impact of using multiple outcome measures can readily be determined. Consider the case of continuous outcome measures where the objective is to assess the differences in the underlying means on the two arms. For a single outcome measure, the sample size required per arm for a two-sided level $\alpha = 0.05$ test to achieve power $1-\beta = 0.80$ is $n/2 = 15.7/\Delta^2$. Now suppose that $J - 1$ other outcome measures are also to be assessed. The cut-off value $z_{\alpha/2}$ is then replaced by $z_{\alpha/2J}$, and the power of the comparison based on this first outcome using the unadjusted sample size n can be calculated. Of greater relevance for the purpose of designing the clinical trial is the sample size now required to maintain the power of the comparison on this first outcome measure at the desired value of $1 - \beta$; this can be obtained by replacing the cut-off value $z_{\alpha/2}$ by $z_{\alpha/2J}$ in the general sample size formula. These quantities are tabulated in Table 4.4, where the case $J = 1$ is included to provide the basis of comparison. As should be expected, with no adjustment of the sample size, the power decreases as the number of additional outcome measures increases. The rate of decrease may appear to be modest but, as the table shows, substantial increases in sample size are required to recover these losses in power: roughly 20%, 45% and 80% with the inclusion of one, four and 19 additional outcome measures ($J = 2$, $J = 5$ and $J = 20$, respectively).

When designing a study in which this approach to the analysis will be taken, the sample size required can be evaluated for each of the outcomes separately. If the sample size for the study is taken to be the maximum of these individual sample sizes, then the power specified for the comparison based on each of the outcomes will be achieved. Note, however, that this does not refer to the overall power of the procedure, namely, the probability that one or more of the comparisons results in a significant difference. The overall power would be larger than that of any one of the individual comparisons and, in certain circumstances, it can be substantially larger. The overall power of the Bonferroni procedure is evaluated for a few specific circumstances below.

For designing a study, knowledge of the underlying variances is required to allow the change in the means that is to be detected to be related to the magnitude of the underlying standard deviation. On the other hand, no knowledge of the correlations between the outcome measures is required either for designing

Table 4.4. Power and sample size for a single Bonferroni adjusted comparison with $\alpha = 0.05$

	J = total no. outcome measures						
	1	2	3	4	5	10	20
Power with unadjusted sample size	0.80	0.71	0.66	0.62	0.59	0.50	0.41
Sample size[a] to achieve power of 0.80	15.7	19.0	20.9	22.3	23.4	26.6	29.9
Power with unadjusted sample size	0.90	0.84	0.80	0.77	0.75	0.67	0.59
Sample size[a] to achieve power of 0.90	21.0	24.8	27.0	28.6	29.8	33.4	37.1

[a]Divide each entry by Δ^2, where $\Delta = (\mu_1 - \mu_2)/\sigma$ is the standardized difference in the underlying population means on the two arms.

the study or for the final analysis. This indicates the main limitation of this approach: the relationships among the outcome measures are not taken into account. Attention is focused on the smallest of the *P*-values obtained from the assessments provided by the different outcomes. Thus, this approach is best suited to the situation where a single outcome measure is expected to reveal a difference between the two arms but it is not known in advance which measure this might be. In the typical situation leading to the use of multiple outcome measures in clinical trials, however, several measures are each expected to reveal some aspect of treatment efficacy, albeit perhaps modest in magnitude. Methods that combine the evidence provided by the different outcome measures into a global statistic that provides an overall assessment of the relative efficacy of the two arms at the desired level α of Type 1 error will often be considerably more powerful in this situation.

Hotelling's T^2 Statistic

The classical method of comparing two samples on several continuous outcome measures simultaneously is based on the multivariate extension of Student's *t* statistic known as Hotelling's T^2 statistic (Johnson and Wichern 1982). This procedure is particularly easy to describe when the different outcome measures are uncorrelated. In that case

$$T^2 = Z_1^2 + Z_2^2 + \ldots + Z_J^2$$

where Z_j is the Z-statistic for comparing the two arms on the jth outcome measure. When the outcome measures are correlated, the form of Hotelling's T^2 depends on these correlations and, as will be illustrated below, these correlations play a key role in determining the performance of this procedure.

If the underlying data are multivariate normally distributed and the variances and correlations are known, then T^2 has a $\chi^2_{(J)}$ distribution, so *P*-values can be readily obtained. If, as would usually be the case, the underlying data is not normally distributed and the variances and correlations are unknown and have to be estimated from the data, then the $\chi^2_{(J)}$ will usually be an adequate approximation provided the sample sizes on the two arms are reasonably large. In what follows, we assume this to be the case. Power and sample size calculations are then straightforward. For designing a study, knowledge of not only the underlying variances but also the underlying correlations is required.

Hotelling's T^2 statistic combines the evidence of differences between the two arms from the individual outcome measures into an overall assessment. In contrast to the Bonferroni approach, this allows the possibility that modest amounts of evidence on each of several outcomes will combine to yield convincing evidence of an overall difference between the two arms. The main limitation of this procedure for application to clinical trials is the omnibus nature of the comparison provided; because the individual Z-statistics are squared before being summed, the evidence of differences between the two arms is combined without regard to the direction of the differences on the individual outcome measures. The procedure addresses the question of whether there is a difference between the two arms but not whether one arm is better than the other in an overall sense. Thus, if an overall difference is identified, the individual Z-statistics would have to be examined subsequently to identify the nature of the evidence provided by the different outcome measures. More fundamentally, in the clinical trials context, the alternatives of main interest would usually relate to consistent, albeit perhaps modest, differences in favor of one arm, and procedures that focus on these types of alternatives would provide more powerful overall assessments.

Linear Combinations of Z-Statistics

The limitations of the approach based on Hotelling's T^2 prompted O'Brien (1984) to suggest two alternative statistics. The first, motivated by ordinary least squares (OLS) considerations, is simply the average of the Z-statistics for comparing the two arms on the individual outcome measures, namely,

$$\mathrm{OLS} = (Z_1 + Z_2 + \ldots + Z_J)/J$$

If the underlying data are multivariate normally distributed and the variances are known, this statistic is normally distributed, and this will usually be an adequate approximation in other cases, provided that the sample sizes on the two arms are reasonably large. The mean value of this statistic is given by

$$\bar{\Delta}\sqrt{n/2}$$

where $\bar{\Delta}$ is the average of the standardized differences in the underlying means on the two arms, and its variance is given by $[1 + (J - 1)\bar{\rho}]/J$, where $\bar{\rho}$ is the average pairwise correlation among the multiple outcome measures. Thus, differences between the means affect the properties of OLS only through $\bar{\Delta}$ and correlations among the multiple outcomes affect its properties only through $\bar{\rho}$. Power and sample size calculations are straightforward. For designing a study, knowledge of $\bar{\rho}$ as well as the variances is required.

This OLS statistic sums the individual Z-statistics, so the direction of the differences on the individual outcome measures is taken into account. However, OLS does not take the correlations among the outcomes into account; the evidence from each outcome is simply weighted equally on the Z-statistic scale, though this will often not be the best way to proceed. For example, if two outcome measures are highly correlated, they convey essentially the same information concerning the relative efficacy of the two arms and their contributions to the overall assessment should be somewhat down-weighted.

Such considerations prompted O'Brien (1984) to propose a generalized least squares (GLS) statistic, which is also a linear combination of the individual Z-statistics but with coefficients depending upon the correlations among the multiple outcomes. It can be shown that O'Brien's GLS statistic is equivalent to his OLS statistic when the multiple outcomes are equally correlated. Therefore, the performance of the two procedures will be similar unless these correlations vary considerably, when the GLS statistic would be expected to provide a more sensitive overall assessment. However, in the clinical trials context, the correlations among the different outcomes should typically be modest because, if two outcome measures are known to be highly correlated, then it would be most sensible to choose one, or perhaps a prespecified combination, as a new outcome measure to be employed. Thus, for the clinical trials context, the improvement provided by GLS over OLS might generally be expected to be modest. With either OLS or GLS, if an overall difference is identified, the individual Z-statistics could subsequently be examined for a better understanding of the nature of the overall difference.

Comparison of Approaches

It is difficult to provide a comprehensive comparison of these approaches to dealing with multiple outcome measures, due to the many possibilities that could be considered. The objective here is to examine a few special cases to highlight the main differences in their statistical properties. Restricting to the case when the joint distribution of the multiple outcome measures can reasonably be approximated as multivariate normal allows a focus on the essential features of the problem, namely, the configuration of the standardized differences in the underlying means and the pattern of the correlations among the different outcome measures.

For a single outcome measure, the three approaches are equivalent provided all tests are two-sided. Suppose at least one effective outcome measure is available and that the difference in the underlying mean responses on the two arms on this outcome measure is such that 100 patients per arm yields a power of 0.80. From the general sample size formula, it follows that, for a two-sided test at level $\alpha = 0.05$, this standardized difference in the underlying means is $\Delta = 0.4 = \Delta^*$, say. The special cases to be presented correspond to an examination of the performance of the three approaches when additional outcome measures with varying properties are included in the final analysis.

Let Δ_j denote the standardized difference in the underlying means on the jth outcome measure. Three configurations of these standardized differences will be considered:

A. $\Delta_1 = \Delta^*, \Delta_2 = \ldots = \Delta_J = 0$. In this configuration, there is a difference in the underlying means on the first outcome measure only. The performance of these procedures for this configuration will indicate the penalty for including component outcome measures that do not effectively compare the two arms.

B. $\Delta_1 = \Delta^*, \quad \Delta_2 = \Delta^*/2, \ldots, \quad \Delta_J = \Delta^*/J$. This configuration of decreasing standardized differences will indicate the benefit arising from including additional outcome measures of diminishing effectiveness in comparing the two arms.

C. $\Delta_1 = \Delta_2 = \ldots = \Delta_J = \Delta^*$. In this configuration, the individual outcome measures are all equally effective in comparing the two arms.

Cases B and C, where all the outcome measures have some degree of effectiveness in comparing the two arms are presumably of greatest relevance to the clinical trials context.

To examine the performance of these procedures, the correlation among the outcome measures must also be specified. For the sake of brevity, we will consider only equally correlated outcome measures, with common correlation of $\rho = 0$, 0.3 or 0.5. As already mentioned, O'Brien's OLS and GLS statistics are equivalent in this case.

For the special case of uncorrelated outcomes, the power of the appropriate level $\alpha = 0.05$ two-sided tests in a two-armed clinical trial with $n/2 = 100$ patients per arm is provided in Table 4.5. For Case A, the power of all procedures decreases as additional outcomes are included in the analysis. The inclusion of even a single such additional outcome has a dramatic deleterious effect on O'Brien's OLS procedure. The decrease in power is considerably more gradual for both the Bonferroni and Hotelling's T^2 procedures, but still substantial. The latter are quite comparable, although Bonferroni adjustment has a slight advantage, which becomes more pronounced as the number of outcomes increases. The main message should be clear: a substantial penalty is incurred due to the inclusion of outcome measures which do not effectively compare the two arms.

Case C represents the opposite extreme, where all outcome measures are equally effective in comparing the two arms. In this case, all procedures benefit considerably from the inclusion of each additional outcome measure. All have excellent power properties, but O'Brien's OLS has a clear advantage over Hotelling's T^2, which in turn has a clear advantage over Bonferroni adjustment.

The results in Case B deserve careful attention. With the exception of the first additional outcome measure, which provides a slight increase in power for both T^2 and OLS, inclusion of additional outcomes has a negative impact on all three procedures. The impact on Bonferroni adjustment is considerably larger than on T^2 and OLS, where the impact is modest until the number of outcomes becomes large, but it may seem surprising that the inclusion of additional uncorrelated out-

Table 4.5. Power of procedures with uncorrelated multiple outcome measures (Two-sided level $\alpha = 0.05$ tests for a two-armed clinical trial with 100 patients on each arm)

Case	Procedure	J = total no. outcome measures						
		1	2	3	4	5	10	20
A	Bonferroni	0.80	0.72	0.67	0.63	0.61	0.52	0.44
	Hotelling's T^2	0.80	0.71	0.64	0.60	0.56	0.43	0.31
	O'Brien's OLS	0.80	0.51	0.37	0.29	0.24	0.14	0.10
B	Bonferroni	0.80	0.77	0.73	0.70	0.68	0.58	0.49
	Hotelling's T^2	0.80	0.81	0.79	0.77	0.75	0.65	0.51
	O'Brien's OLS	0.80	0.84	0.84	0.83	0.82	0.74	0.62
C	Bonferroni	0.80	0.92	0.96	0.98	0.988	0.999	1.000
	Hotelling's T^2	0.80	0.95	0.990	0.998	1.000	1.000	1.000
	O'Brien's OLS	0.80	0.98	0.998	1.000	1.000	1.000	1.000

Case A: $\Delta_1 = \Delta^* = 0.4$, $\Delta_2 = \ldots = \Delta_J = 0$; only the first outcome measure is effective in comparing the two arms.

Case B: $\Delta_1 = \Delta^* = 0.4$, $\Delta_2 = \Delta^*/2, \ldots, \Delta_J = \Delta^*/J$; successive outcome measures are of diminishing effectiveness.

Case C: $\Delta_1 = \Delta_2 = \ldots \Delta_J = \Delta^* = 0.4$; all outcome measures are equally effective.

comes, each of which has some degree of effectiveness in comparing the two arms, actually leads to a deterioration in performance. This illustrates the subtle nature of such multivariate problems.

The results of Case C indicate that procedures like Hotelling's T^2 and O'Brien's OLS, which combine the evidence provided by the different outcome measures into a global statistic to provide an overall assessment of the relative efficacy of the two arms, have considerable potential. However, Cases A and B demonstrate that care is required in the implementation of this general approach; the inclusion of ineffective outcome measures will substantially degrade the performance of all these procedures, as will the inclusion of too many weakly effective outcome measures.

Taken together, Cases B and C indicate that, in terms of power, Bonferroni adjustment is not a competitive approach when the available outcome measures are uncorrelated and all have some degree of effectiveness in comparing the two arms. Therefore, we now focus on Hotelling's T^2 and O'Brien's OLS in the possible presence of correlation among the outcome measures. Table 4.6 provides the sample sizes required to achieve a power of $1 - \beta = 0.80$ when $\rho = 0$, 0.3 or 0.5. The results for $\rho = 0$ translate the impact on power illustrated in Table 4.5 into corresponding sample size requirements, which are of more direct relevance for the purpose of designing trials; for these cases, the sample sizes required for the Bonferroni adjustment procedure are also included.

The results for $\rho = 0$ demonstrate that even modest differences in power correspond to substantial differences in required sample sizes (see the results for T^2 and OLS for Cases B and C, for example). Thus, even modest gains in power that may be available via improved methods of statistical analysis can be very important. Substantial differences in power cannot be tolerated (see the differences in required sample sizes between OLS and the other two procedures in Case A).

Positive correlation among the multiple outcomes has a negative impact on O'Brien's OLS procedure: for any configuration of the J standardized differences, the required sample size is directly proportional to $1 + (J - 1)\overline{\rho}$. As can be seen in Table 4.6, this effect becomes substantial with a large number of outcomes. With O'Brien's OLS procedure, any positive correlation among the multiple outcomes dilutes the information available on the comparison of the two arms. Because only $\overline{\rho}$ plays a role, the properties of OLS would be identical to those tabulated in Tables 4.5 and 4.6 for any pattern of correlations of varying strength with the same value of $\overline{\rho}$. (Of course, if the correlations are expected to vary substantially, use of GLS in place of OLS should be considered.) Similarly, as should be clear from the form of OLS, the pattern of standardized differences affects the properties of this procedure only through their average, $\overline{\Delta}$.

The effects of correlation among the multiple outcomes on Hotelling's T^2 are complicated, even in this simple situation of equally correlated outcomes. In Case A, the additional outcome measures are not effective in comparing the two arms but positive correlation enables Hotelling's T^2 to make better use of the information provided by the first outcome, with resulting increased power and reduced sample size as the correlation increases. In Case C, where all outcomes are equally effective, any positive correlation among the multiple outcomes dilutes

Table 4.6. Sample size required to achieve power of $1 - \beta = 0.80$ with equally correlated outcomes (two-sided level $\alpha = 0.05$ tests for a two-armed clinical trial)

Case	ρ^a	Procedure	J = total no. outcome measures						
			1	2	3	4	5	10	20
A	0.0	Bonferroni	100	120	132	140	147	167	187
		Hotelling's T^2	100	123	139	152	163	207	267
		O'Brien's OLS	100	200	300	400	500	1000	2000
	0.3	Hotelling's T^2	100	112	120	126	132	158	196
		O'Brien's OLS	100	260	480	760	1100	3700	13400
	0.5	Hotelling's T^2	100	92	93	95	98	114	140
		O'Brien's OLS	100	300	600	1000	1500	5500	21000
B	0.0	Bonferroni	100	108	116	123	129	150	172
		Hotelling's T^2	100	95	102	107	112	134	167
		O'Brien's OLS	100	89	89	92	96	117	155
	0.3	Hotelling's T^2	100	118	133	144	152	170	184
		O'Brien's OLS	100	116	143	175	211	431	1035
	0.5	Hotelling's T^2	100	123	133	137	137	134	136
		O'Brien's OLS	100	133	179	230	288	641	2900
C	0.0	Bonferroni	100	72	61	55	50	40	33
		Hotelling's T^2	100	61	46	38	33	21	13
		O'Brien's OLS	100	50	33	25	20	10	5
	0.3	Hotelling's T^2	100	80	74	72	72	77	89
		O'Brien's OLS	100	65	53	48	44	37	34
	0.5	Hotelling's T^2	100	92	93	95	98	114	140
		O'Brien's OLS	100	75	67	63	60	55	53

Case A: $\Delta_1 = \Delta^* = 0.4, \Delta_2 = \ldots = \Delta_J = 0$; only the first outcome measure is effective in comparing the two arms.
Case B: $\Delta_1 = \Delta^* = 0.4, \Delta_2 = \Delta^*/2, \ldots, \Delta_J = \Delta^*/J$; successive outcome measures are of diminishing effectiveness.
Case C: $\Delta_1 = \Delta_2 = \ldots = \Delta_J = \Delta^* = 0.4$; all outcome measures are equally effective.
[a] ρ = common correlation between the multiple outcome measures.

the information available on the comparison of the two arms; the effect on the required sample size for T^2 is essentially identical to that for OLS. Case B is intermediate and it can be shown that, for each fixed number of outcomes in Table 4.6, there is a particular value below which positive correlation has a detrimental effect on T^2, but above which the effect is beneficial. With $J = 5$ outcomes, for example, correlations above about $\rho = 0.30$ are beneficial, as the pattern of required sample sizes reflects.

These effects of increasing correlation underlie the patterns of performance as additional correlated outcome measures are included in the final analysis. In Case A, the detrimental effect on OLS of including additional outcomes is even more dramatic when the outcomes are correlated. For large enough correlation, the inclusion of a few such correlated outcomes actually improves the performance of Hotelling's T^2 slightly, despite the fact these additional outcome measures are not effective in comparing the two arms. In Case C, OLS continues to benefit as additional correlated and equally effective outcomes are included, but the marginal benefit for including more than the first few is small when ρ is as large as 0.5. For Hotelling's T^2, the inclusion of more than a few such correlated outcomes results in a deterioration in performance.

The complicated nature of this problem is perhaps best illustrated by Case B, where all the outcome measures have some degree of effectiveness in comparing the two arms and O'Brien's OLS procedure has a clear advantage over Hotelling's T^2 when the outcomes are uncorrelated. For the relatively modest $\rho = 0.3$, the performance of both procedures deteriorates slightly with the addition of the first additional outcome measure, and OLS has a slight advantage over T^2. With the inclusion of more outcomes, OLS deteriorates more rapidly in performance and T^2 has the advantage. The overall pattern is similar for $\rho = 0.5$, but T^2 has a clear advantage over OLS irrespective of how many additional outcomes are included. As the required sample sizes indicate, this advantage becomes substantial with a large number of outcome measures, but the most important point to note is that neither procedure is very effective in these circumstances.

Discussion

Despite their limited scope, the results in Tables 4.5 and 4.6 allow several general conclusions. First, a substantial penalty results from the inclusion of outcome measures that are not effective in comparing the two arms. Case A illustrates there is no statistical magic that can overcome a lack of sensitive measures for assessing the relative efficacy of the two arms. In such a situation, it would be counterproductive to combine the evidence from the different outcome measures; it is essential to identify the single effective outcome measure for use as the primary endpoint. If several primary endpoints must be included because it is not clear which is the effective outcome measure, the simplest approach of Bonferroni adjustment will be the best way to proceed. Every effort should be made to keep the number of primary endpoints to a minimum.

Secondly, when several roughly equally effective outcome measures are available, approaches based on combining the evidence from the different outcome measures can provide a considerably more sensitive overall assessment of the relative efficacy of the two arms. The results for Case C indicate that O'Brien's OLS procedure should be preferred to the approach based on Hotelling's T^2, but, with correlated outcome measures, the gains due to including more than a small number of measures can be quite modest. Taken together with the extreme danger associated with the inclusion of ineffective outcome measures when using O'Brien's OLS procedure, this again indicates it would be wise to limit the number of outcome measures to be included.

Thirdly, the decision on how to proceed in clinical trials of therapy in MS will invariably be difficult, as it will often not be clear which situation pertains. In particular, the potential beneficial effects of a proposed new therapy may not be well understood, so it may not be clear which of the component outcome measures describing the effects of therapy on the most relevant clinical dimensions of MS will be effective in comparing the two arms. Further, it may be difficult to determine in advance whether the component outcome measures selected for inclusion as multiple primary endpoints will be equally effective in comparing the two arms (Case C) or will vary considerably in their effectiveness (Case B). Yet, in contrast to Case C, O'Brien's OLS procedure provides a more sensitive overall assessment in Case B only if a small number of weakly correlated outcome measures are included. Thus, the decision to base the design and analysis of a clinical trial on a global statistic like O'Brien's OLS can only be made after detailed consideration of the statistical properties of the component outcome measures in the context of the specific clinical trial under consideration. The dearth of high quality information on the properties of some of the outcome measures in current use in MS, and particularly on the relationships among these outcome measures, is a major limitation to determining which of these statistical approaches to multiple outcome measures might be most appropriate for a particular MS clinical trial under consideration, as well as for the construction of prespecified composite outcomes (Goodkin et al. 1992). More empirical work based on high quality data is urgently needed to shed light on these critical issues.

In some circumstances, it may not be reasonable to consider an approach based on combining the evidence provided by the component outcome measures into a global statistic to provide an overall assessment. If the components reflect quite distinct aspects of treatment efficacy, each may be considered important in its own right. In this case, the approach based on Bonferroni adjustment might be the most suitable, as it maintains the individuality of the components. The decision of how to approach the design of a particular trial ultimately rests with the clinical investigators; the discussion in this section has attempted to describe some of the statistical ramifications of this decision. As noted by Pocock et al. (1987), in some circumstances, the main value of approaches based on a global statistic may be in providing an overall assessment for a battery of secondary endpoints.

The discussion in this section has focused on the case of normally distributed data, but all three approaches can be applied quite generally. Indeed, due to particular concern with small samples and outlying data values, O'Brien (1984) originally recommended converting quantitative data to ranks before applying his approach. The key requirement for application of both the approach based on Hotelling's T^2 and that of O'Brien's is that the joint distribution of the Z-statistics based on the different outcome measures can be approximated as multivariate normal. Thus, the underlying data could be binary on one endpoint, ordinal on another, continuous on a third, and so on. Pocock et al. (1987) explore this issue in some detail and Tang et al. (1989a, 1993) investigate several refinements and generalizations of the O'Brien approach.

Designs for interim analyses are available for all three approaches. With Bonferroni adjustment, the standard designs of the previous section can be applied to the component outcome measures separately. For O'Brien's approach, those same designs can be applied to the global statistic (Tang et al. 1989b). Designs for the approach based on Hotelling's T^2 statistic are less familiar, but can be based on the results of Jennison and Turnbull (1991).

Finally, it is worth emphasizing that our discussion has been limited to the case where all outcomes are concerned with the assessment of efficacy. An extreme example of a situation where a global statistic would not be suitable occurs when some outcomes are concerned with efficacy while others are concerned with toxicity. Toxicity outcomes are often not formally considered when designing clinical trials but the need formally to monitor such outcomes could arise in MS therapy trials if a comprehensive evaluation of toxicity was not completed prior to undertaking a Phase III trial. Motivated by this context, Cook (1994) and Cook and Farewell (1994) have developed a design for the interim monitoring of two outcomes, which can be viewed as a sophisticated generalization of the Bonferroni adjustment approach. Extension to the case of multiple outcomes is straightforward, in principle, and their approach could equally well be employed when all outcomes relate to efficacy.

Other Design Issues

Multiple Treatment Arms

Some clinical trials involve more than two arms. This can occur, for example, when there is an interest in increasing doses of an experimental therapy. In this case, three arms would often be included: standard treatment (in the past, this was invariably a placebo in MS clinical trials), low dose and high dose arms. For situations where the standard therapy is an active treatment (e.g. interferon beta-1b for mild to moderate relapsing–remitting MS), combination therapy can be of interest. In this case, there might again be three arms: standard treatment A, experimental therapy B, and standard treatment A combined with experimental therapy B. Alternately, if two experimental therapies are to be investigated, a factorial design may be of interest: standard treatment A, experimental therapy B alone, experimental therapy C alone, and a combination of experimental therapies B and C.

The most common of these scenarios for clinical trials in MS to date appears to have been the first, involving low and high dose arms of an experimental therapy and a placebo arm. The primary reason for multiple arms may simply have been an interest in collecting dose response information. Alternatively, as in the planning of the interferon beta-1b trial, there could be a concern that the high dose arm might be somewhat toxic, potentially leading to a large number of dropouts or even termination of that arm. The comparison of the high dose and placebo arms would then be compromised, but inclusion of a low dose arm might still allow an evaluation of the efficacy of the experimental therapy. The increasing availability of agents with demonstrated efficacy leads to a related concern: in ongoing and future placebo-controlled trials, patients may be inclined either to drop out or to violate the protocol once they become convinced they are on the placebo arm. Comparisons with placebo might then be compromised, but inclusion of low and high dose arms might still allow an assessment of evidence for increased efficacy associated with increased dose of the experimental therapy.

The decision to include more than two arms will not be taken lightly, as there are obvious sample size implications, but, given the manner in which such a trial is usually designed, is a third arm likely to be useful in this context of increasing doses? To provide a concrete illustration of the statistical properties of such designs, suppose that the standardized difference in means between the high dose and placebo arms is again given by $\Delta = 0.4 = \Delta^*$ say, so that, with 100 patients per arm, a level $\alpha = 0.05$ two-sided comparison of these two arms will achieve a power of $1 - \beta = 0.80$.

Now, suppose a low dose arm, only half as effective as the high dose arm (the standardized difference in means between the low dose and placebo arms is $\Delta^*/2 = 0.2$), is to be included in the trial. With the usual approach of also including 100 patients on the low dose arm, then the resulting power of the comparison of the low dose and placebo arms is only 0.29. However, if the trial is now intended to carry out comparisons of both high and low dose to placebo, then a Bonferroni adjustment should probably be made. In this case, the power of the comparison of high dose to placebo is only 0.71 (Table 4.4) and that of low dose to placebo is only 0.20. Restoring the power of the high dose versus placebo comparison to 0.80 would require a sample size of 122 patients per arm (Table 4.4), but the low dose versus placebo comparison would still have a power of only 0.24.

The inclusion of such a low dose arm cannot be justified on the grounds that it might serve as the basis for an efficacy comparison. If the concern is with the possible toxicity of the high dose arm, a hope that the comparison of low dose to placebo might still provide a useful assessment of the efficacy of the experimental therapy is misplaced; the power is totally inadequate. (In this scenario, some allowance for the anticipated rate of dropouts on the high dose arm would be incorporated into these sample size calculations, but that should not change the qualitative nature of these conclusions.) Similarly, if the concern is with dropouts on the placebo arm, a hope that the comparison of low dose to high dose might still provide a useful assessment of efficacy is also misplaced; the power of this comparison is identical to that of low dose to placebo.

When the experimental therapy has known side effects, a possible justification for the inclusion of such a low dose arm would be the expectation that it could improve the blinding and thereby enhance the integrity of the trial; this benefit appears to have been realized in the interferon beta-1b trial. In addition, even if comparisons of the low dose arm to placebo do not provide convincing evidence of a difference, the low dose arm might still provide an indication of a dose response relationship that could be valuable.

If the concern is with the possible toxicity of the high dose arm, elimination of this arm to allow a concentration of resources on the comparison of the low dose and placebo arms might be contemplated. Unfortunately, allocating all 366 patients to these two arms (183 per arm) leads to a power of only 0.47; to achieve a power of 0.80 would require 400 patients on each of these arms (with one-half the standardized difference, four times the sample size is required for the same power). Another strategy would be to allocate all 366 patients to the high dose and placebo arms, thereby providing greater allowance for dropouts; the obvious difficulty with this strategy is the serious complications associated with a high rate of dropouts. Perhaps the best strategy would be to plan a two-armed placebo controlled trial, but with a lower dose than originally contemplated for the high dose arm. Allocating all 366 patients to the two arms would allow the smaller standardized difference of $\Delta = 0.29$, or about 75% of Δ^*, to be detected with a power of 0.80. The key question is whether such a reduction in the dose would reduce the rate of dropouts to such a level that one could be confident the trial would be successfully completed. Unfortunately, strategies for coping with anticipated dropouts on the placebo arm are much more difficult to develop.

Interim monitoring is considerably more complicated for trials involving multiple treatment arms. As Geller and Pocock (1987) point out, the first question is whether the monitoring is to be of the separate treatment comparisons of interest or of all arms simultaneously. In the three-arm trial discussed above, for example, do we want to monitor the separate comparisons of low and high dose to placebo (or perhaps a comparison of both doses to placebo and a separate comparison of the two doses) or simply whether there is any difference among the three arms? Jennison and Turnbull (1991) provide cut-off values for group sequential designs for the latter case, but monitoring plans based on such procedures could call for termination without any of the treatment comparisons of interest exhibiting a difference. Thus, monitoring each of the separate comparisons of interest seems a more reasonable approach. In this case, one must consider whether exceeding a monitoring guideline is intended to result in the termination of the entire trial or simply the elimination of one or more of the arms. The development of plans with the latter objective is an active area of current research. Hughes (1993), Follmann et al. (1994) and Proschan et al. (1994) present recent developments and further discussion of these issues.

Active Control Trials

The increasing availability of therapies of demonstrated efficacy raises a variety of issues for the conduct of clinical trials in MS. As already mentioned, placebo-controlled trials may now experience greater dropout and protocol violation rates. Similarly, investigators may now experience greater difficulty in recruiting patients to placebo-controlled trials. The question of whether placebo or active controls should be used is primarily an ethical one, related to the current standard of care for the patient population to be investigated (see Goodkin and Kanoti 1994, for a detailed discussion of the ethical issues). The objective here is simply to highlight a specific issue that arises in connection with active control trials.

Placebo-controlled trials are efficacy trials; that is, the purpose of the trial is to investigate whether an experimental therapy can be demonstrated to provide a clinically meaningful benefit (over placebo). Active control trials, on the other hand, may be either efficacy trials or equivalence trials; this distinction has implications for the design of the trial. When an effective standard therapy is available, a trial may be undertaken to investigate an experimental therapy that promises to provide benefits not directly related to efficacy: perhaps less toxicity, lower cost or easier administration. In this case, the experimental therapy would presumably be recommended for future use, provided it could be established to be have efficacy equivalent to the standard. The usual approach to designing trials is not well suited to this objective.

Failure to reject the null hypothesis of no difference is often interpreted as establishing equivalence, thereby leading to the adoption of the experimental therapy, but, if the power of this test is low for clinically meaningful differences, then an inferior treatment is quite likely to be adopted. Failure to reject such a null hypothesis indicates only an absence of evidence of a difference, it provides no indication of how large a difference might still exist. The size of the *P*-value does not provide such an indication. The difficulty is that it is the Type 2 error of accepting equivalence when the two therapies are not equivalent that should be controlled in this situation. What is really needed is definitive evidence against any clinically meaningful advantage for the standard treatment.

An approach based on hypothesis testing would be to set as the null hypothesis that the standard therapy has a modest advantage over the experimental therapy, with the alternative being that of no difference. The magnitude of the advantage specified in the null hypothesis should be the smallest clinically meaningful difference. The more important error would then be explicitly controlled and the sample size calculation would be based on having adequate power to reject the null hypothesis when the two therapies are equivalent.

A more natural approach is based on confidence intervals for the difference in the efficacy of the two treatments. This has the advantage that the magnitude of the treatment difference, and the precision with which that difference is determined, are very explicitly described. At the end of the trial, if the upper limit of a confidence interval for the advantage of the standard over the experimental was less than the smallest clinically meaningful difference, then equivalence would be claimed. Repeated confidence interval methods provide natural monitoring plans. Fleming (1987, 1992), Jennison and Turnbull (1989, 1990) and Durrleman and Simon (1990) provide further discussion of this approach.

Although perhaps well understood, it is worth emphasizing that, when active controls become ethically required for efficacy trials in MS, then substantially larger trials may be required. This point can be made by a simple example. Suppose that in a population of secondary progressive MS patients to be investigated, approximately 40% exhibit progression of at least one confirmed EDSS point within a 2-year period. Consider a placebo-controlled trial designed to detect a 50% improvement in the proportion progressing, that is, a reduction from 40% to 20%. If the trial is planned as a two-sided level $\alpha = 0.05$ test, then a sample size of about 110 patients per arm yields a power of $1 - \beta = 0.90$. This calculation results from using $\mu_1 = 0.4$, $\mu_2 = 0.2$ and $\sigma^2 = \overline{pq}$, where $\overline{p} = (0.4 + 0.2)/2 = 0.3$ in the general sample size formula.

Now, suppose this therapy has been demonstrated to exhibit this effectiveness and patients treated with this therapy will be the active controls in the trial of a new experimental therapy. To demonstrate a 50% improvement of this new experimental therapy, a sample size of about 270 patients per arm would now be required to achieve a power of $1 - \beta = 0.90$. The details of such calculations will vary, depending on the nature of the patient population to be investigated and the outcome measure to be employed, but the overall conclusion will inevitably be the same.

Issues Concerning Analysis

Covariance Analysis

Covariance or regression analysis can be used for a variety of purposes in the context of clinical trials. Least squares and weighted least squares methodology for continuous outcome measures have long been employed. Logistic regression is particularly useful because many clinical outcome measures are either binary, or are reduced to this form. The proportional hazards model provides a corresponding methodology for censored time-to-event response data. Koch et al. (1982) provide a comprehensive review of available methodology for covariance analysis of categorical outcome measures. These methods seem much less well known and much less frequently used in the analysis of data collected in clinical trials. Despite the considerable loss of information this can entail, perhaps the most common approach to such outcome measures is to reduce them to binary outcomes (perhaps in several different ways) and use logistic regression on these derived responses.

Despite widespread knowledge of these methodologies, they are often not fully utilized in the analysis of data collected in clinical trials. For example, a primary use of covariance analysis is to induce closer equivalence between the treatment and placebo arms. Despite the use of randomization, some degree of imbalance on covariates will always exist and covariance analysis can offset such imbalances. Yet an approach that is often used is to carry out tests of homogeneity on prognostic factors and, if no difference is detected, to ignore that covariate when assessing the relative efficacy of the two arms. This practice was criticized by Altman (1985) on the basis that covariate imbalance is not sensibly determined by significance tests. For simple randomization, Senn (1989) was able to demonstrate that covariate imbalance is as much a problem for assessing the relative efficacy of the two arms in large trials, as in small trials, and that tests of significance do not adequately indicate when there is a problem. Thus, a covariance analysis including all important prognostic factors identified in advance is most appropriate. A complementary approach is the use of more sophisticated randomization schemes, which are capable of inducing a greater degree of balance than conventional permuted block methods (see Kalish and Begg 1985, for a review of these approaches).

A second use of covariance analysis is to examine the degree to which treatment effects are consistent across different subgroups of patients by means of interaction tests. Here, the approach of assessing the relative efficacy of the two arms within the subgroups is sometimes employed. Depending on the number of subgroups, a serious multiple comparisons problem can arise. Further, the clinical trial has been designed to achieve a specified power for the overall comparison, so the power to detect treatment effects within subgroups is usually quite limited. Consequently, false positives and false negatives are rather likely. Such subset analyses should probably not be undertaken unless the corresponding overall interaction test provided by the covariance analysis indicates an effect; even in this case, these subset analyses should be viewed strictly as exploratory.

Reports of MS clinical trials often utilize covariance analysis to clarify the extent to which detected differences between the two arms are due to treatment rather than to other factors associated with response. However, the potential of covariance analysis to generate a more powerful assessment of the relative efficacy of the two arms through the variance reduction that results from taking into account covariates which are highly associated with response does not appear to be often utilized or explored. Perhaps this is because the primary prognostic factor in the MS context might be the baseline EDSS, and the ordinal nature of this measure does not immediately lend itself to inclusion in a covariance analysis. Transforming the baseline EDSS into a simpler categorical variable for inclusion in such covariance analyses could be considered. For a trial in relapsing-remitting MS, for example, dichotomizing the baseline EDSS according to EDSS ≤3.5 and EDSS >3.5 might be adequate, but, for a trial in chronic progressive MS, a further breakdown of the higher baseline EDSS values would seem desirable. Ideally, categorization of the baseline EDSS values should be based on the knowledge of differences in prognosis according to the levels of baseline EDSS, as demonstrated by Weinshenker et al. (1991), Ellison et al. (1994) and Weinshenker (1994). This once again emphasizes the need for empirical work on high quality data to obtain a better understanding of the influence of various factors on progression in MS which in turn allows not only better trial design but also more focused and enhanced analyses. Cox and McCullagh (1982) provide a valuable review of the principles and methodology of covariance analysis.

Longitudinal Analysis

A basic feature of most clinical trials, not only in MS, is the longitudinal nature of the data collection process. Of course, time-to-event data is by definition longitudinal, but often outcome measures will be recorded regularly throughout the period that the patient is on the study. One approach to the analysis of such data would begin by replacing such longitudinal data by a suitable univariate summary over time. For a quantitative outcome measure, this might be the average of all values recorded during treatment and follow-up periods, for example. Extreme forms of this approach seem often to be employed in the analysis of data from MS clinical trials; typically the summary consists simply of the value recorded on the outcome measure at the end of planned follow-up, or perhaps the change in value from baseline to the end of planned follow-up. The assessment of the relative efficacy of the two arms would then be addressed by comparing these summaries for the individual patients across the treatment groups using standard methods of univariate analysis. Even with this simple approach there are questions of design and analysis that are often not considered (see Frison and Pocock 1992, for example).

This approach of summarizing the longitudinal data as summary measures that no longer depend explicitly upon time since entry to the study is a valid approach, but prevents any examination of possible patterns over time. Thus, the approach amounts to throwing away some of the information collected in the study. Depending on the behavior of the original outcome measure and the nature of the summary measure, the approach could amount to throwing away a very large fraction of the information collected. The patterns over time may contain important information concerning the action of the treatment. Further, the longitudinal data will allow an improved estimation of change over time and therefore provide a more sensitive assessment of the differences between the arms. Methods of analysis that allow examination of patterns over time, as well as differences between treatment arms, should be employed in the analysis; such methods will extract more information from the data collected at great expenditure of financial and human resources.

Traditional statistical methodology for dealing with longitudinal data, such as growth curves models and repeated measures analysis of variance, are not well suited to the clinical trials context. The former requires a rigid schedule of data collection and the latter, in addition, requires strong and unrealistic assumptions concerning the variance and correlation structure in the longitudinal data. Further, neither can easily handle the missing data that inevitably arise in the context of clinical trials. However, a variety of flexible methodologies designed specifically for such analyses have become available in the last 10 years. The methodology can accommodate baseline covariates as well as time-varying covariates. Rather general patterns of variances and correlations over time are allowed. One particularly attractive feature is that, in principle, the analysis is no more difficult if different patients are observed at different times; an immediate consequence is that missing data create no particular difficulty for the analysis.

One general approach, initially developed by Liang and Zeger (1986), Zeger and Liang (1986) and Zeger et al. (1988), is based on extensions of the equations used for regression analysis referred to as *generalized estimating equations* (GEE). Because the focus in the GEE approach is on the relationship of the outcome measure for the patients in each arm, as a group, to the various prognostic factors, the approach is sometimes referred to as *population-average modeling*. This approach can be used for binary, count and continuous outcome measures; several authors have recently applied the approach to ordinal outcome measures (see Lipsitz et al. 1994, for example). Thus, the GEE approach provides a unified method for the analysis of longitudinal data collected in clinical trials of therapy in MS.

The limitations of the traditional statistical methods for the analysis of longitudinal data on continuous outcome measures prompted Laird and Ware (1982) to develop an approach based on *random effects models*. Because the focus here is on the relationship of the outcome measure for each individual patient to the various prognostic factors, the approach is sometimes referred to as *subject-specific modeling*. This approach represented a major advance, due to the greatly increased flexibility of the modeling possible; this class of models has been successfully used in a wide variety of applications (see Waternaux et al. 1989, for example). This general approach is still not very well developed for other than continuous outcome measures. For a detailed discussion of this approach directed to a non-statistical audience, see Gibbons et al. (1993).

Diggle et al. (1994) provide an excellent introduction to both these general approaches, as well as many other models and methods for the analysis of longitudinal data. Interim monitoring based on longitudinal data may require specialized techniques; Lee (1994) provides a survey of recent developments in this area. All clinical studies tend to be affected by problems of missing data, but this is highlighted in longitudinal studies due to the greater difficulty of obtaining a complete set of observations for each patient. Laird (1988) discusses the concepts of "ignorable" and "non-ignorable" non-response in the context of longitudinal studies, distinguishes these from the more common concept of data which is "missing completely at random", and provides a detailed description of the ramifications of these types of incomplete data for longitudinal studies.

Summary

The focus of this chapter has been on statistical issues of particular current relevance to clinical trials of therapies in MS. The 1993 FDA approval of interferon beta-1b for the treatment of relapsing–remitting MS signaled the beginning of a new era for clinical trials in MS, with a clear ethical requirement for designs incorporating interim analyses of accumulating efficacy data. A fundamental principle is that early interim analysis should be based on fairly stringent nominal significance levels. A variety of approaches are available for developing such designs; all approaches require an accurate specification of the sequence of information fractions corresponding to the times of the interim analyses to allow the determination of the appropriate corresponding cut-offs. Clinical trials are complex undertakings, so data monitoring committees have to weigh many factors when considering the termination of a trial, but formalized plans for the interim analyses, specified in advance but with adequate flexibility to accommodate complications that might arise, provide a valuable objective guideline to assist in these deliberations.

For MS clinical trials, the consensus seems to be that several outcome measures are essential adequately to describe the effects of a therapy on the most relevant clinical dimensions of this complex disease. At present, there seems to be no general agreement concerning how these component outcome measures might be combined into a single prespecified composite (or on which components should be used). Three possible statistical approaches to the design of clinical trials where the efficacy of a therapy is to be measured by a battery of primary endpoints were described and compared. While the detailed results are somewhat complicated, a general conclusion for situations that appear to be of greatest relevance to MS clinical trials is that approaches based on combining evidence from the different outcome measures via a global statistic can provide a considerably more sensitive overall assessment of the relative efficacy of the two arms. Among the three approaches considered, O'Brien's OLS procedure was the most sensitive. However, when the component outcome measures are correlated, the gains due to including more than a small number of components can be quite modest even if the components are equally effective in comparing the two arms. Perhaps the most important conclusion is that a substantial penalty results from the inclusion of outcome measures that are not, or are only slightly, effective. Thus, just as is the case when using a single primary endpoint, the choice of outcome measures is absolutely crucial. Our results provide qualitative guidance for the context of clinical trials in MS, but specific recommendations would require considerable additional information on the properties of the outcome measures in current use, particularly on their interrelationships.

Several other topics were discussed very briefly. These included some issues arising in MS clinical trials involving more than two arms, the importance of the distinction between equivalence and efficacy trials for the design of active control trials, the many uses of covariance analysis for the comprehensive analysis of data collected in clinical trials, and the need for longitudinal analysis of data collected in MS clinical trials.

A recurring theme throughout the chapter was the need for more empirical work, to validate outcome measures in current use, and in development, to provide information on the relationships among different outcome measures, and to shed additional light on the natural history of this complex disease. Such work is essential not only to allow better design of MS clinical trials but also to allow more focused and enhanced statistical analysis of the data collected.

Acknowledgements

This work was partially supported by a research grant from the Natural Sciences and Engineering Research Council (NSERC) of Canada. The detailed comments of the Editors led to a substantially improved version of this chapter and are gratefully acknowledged. The chapter was written and revised while the author was on leave in the Department of Statistics at the University of Auckland, and the hospitality and facilities provided are gratefully acknowledged.

APPENDIX A

For the very simple clinical trial described, the parameter of interest is the difference in the underlying population means $\mu_1 - \mu_2 = \theta$, say. At the end of the trial, this parameter can be estimated by the difference in the corresponding sample means

$$\overline{X}_1 - \overline{X}_2 = \hat{\theta}, \text{ say}$$

and an approximate $1 - \alpha$ confidence interval for $\theta = \mu_1 - \mu_2$ is given by

$$\overline{X}_1 - \overline{X}_2 \pm z_{\alpha/2}\mathrm{SE}(\overline{X}_1 - \overline{X}_2),$$

where

$$\mathrm{SE}(\overline{X}_1 - \overline{X}_2) = \sqrt{\sigma_1^2 / n_1 + \sigma_2^2 / n_2}\,,$$

with σ_1^2 the variance in the first population and σ_2^2 in the second. In the special case described where these variances are known to be equal, we have

$$\mathrm{SE}(\overline{X}_1 - \overline{X}_2) = \sigma\sqrt{1/n_1 + 1/n_2},$$

where σ is the common underlying standard deviation. In either case, the approximate *Z*-statistic for testing the null hypothesis of no difference in the underlying population means, H_0: $\mu_1 - \mu_2 = 0$, is given by

$$Z = (\overline{X}_1 - \overline{X}_2)/\mathrm{SE}(\overline{X}_1 - \overline{X}_2)$$

Provided both n_1 and n_2 are reasonably large, the Central Limit Theorem justifies use of these techniques, even if the underlying response variable is not normally distributed; the key requirement is that the distribution of $\hat{\theta} = \overline{X}_1 - \overline{X}_2$, the difference in the sample means (which is used to estimate the parameter of interest, $\theta = \mu_1 - \mu_2$), can be well approximated by the normal distribution. The quality of the approximations will depend on the extent of the departures from the normal distribution, but, for the sample sizes typically employed in large-scale clinical trials, this would usually not be a serious concern. Further, if as would almost always be the case, σ_1 and σ_2, the underlying standard deviations in the two populations are not known, then they can be replaced by the sample standard deviations in the above formulas and the techniques are still valid.

For two-armed clinical trials involving other than continuous response variables, these techniques would often still apply. A parameter of interest, θ, is the basis of the comparison of the two arms and an estimate $\hat{\theta}$ of this parameter of interest is based on the data collected in the trial. The approximate $1 - \alpha$ confidence interval for the parameter of interest would be given by $\hat{\theta} \pm z_{\alpha/2}\mathrm{SE}(\hat{\theta})$, and the approximate *Z*-statistic for the null hypothesis, H_0: $\theta = 0$, would be given by $Z = \hat{\theta}/\mathrm{SE}(\hat{\theta})$. The fundamental requirement is that the distribution of the estimate $\hat{\theta}$ can be well approximated by the normal distribution. Provided both n_1 and n_2 are reasonably large, this would almost always be the case, although the advice of a statistician should be sought when the clinical trial is being planned to insure that the technical issues concerned with how best to make such approximations are carefully addressed.

APPENDIX B

Suppose the relative efficacy of the two arms at the planned end of the clinical trial, when responses will be available from $n = n_1 + n_2$ patients, will be estimated by a statistic $S(n)$, with variance given by $\mathrm{var}[S(n)]$. Then the Z-statistic for the final analysis would be $Z = S(n)/\sqrt{\mathrm{var}[S(n)]}$. In statistical terminology, the total information available for estimating the relative efficacy of the two arms will be $1/\mathrm{var}[S(n)]$. At a time during the trial when responses from $m = m_1 + m_2$ patients are available, the information currently available is $1/\mathrm{var}[S(m)]$. As more data accumulate, m increases, var[$S(m)$] decreases, and the information currently available increases to its eventual maximum value of 1/var[$S(n)$]. The information fraction is var[$S(n)$]/var[$S(m)$], which increases from 0 to 1 as data accumulate.

This concept is easiest to illustrate in the special case of continuous responses having equal variances on the two arms of the clinical trial, where the relative efficacy of the two arms is estimated by $\overline{X}_1 - \overline{X}_2$, the difference in the sample means. At the planned termination of the trial, we would have

$$\mathrm{var}(\overline{X}_1 - \overline{X}_2) = \sigma^2 (1/n_1 + 1/n_2).$$

At a time during the trial when observations are available from m_1 and m_2 patients, we have

$$\mathrm{var}(\overline{X}_1 - \overline{X}_2) = \sigma^2 (1/m_1 + 1/m_2).$$

At such a time the information fraction, f say, would be given by

$$f = (1/n_1 + 1/n_2)/(1/m_1 + 1/m_2).$$

If we let $n = n_1 + n_2$, the total sample size at the planned termination of the trial, and $\lambda = n_1/n$, the proportion of the total sample on arm 1, and similarly $m = m_1 + m_2$ and $\gamma = m_1/m$, then

$$f = [\gamma(1 - \gamma)/\lambda(1 - \lambda)](m/n)$$

where m/n is the fraction of the total planned responses currently available. In two-armed trials, the design would usually call for $n_1 = n_2$, so that $\lambda = 1/2$; in this case

$$f = 4\gamma(1 - \gamma)(m/n).$$

Now $4\gamma(1 - \gamma) \leq 1$, with equality only if $\gamma = 1/2$; that is, if an equal number of responses are currently available on each arm. However, a rather substantial lack of balance is required before $4\gamma(1 - \gamma)$ deviates a great deal from 1; for example, when $\gamma = 0.4$ or 0.6, we have $4\gamma(1 - \gamma) = 0.96$. Thus, in this simple example, unless there is a substantial lack of balance in the number of responses currently available on the two arms, the information fraction will be very close to the fraction of the total planned responses currently available.

References

Alling DW (1963) Early decision in the Wilcoxon two-sample test. J Am Stat Assoc 58:713–720
Altman DG (1985) Comparability of randomized groups. Statistician 34:125–136
Armitage P (1975) Sequential medical trials. Blackwell, Oxford
Armitage P, McPherson CK, Rowe BC (1969) Repeated significance tests on accumulating data. J R

Stat Soc A 132:235–244

Cook RJ (1994) Interim monitoring of bivariate responses using repeated confidence intervals. Controlled Clin Trials 15:187–200

Cook RJ, Farewell VT (1994) Guidelines for monitoring efficacy and toxicity responses in clinical trials. Biometrics 50:1146–1152

Cox DR, McCullagh P (1982) Some aspects of covariance. Biometrics 38:541–561

Davis BR, Hardy RJ (1994) Data monitoring in clinical trials: the case for stochastic curtailment. J Clin Epidemiol 47:1033–1042

DeMets DL, Gail MH (1985) Use of logrank tests and group sequential methods at fixed calendar times. Biometrics 41:1039–1044

Diggle PJ, Liang KY, Zeger SL (1994) Analysis of longitudinal data. Clarendon Press, Oxford

Durrleman S, Simon R (1990) Planning and monitoring of equivalence studies. Biometrics 46:329–336

Ellison GW, Myers LW, Leake BD et al. (1994) Design strategies in multiple sclerosis clinical trials. Ann Neurol 36:S108–S112

Fleming TR (1987) Treatment evaluation in active control studies. Cancer Treat Rep 17:1061–1065

Fleming TR (1992) Evaluating therapeutic interventions: some issues and experiences (with discussion). Stat Sci 7:428–456

Follmann DA, Proschan MA, Geller NL (1994) Monitoring pairwise comparisons in multi-armed clinical trials. Biometrics 50:325–336

Frison L, Pocock SJ (1992) Repeated measures in clinical trials: analysis using mean summary statistics and its implications for design. Stat Med 11:1685–1704

Gail MH, DeMets D, Slud E (1982) Simulation studies on increments of the two-sample logrank score test for survival data, with application to group sequential boundaries. In: Crowley J, Johnson RA (eds) Survival analysis. Institute of Mathematical Statistics, Hayward CA, pp 287–301 (IMS Lecture notes: monograph series, vol 2)

Geller NL, Pocock SJ (1987) Interim analysis for randomized clinical trials: ramifications and guidelines for practitioners. Biometrics 43:213–223

Gibbons RD, Hedeker D, Elkin I et al. (1993) Some conceptual and statistical issues in analysis of longitudinal psychiatric data. Arch Gen Psychiatry 50:739–750

Goodkin DE, Kanoti GA (1994) Ethical considerations raised by the approval of interferon beta-1b for the treatment of multiple sclerosis. Neurology 44:166–170

Goodkin DE, Rudick RA, VanderBrug Medendorp S et al. (1992) Low dose (7.5 mg) oral methotrexate for chronic progressive multiple sclerosis: design of a placebo-controlled trial with sample size benefits from a composite outcome variable including preliminary data on toxicity. Online J Curr Clin Trials Sep 25 (Doc no. 19)

Goodkin DE, Rudick RA, VanderBrug Medendorp S et al. (1995) Low dose (7.5 mg) oral methotrexate reduces the rate of progression in chronic progressive multiple sclerosis. Neurology 37:30–40

Halperin M, Ware JH (1974) Early decision in a censored Wilcoxon two-sample test for accumulating survival data. J Am Stat Assoc 69:414–422

Halperin M, Lan KKG, Ware JH, Johnson NJ, DeMets D (1982) An aid to data monitoring in long-term clinical trials. Controlled Clin Trials 3:311–323

Haybittle JL (1971) Repeated assessment of results in clinical trials of cancer treatment. Br J Radiol 44:793–797

Hughes MD (1993) Stopping guidelines for clinical trials with multiple treatments. Stat Med 12:901–913

Hughes MD, Pocock SJ (1988) Stopping rules and estimation problems in clinical trials. Stat Med 7:1231–1242

Jennison C, Turnbull BW (1984) Repeated confidence intervals for group sequential clinical trials. Controlled Clin Trials 5:33–45

Jennison C, Turnbull BW (1989) Interim analyses: the repeated confidence interval approach (with discussion). J R Stat Soc B 51:305–361

Jennison C, Turnbull BW (1990) Statistical approaches to interim monitoring of medical trials: a review and commentary. Stat Sci 5:299–317

Jennison C, Turnbull BW (1991) Exact calculations for sequential t, χ^2 and F tests. Biometrika 78:133–141

Johnson RA, Wichern DW (1982) Applied multivariate statistical analysis. Prentice-Hall, Englewood Cliffs, New Jersey

Kalish LA, Begg CB (1985) Treatment allocation methods: a review. Stat Med 4:129–144

Kim K, DeMets DL (1987) Design and analysis of group sequential tests based on the Type I error spending rate function. Biometrika 74:149–154

Kim K, DeMets DL (1992) Sample size determination for group sequential clinical trials with immediate response. Stat Med 11:1391–1399

Koch GG, Amara IA, Davis GW, Gillings DB (1982) A review of some statistical methods for covariance analysis of categorical data. Biometrics 38:563–595

Kurtzke JF (1983) Rating neurologic impairment in multiple sclerosis: an expanded disability scale (EDSS). Neurology 33:1444–1452

Laird NM (1988) Missing data in longitudinal studies. Stat Med 7:305–315

Laird NM, Ware JH (1982) Random-effects models for longitudinal data. Biometrics 38:963–974

Lan KKG, DeMets DL (1983) Discrete sequential boundaries for clinical trials. Biometrika 70:659–663

Lan KKG, DeMets DL (1989) Changing frequency of interim analysis in sequential monitoring. Biometrics 45:1017–1020

Lan KKG, Wittes J (1994) Data monitoring in complex clinical trials: which treatment is better? J Stat Planning Inference 42:241–245

Lan KKG, Zucker DM (1993) Sequential monitoring of clinical trials: the role of information and Brownian motion. Stat Med 12:753–765

Lan KKG, Simon R, Halperin M (1982) Stochastically curtailed tests in long-term clinical trials. Sequential Anal 1:207–219

LaRocca NG (1989) Statistical and methodological considerations in scale construction. In: Munsat TL (ed) Quantification of neurologic deficit. Butterworths, Boston, pp 49–67

Lee JW (1994) Group sequential testing in clinical trials with multivariate observations: a review. Stat Med 13:101–111

Liang KY, Zeger SL (1986) Longitudinal data analysis using generalized linear models. Biometrika 73:13–22

Lipsitz SR, Kim K, Zhao L (1994) Analysis of repeated categorical data using generalized estimating equations. Stat Med 13:1149–1163

Miller RG (1981) Simultaneous statistical inference, 2nd edn. Springer-Verlag, New York

O'Brien PC (1984) Procedures for comparing samples with multiple endpoints. Biometrics 40:1079–1087

O'Brien PC, Fleming TR (1979) A multiple testing procedure for clinical trials. Biometrics 35:549–556

Peto R, Pike MC, Armitage P et al. (1976) Design and analysis of randomized clinical trials requiring prolonged observation of each patient: I. Introduction and design. Br J Cancer 34:585–612

Pocock SJ (1977) Group sequential methods in the design and analysis of clinical trials. Biometrika 64:191–199

Pocock SJ (1982) Interim analyses for randomized clinical trials: the group sequential approach. Biometrics 38:153–162

Pocock SJ, Hughes, MD (1989) Practical problems in interim analyses, with particular regard to estimation. Controlled Clin Trials 10:209S–221S

Pocock SJ, Geller NL, Tsiatis AA (1987) The analysis of multiple endpoints in clinical trials. Biometrics 43:487–498

Proschan MA, Follmann DA, Waclawiw MA (1992) Effects of assumption violations on Type I error rate in group sequential monitoring. Biometrics 48:1131–1143

Proschan MA, Follmann DA, Geller NL (1994) Monitoring multi-armed trials. Stat Med 13:1441–1452

Senn SJ (1989) Covariate imbalance and random allocation in clinical trials. Stat Med 8:467–475

Slud E, Wei LJ (1982) Two-sample repeated significance tests based on the modified Wilcoxon statistic. J Am Stat Assoc 77:862–868

Tang DI, Gnecco C, Geller NL (1989a) An approximate likelihood ratio test for a normal mean vector with non-negative components with application to clinical trials. Biometrika 76:577–583

Tang DI, Gnecco C, Geller NL (1989b) Design of group sequential clinical trials with multiple endpoints. J Am Stat Assoc 84:776–779

Tang DI, Geller NL, Pocock SJ (1993) On the design and analysis of randomized clinical trials with multiple endpoints. Biometrics 49:23–30

Tsiatis AA (1982) Repeated significance testing for a general class of statistics used in censored survival analysis. J Am Stat Assoc 77:855–861

Waternaux C, Laird NM, Ware JH (1989) Methods for the analysis of longitudinal data: Blood lead concentrations and cognitive development. J Am Stat Assoc 84:33–41

Weinshenker BG (1994) Natural history of multiple sclerosis. Ann Neurol 36:S6–S11
Weinshenker BG, Rice GPA, Noseworthy JH et al. (1991) The natural history of multiple sclerosis: a geographically based study: 4. Applications to planning and interpretation of clinical therapeutic trials. Brain 114:1057–1067
Weiss W, Stadlan EM (1992) Design and statistical issues related to testing experimental therapy in multiple sclerosis. In: Rudick RA, Goodkin DE (eds) Treatment of multiple sclerosis: trial design, results, and future perspectives. Springer-Verlag, London, pp 91–122
Whitaker JN, McFarland HF, Rudge P, Reingold SC (1995) Outcomes assessment in multiple sclerosis clinical trials: a critical appraisal. Multiple Sclerosis 1:37–47
Zeger SL, Liang KY (1986) Longitudinal data analysis for discrete and continuous outcomes. Biometrics 42:121–130
Zeger SL, Liang KY, Albert PS (1988) Models for longitudinal data: a generalized estimating equation approach. Biometrics 44:1049–1060

5 Clinical Outcome Measures for Multiple Sclerosis

Brian G. Weinshenker

Historical Perspective

The first rating scales designed to quantitate disability due to multiple sclerosis (MS) were developed to characterize the natural history of the disease. McAlpine's scale (McAlpine and Compston 1952) is an example, but similar scales have been devised by others. These instruments were ordinal scales oriented to mobility and had a few large steps. They could reasonably categorize patients over the broad range of disabilities encountered in MS and were satisfactory to describe the evolution of MS over decades in retrospective or cross-sectional surveys. Alexander (1951) developed a rating scale based on a weighted scoring of the formal neurologic examination, including deep tendon reflexes and Babinski signs. Mobility was one of a number of factors weighted into the composite score. These rating scales illustrate the dichotomy between rating neurologic impairment, emphasizing mobility and scoring the formal neurologic examination, including reflexes and other elements not directly linked to impairment.

The advent of controlled clinical trials required fine instruments to measure disability, sufficiently sensitive to change that is encountered over the short term of a clinical trial. In the context of a clinical trial of isoniazid, Kurtzke (1955, 1961, 1983) developed a set of scales, which, in their simplicity and wide applicability, became the standard for quantitating disability resulting from MS over the last 40 years. Kurtzke's Disability Status Scale (DSS) and Functional System (FS) scores have undergone expansion (Expanded Disability Status Scale, EDSS) and modification in the guidelines for scoring over the years, but remain remarkably close to the original concept. The FS scores are based primarily on the findings on neurologic examination. The DSS, a composite measure of neurologic impairment, is determined by the FS score at the low range and by an assessment of ambulation, ability to transfer (as in from bed to wheelchair), upper extremity function and bulbar function at successively higher levels.

In parallel with the development of ordinal ranking scales developed by Kurtzke, others, especially Tourtellotte et al. (1965), have explored quantitative timed measures of neurologic function as finer, more precise and sensitive methods to quantitate the burden of MS. Kurtzke (1965) refers to this alternative approach and expresses concern that:

> The precision of these data might possibly be misleading, as the patient's attitude to the test undoubtedly influences performance. Furthermore, each scale has to be considered individually, since there is no method of overall assessment and obviously not all deficits attributable to the disease are measured...whether such emphasis on fine testing might be more misleading than reliance upon the coarse steps in the scales presented (in this paper) will be determined by future experience.

The same debate continues until the present time.

The DSS and its successor, the EDSS, and FS have been extensively field tested over the last 10–20 years. Kurtzke's initial observation that patients are distributed normally over the range of DSS disability (Kurtzke 1961) has been disputed. Prospective and longitudinal studies reveal that staying times at different levels of the DSS vary sufficiently to alter the probability of worsening by one (E)DSS point over the course of the 2–3-year clinical trial (Ellison et al. 1994; Weinskenker et al. 1991). Some more recent competitors to the EDSS and FS, the Scripps Neurologic Rating Scale (NRS) (Sipe et al. 1984), the Troiano Scale (TS) (Cook et al. 1986) and the Harvard Ambulation Index (AI) (Hauser et al. 1983), offer some advantages and disadvantages, but have not achieved the widespread acceptance of the EDSS and FS.

The International Federation of Multiple Sclerosis Societies, following the lead of the World Health Organization (WHO), developed a Minimal Record of Disability (MRD) based on a three-tier classification of dysfunction: impairment, disability and handicap. (International Federation of Multiple Sclerosis Societies 1985) Impairments are rated according to signs and symptoms. The EDSS and FS are the scales approved to measure impairment. Disability, which reflects the impact of impairments on activities of daily living, is measured by the Incapacity Status Scale (ISS) also developed by Kurtzke and others. Finally, the Environmental Status Scale (ESS), developed by Mellerup and Fog, quantitates social consequences of MS. The MRD reflects the need to assess the impact of neurologic impairment from a patient and societal point of view, taking the issue of clinical outcomes beyond physician-centered assessment.

The equivocal results of clinical trials of immunosuppression and concern about Type II errors has highlighted concern over the sensitivity of clinical outcome measures in MS. The use of quantitative testing has been increasingly advocated and functional tests have been incorporated in several recent clinical trials in MS, in some cases as part of or the entire primary outcome measure. Nonetheless, concerns over its use, very similar to those expressed by Kurtzke in 1965, still persist.

There has been increasing awareness of some aspects of MS-related dysfunction to which formerly little attention was paid. Neuropsychologic dysfunction, which may or may not be apparent on neuropsychologic screening tests, such as the mini mental status examination, has been recognized as being more frequent and disabling than previously realized. More sensitive batteries of testing, which assess higher order dysfunction in information processing, have been developed to detect the mild degrees of impairment of which MS patients, even those mildly impaired according to the EDSS, frequently complain. The excellent correlation observed between neuropsychologic dysfunction, as assessed by sensitive testing batteries to MS-specific dysfunction and magnetic resonance imaging (MRI) burden of disease (Filippi et al. 1993; Rao et al. 1989) have led many to suggest that neuropsychologic testing should be incorporated in all clinical trials. Fatigue is a major and disabling symptom that is weakly associated with DSS-rated disability. Assessments appropriate to these symptoms have been proposed. The imperfect relationship of impairment measures to patient perception of quality of life has been acknowledged. Various MS-specific and non-disease-specific measurements have been identified to quantitate the perception of general health and quality of life.

Given the issues raised above, coupled with the new and apparently independent measure of disease activity in the form of MRI and related methodologies (e.g. magnetization transfer, magnetic resonance spectroscopy), the National MS Society, in collaboration with the International Federation of MS Societies, held a workshop on outcomes assessment in Charleston, South Carolina, 23–27 February, 1994. As a result of discussions held at that meeting, a task force to further explore clinical outcomes was established under the chairmanship of Dr R. Rudick. The work of this task force is anticipated to span the next 1–2 years. The task force will have the advantages of incorporating the views of individuals representing many disciplines: neurology, neuropsychology, neuroimmunology, industry and biostatistics. Its recommendations should be unrelated to any individual agenda and reflect a broad consensus of opinion.

This chapter will review critically the characteristics of an ideal outcome measure. The DSS and EDSS impairment scales, the standards for clinical assessment in MS as well as the MRD, which also incorporates disability and handicap scales, will be reviewed. Proposals advanced to enhance the precision and sensitivity of the FS and EDSS will be discussed. The AI, NRS, TS and Cambridge Multiple Sclerosis Basic Score (CAMBS) will be reviewed, comparing and contrasting these scales to the DSS. Fatigue assessment will be briefly discussed. Finally, quantitative functional tests will be reviewed. The emphasis of the chapter will be on application to clinical therapeutic trials. Neuropsychologic dysfunction and quality of life assessment will be discussed in Chapters 6 and 7.

The Ideal Outcome Measure

A single outcome measure is unlikely to suffice for all MS clinical trials. For trials of progressive MS, a broad scale, one that reflects all relevant outcomes, is required. For example, if a patient were to be stable in terms of ambulation, but developed progressive dementia or blindness due to MS, the composite score or primary outcome measure should reflect the change, albeit that this is an unusual occurrence. Others, such as Kurtzke (1989a), have argued that impairments that reflect a greater extent of pathologic involvement of the neuraxis should be more heavily weighted.

In the context of a clinical trial, it is important to measure changes that occur frequently and to avoid measuring changes that occur infrequently, as the additional "noise" that they contribute to the composite outcome measures may compromise power, as will be discussed by Petkau in Chapter 4. Some parameters, such as visual dysfunction and cognitive impairment, are clinically relevant and likely to occur at a significant rate, but the impact of their inclusion in a multidimensional composite outcome measure has not been extensively studied and is uncertain.

For symptomatic treatments or for treatment trials of agents designed to enhance recovery from specific neurologic deficits, a scale more targeted to the problem being addressed (e.g. fatigue, right leg weakness) is preferable. This chapter will concentrate on scales that assess overall neurologic function, as would apply to trials of progressive MS.

Choosing a scale broadly applicable to the spectrum of MS disabilities assumes that it is desirable to be inclusive rather than exclusive in patient selection for clinical trials, and that the MS process is homogeneous over the course of the disease. This may not be true; mounting evidence has been interpreted to suggest that, once sufficient inflammatory demyelination has taken hold, secondary axonal degeneration, which may be more refractory to immune modulation, may become the predominant pathologic process (Arnold et al. 1992). If this were to be proven, it may be desirable to "split" patients according to the mechanism for worsening and not attempt to "lump" them together in treatment trials. This is currently not feasible, though magnetic resonance spectroscopy is promising in this regard.

The characteristics of the optimal MS clinical outcome measure, as outlined in a consensus statement at the Charleston conference on outcome measures are shown in Table 5.1. An additional item might be included in the list, as was discussed at a subsequent task force meeting, namely predictive criterion validity. Validity refers to success at measuring what one intends to measure. Predictive criterion validity refers to the ability of a sensitive, but not clearly relevant, outcome to predict future clinically meaningful change. The term "surrogate measures" in MS clinical trials has traditionally referred to paraclinical tests, such as evoked potentials and magnetic resonance imaging. In a sense, the clinical measures in a clinical trial are also surrogate measures, in that they serve as predictors of clinically meaningful change in MS over the long term

Table 5.1. Criteria for optimal outcome measures for MS (per consensus statement reached at the Workshop on Outcome Assessment sponsored by the National MS Society, Charleston, South Carolina, 23–27 February, 1994)

Criteria	Explanation
Sensitive	The measure should be sensitive to disease worsening over a relatively short time interval
Reliable	The score should be derived using objective criteria and should have high intra- and inter-rater reproducibility
Valid	Test instrument measures impairment caused directly by the disease and disability that is clinically relevant
Measure contains components that reflect the independent dimensions of MS	Test instrument measures the principal independent dimensions of the disease, but contains minimally redundant components
Measure is applicable to the range of MS impairment	Available scores should allow classification of all patients and avoid ceiling effects
Easy to administer	The measurement instrument should be easy and quick to administer
Cost effective and efficient	The measurement instrument should be conservative of time and resources

of decades. One point in deterioration on the EDSS scale, often used as the standard primary outcome in clinical trials of progressive MS, is pertinent only if a one-point deterioration over the short term predicts subsequent deterioration. One item that is conspicuously absent from the list of characteristics of an optimal MS clinical outcome measure is specificity, which implies that stability of the outcome score should mean that the disease is stable. However, given the frequent subclinical occurrence of asymptomatic MRI lesions (Wiebe et al. 1992), this may be an unrealistic objective.

Predictive validity has been considered in the context of several natural history studies. Specifically, attack frequency, first interattack interval and time to reach DSS 3 have been studied as clinical predictors of the time to reach DSS 6 (the need for a cane to walk a distance of half a block). The association between attack frequency and time to DSS 6 will be discussed further under the next heading. It appears that a majority of authors find that MS tends "to declare itself" early in most cases and an aggressive early course, defined by Kurtzke et al. (1977) according to the DSS score at 5 years and by Weinshenker et al. (1989) according to the time to reach DSS 3, all predict a more severe course. Predictive validity has also been examined in relationship to quantitative neuro-performance measures; this will be addressed in a later section.

Attack Frequency

A seemingly straightforward clinical outcome measure is counting attacks. Attacks of MS are generally defined as new or worsening symptoms attributable to MS lasting longer than 24 hours, although variation exists in the precise duration of symptoms required. The requirement for at least 24 hours' duration is designed to eliminate "pseudoexacerbations", which are precipitated by heat exposure, fever or fatigue, and are often reversible within hours. The frequency of attacks of MS in the first 2 years from onset has been negatively associated with the time to reach DSS 6 in some (Weinshenker et al. 1989) but not all studies (Runmarker et al. 1994). The measure is open to parametric statistics when comparing mean group attack rates in clinical trials and thus provides the opportunity to use more statistically powerful tools than those that are applicable to the EDSS, for which parametric statistical tests are inappropriate. Despite these apparent strengths, there are several drawbacks to the use of attack frequency as a primary outcome. First, attacks decrease in frequency with time in all MS patients. This phenomenon is exaggerated in clinical trials in which patients selected for relatively high attack frequency tend to "regress to the mean" (Weinshenker 1995). Attacks vary in severity and degree of recovery and these factors are hard to compare between patients. For example, it is difficult to say how a severe optic neuritis, with an excellent chance of full recovery, should be compared with a more insidious exacerbation of chronic myelopathy, with a lesser chance of full recovery. Furthermore, while there is an association between attack frequency and time to DSS 6, the association is weak (Weinshenker et al. 1989). Finally, most would agree that impairment is the most critical factor to be influenced in an MS clinical trial.

Extended Disability Status Scale and Functional Systems

Kurtzke introduced the DSS in 1955, and the FS in 1961. These scales were designed to capture the degree of impairment on independent measures of neurologic function felt to characterize all those relevant to MS. The scores are determined based on neurologic examination and not history, although bladder and bowel dysfunction are based on self report. The FS scores include the following: pyramidal (P), cerebellar (Cll), sensory (S), brainstem (BS), bowel and bladder (B/Bl), cerebral (C), visual (V) and other (O). Kurtzke classified the FS as major (P, Cll, S, BS) and minor (B/Bl, V, C, O), based on the frequency with which these systems were affected. Kurtzke (1989b) points out that only a fraction of the possible permutations and combinations of theoretical FS involvement are actually represented in MS population samples. Recognizing that the FS usually "peaked" at scores much lower than the maximum impairment for a given subscale and a summed score did not adequately represent the patient's impairment, the DSS was left as the composite measure of impairment. The DSS was later expanded by adding 0.5 points at all levels except 1.0 to generate a 20-point scale with finer steps, the EDSS (Kurtzke 1983). The scoring of the (E)DSS was clearly designed to reflect the pattern of worsening of MS. Initially, patients experience one or more neurologic impairments reflected on the FS but do not have impaired mobility or upper extremity dysfunction. The (E)DSS scores up to 4.0 were designed to reflect the FS, especially the severity of individual FS scores. Minor additional weighting is given for the number of systems involved. For example, a score of 3.0 on two FS rather than on one FS elevates the score from 3.0 to 3.5. From (E)DSS 4.0 to 8.0, the scale was designed to reflect the most common problem encountered by MS patients: difficulty with ambulation. Initially, this is based on the distance a patient can reasonably walk without having to stop. Beginning with (E)DSS 6.0, the scale makes use of both distance and the aids necessary for ambulation. Kurtzke emphasizes the distinction between the need for a cane and the use of a cane. Assessments are based on the physician's best assessment of a patient's best reasonable performance without requiring supramaximal performance. All scores are rated according to the principle of "closest" to the most appropriate score (Kurtzke 1989a). At EDSS 7.5, the ability to walk is essentially lost, and worsening from 8.0 to 9.0 is based primarily on upper extremity dysfunction. From EDSS 9.0 to 9.5, rating is based on bulbar dysfunction. EDSS 10 is arbitrarily assigned as death due to MS.

The EDSS is a rank order (ordinal) scale to which parametric statistics do not apply. Thus, the change from 2.0 to 3.0 is not equivalent to change from 3.0 to 4.0. A four-point deterioration is not "twice as bad" as a two-point deterioration. Kurtzke found that a cross-section of MS patients were distributed in a normal (Gaussian) distribution according to the scale, but this has not been the experience of several other cross-sectional population-based studies. There is a relative dearth of patients at EDSS 4.0–5.5, which is likely to be due to the fact that the staying time at these levels is significantly shorter, as has been discovered in both combined retrospective and prospective longitudinal (Weinshenker et al. 1991), and in entirely prospective series (Ellison et al. 1994). Kurtzke has argued that this may be an artifact resulting from misuse of the

EDSS, wherein patients are assigned a score of 6.0 if they use a cane, without assessing their ability to walk the distance that must be observed without walking aids for grades 4.0–5.5. As appreciated by most MS investigators, this is not likely to be the sole explanation for this phenomenon.

The EDSS and FS have been extensively investigated for inter-rater agreement at both the upper range and the lower range (Amato et al. 1988; Francis et al. 1991; Goodkin et al. 1992; Noseworthy et al. 1990; Verdier-Taillefer et al. 1991). Although inter-rater agreement is not perfect, it is better than 80% when ±0.5 EDSS points or ±1.0 FS points is allowed (Noseworthy et al. 1990). The inter-rater agreement on EDSS is not as good in the lower range, being approximately 60%–70% within ±1.0 EDSS point (Goodkin et al. 1992). Exact intra-rater agreement in apparently stable patients rated on two occasions 90 days apart was approximately 75% using the 10-step DSS, which is likely to be comparable to allowing a ±0.5 EDSS point variation in the EDSS (Myers et al. 1993).

The EDSS has been reviewed critically by Willoughby and Paty (1988). The major criticisms have been the following:

1. Officially, it is named an impairment scale by the WHO criteria.
2. The deficits are not specific to neuroanatomic structures; for example, a brainstem lesion could produce pyramidal involvement.
3. Certain FS scores are not objectively verifiable, such as bladder and bowel involvement.
4. Precision is poor for the descriptors of the FS (mild, moderate and severe). Integration of extent, severity and type of certain functional impairments, especially within the sensory FS, into a small number of steps is arbitrary and leads to difficulty in application.
5. The composite measure fails adequately to account for visual impairment, selective upper extremity dysfunction and dementia.

Kurtzke (1989a) responded to these criticisms. He points out that the scale was named a disability scale before the WHO developed a three-tier classification, under which it is officially an impairment scale. P, Cll and S FS always rate phenomena "below the neck", regardless of the site of pathology. Symptoms that are quantifiable when based on history, such as bladder and bowel dysfunction, are considered as objectively verifiable. Gait can be quantified by observing a patient walk up to 500 meters when necessary. Finally, the ceiling of contribution to the composite EDSS by visual impairment is justified by the fact that even severe visual impairment results from limited involvement of the neuraxis. Kurtzke recognizes the difficulty in grading FS but emphasizes that one should score according to the principle "to which one [step] is [the patient] closer". Within a buffer of ±1 point, he claims that this is feasible.

The arguments are good on both sides. It is important to regard the FS as neurologic functions and not neuroanatomic structures. Specific parts of the neurologic examination should be regarded as pertaining to the scoring of specific FS, regardless of the site of pathology. For example, gait hopping is said to be a cerebellar function. Recognizing that it is untestable if the P FS score is ≥3, an additional grade of "untestable" is added to the C11 FS score in that instance. This is a partial compensation, but it is likely that even patients with mild pyramidal dysfunction have mild impairment of gait hopping in the absence of cerebellar features. Thus, the EDSS is an operational system of scoring with a definite, but imperfect, association with neuroanatomic pathways.

In the official publication of the MRD by the International Federation of Multiple Sclerosis Societies (1985), further descriptions were added and some modifications to the FS were made, presumably to reflect the extensive field testing of this scale by the author. For example, level 2 "mild ataxia" of the Cll FS was further defined by "tremor or clumsy movements easily seen, minor interference with function". The S FS were expanded from five to six levels. Goodkin has proposed further modifications to the rating scores to improve precision (Chapter 12, Appendix). For example, P FS grade 2 is defined as 4 – /5 strength, P FS grade 3 is defined as 4/5 or 4 – /5 hemiparesis or paraparesis, and P FS grade 4 is defined as grade 2–3/5 strength in at least three limbs. A score of 1 on the Cll FS is allowed for abnormality on testing Cll function, which might be attributable to P FS involvement, even though, strictly speaking, the function is testable. This approach does improve precision, but, even with this modification, there are deficiencies. Different variations of involvement of individual muscles are common. Some patients have moderate or greater foot drop with good proximal strength while others have predominantly hip flexor weakness. Should weakness in proximal and distal muscles be rated equally? No rating system for spasticity is given. Incontinence is used to determine bladder and bowel function scoring. However, the occurrence of bladder incontinence is in large part dependent on the pattern of bladder involvement (failure to store versus failure to empty) and the use of medications to control urinary urgency. The rules proposed by Goodkin represent an excellent effort to improve the precision of the EDSS, but a thorough consideration of all permutations clinically encountered should be considered and perhaps integrated into a computer software program that could integrate such items as frequency of incontinence, anticholinergic agent usage, residual volume and intermittent self-catheterization, as well as a measure of urgency, in order to derive a more precise bowel and bladder functional score. Precision is especially important when these measures are applied in the context of the controlled clinical trial. A standard testing format should be imposed to minimize variation in patient interview and examination techniques. This approach has been tried in clinical trials in which sample examinations have been videotaped and sent to each of the investigators, or the investigators have met to improve the consistency of examination and use of rating scales.

The ordinal nature of the scale leaves it open to statistical abuse. Mean change in EDSS is an unacceptable endpoint for clinical trials. A treatment failure endpoint is more acceptable, wherein a degree of broadly accepted change indicative of unequivocal deterioration is defined a priori. However, even with this approach, the probability of treatment failure is dependent on the baseline EDSS score. One approach to bypass the non-linear nature of this scale without modifying the scale itself is to adapt the use of this scale based on the results of field testing. Based on the work of several groups, it has been suggested that a buffer of ±0.5 points should be allowed for baseline EDSS ≤5.5 without declaring treatment failure, but for EDSS greater than or equal to 5.5, 0.5 EDSS worsening should be accepted as meeting the criterion for failure. This recommendation is based on differences in the observed staying times at different levels of the EDSS. It is likely that this approach will successfully bypass the difficulties posed by differing probabilities for treatment failure according to entry EDSS level. It will also substantially improve the sensitivity of the EDSS in a clinical trial by allowing less stringent treatment failure criteria at higher EDSS levels. Goodkin et al. (1991) utilized this approach in defining one of several secondary outcome measures in a clinical trial of azathioprine in relapsing–remitting MS; he based this approach on his own observations of inter-rater reliability at different levels of the EDSS as well as those of others. At approximately the same time, in studies of the natural history of MS, Weinshenker et al. (1991) observed that staying times varied substantially at different DSS levels, and were roughly two to three times longer at DSS 6 and 7 than at DSS 4 and 5. In a meta-analysis of four large randomized clinical trials of progressive MS, Weinshenker et al. found that the proportion of treatment failures using different definitions vary considerably. Over 2–3 years' follow-up, the proportion of treatment failures in the aggregate control group increased from 30% to 50% when allowance was made for a modified definition of treatment failure with a 0.5 EDSS point being the criterion for treatment failure with baseline EDSS ≥6.0 (Weinshenker et al. in press).

Other Clinical Rating Scales

The Ambulation Index

The AI was developed by Hauser et al. (1983) for a clinical trial of cyclophosphamide, plasma exchange and ACTH in progressive MS. It is based only on ambulation and was used as an adjunct to the EDSS in the context of that trial. Some elements are subjective (e.g. step 1 requires patient-reported fatigue with demanding activity and step 2 requires a gait disorder "noted by family and friends"). However, timed walking of a distance of 25 feet is used for most levels of the 10-step scale, making it a hybrid quantitative neuroperformance and impairment scale. This is a significant advantage, as assessment of the time to walk 25 feet is more practical than observing the patient walk 500 meters, as is necessary to score the EDSS at some levels. Francis et al. (1991) found the kappa statistic for inter-rater agreement to be better for the AI than for the EDSS. Although somewhat limited by its restriction to assessment of ambulation, it appears to be a useful adjunct for improving sensitivity and inter-rater reliability in the EDSS 4.0–7.0 range.

The Scripps Neurologic Rating Scale

The NRS is a quasi-impairment scale, which was developed by Sipe et al. (1984) for use in a trial of alpha interferon conducted at the Scripps Clinic. It is a direct translation of the scoring on standard neurologic examination. It rates abnormalities in the following dimensions: mentation and mood (10 points), cranial nerves of vision (21 points), lower cranial nerves (5 points), strength (20 points), deep tendon reflexes (8 points), Babinski signs (4 points), sensory function rated for each limb (12 points), cerebellar function rated separately for upper and lower extremities (10 points) and gait and balance (10 points). The maximum score for a normal individual is 100. Abnormalities lower the score. Up to a further 10 points can be deducted for various combinations of bowel, bladder and sexual dysfunction. The principal advantages are its ready derivation from the neurologic examination and added sensitivity by virtue of a much greater range of scores than the EDSS. Other advantages include the fact that each limb is separately rated for motor and sensory function on a scale of 1–5, and it is more sensitive to vision than the EDSS. The disadvantages are a lack of guidelines on scoring severity, its retention of imprecise descriptive terms such as "mild, moderate and severe" impairment, and its somewhat arbitrary weighting of various neurologic functions, albeit done with due regard to the frequency with which these findings are seen in MS and their impact on neurologic function (i.e. strength has more points than reflexes). It is insensitive to mental status and relatively insensitive to ambulation.

The added sensitivity of this scale resulted in its being chosen to arbitrate the severity of exacerbations in the recent Betaseron® study (IFNB Multiple Sclerosis Study Group 1993) (Chapter 11). In this study, a decline of ≤7 points was regarded as a mild exacerbation, 8–14 points moderate, and ≥15 points severe. Using this classification, the annualized exacerbation rate in the control (placebo) group was 0.54 mild attacks/year and 0.45 moderate and severe attacks/year over the first 2 years. There was imperfect agreement between this "objective" criterion of exacerbation severity and the subjective evaluation of the investigators, however. Goodkin et al. (1988) have expressed concern about the imprecision of descriptive terms used in determining the severity of an exacerbation.

The Troiano Scale

The TS, developed by R. Troiano of Newark, New Jersey, was designed for use in a clinical trial of total lymphoid irradiation in chronically progressive MS (Cook et al. 1986). The TS is a 12-point hybrid impairment and disability scale scored in three subscales: gait, activities of daily living (ADL) and transfers. The gait scale is substantially similar to the AI, but abbreviated to a 6-point scale. The transfer scale is a 4-point scale, of which only the last two steps refer to a significant requirement for assistance in transfers. The ADL subscale is a 5-point disability scale. Its major advantage is simplicity. The drawbacks are insensitivity, and lack of assessment of vision, sphincter, brainstem and mental function. As acknowledged by the authors, it is designed primarily to assess progressive MS and not exacerbations. Work by the authors suggest that the scores are unimodal. It is difficult to accept the independence of the three measures and the assertion that it is more sensitive than the EDSS. For example, there is no attempt to grade ambulation impairment according to either distance or speed, but rather on the requirement for walking aids alone, with the inherent subjectivity of this observation.

The Cambridge Multiple Sclerosis Basic Score

The CAMBS was proposed by Mumford and Compston (1993) of the University of Cambridge. This score is a shorthand method to express disability and impairment, relapse status and severity, degree of progression and patient-perceived handicap using a visual analog scale. Each of these dimensions is graded on an abbreviated 5-point scale, and expressed as a 4-digit score. Reproducibility is claimed to be good but, given its inherent insensitivity, this is not surprising. The authors point out that it is not designed to be an outcome measure for clinical trials. Recording relapse and progression status removes the restriction of other rating scales to assessment when the disease is in a relatively stable state. Its advantages are simplicity and wide applicability. Otherwise, it offers no unique advantages.

Global Opinions

Global opinions are gaining increasing attention as providing enhanced sensitivity despite greater subjectivity and potential inter-rater variability. The successful use and credibility of global opinions is highly dependent on the blinding effectiveness on clinical trials. Global opinions have been widely used in trials of Alzheimer's disease as a supplement to neuropsychologic measures.

Global opinions can be used either to enhance or to limit sensitivity. Noseworthy et al. are conducting a clinical trial of sulfasalazine for active relapsing–remitting or chronically progressive MS at the Mayo Clinic. A secondary outcome is the number of clinically active 3-month quarters over 3 years. Investigators are exploring whether a less rigorous subjective opinion than that required for the strict definition of disease activity on a quarterly basis might improve the sensitivity of determining whether or not MS is active in a given quarter. For example, if a patient reports a credible constellation of symptoms indicating MS worsening, although the disease activity is not reflected on the primary outcome (EDSS score), a second less stringent level of disease activity is recorded (i.e. in the neurologist's global opinion that the disease has been active). It is to be hoped that, by comparison with other measures such as MRI, it will be possible to assess the validity of this approach.

The approach of using a global opinion can also serve to limit sensitivity to detection of only those changes deemed to be of significant functional consequence. It is especially valuable when the targeted deficit can be in one of several neurologic systems and a limited number of scales are insufficient to evaluate all potential targeted outcomes. The rating neurologist is asked whether, as a global opinion, the targeted neurologic deficit is improved to a moderate or greater extent, moderate being defined as having definite functional impact. This approach is being used in two Mayo Clinic trials, one evaluating whether plasma exchange and the second whether intravenous immunoglobulin (IVIg) improves recovery from MS-related neurologic deficits, either in the 3 months following an acute exacerbation (plasma exchange) or in the 3–18 months following an acute exacerbation (IVIg). Using this approach, patients with diverse targeted neurologic deficits, such as coma, encephalopathy, aphasia and quadriparesis, are being included in the plasma exchange trial.

Disability and Handicap Scales

Disability and handicap scales have been less extensively used than the EDSS, largely because neurologists are not generally familiar with them, and paramedical personnel are most often involved in their use. They are assessed by interview, which leads to greater subjectivity than impairment scales, which are based on objective examination. The IFMSS-sanctioned disability scale is the ISS (International Federation of Multiple Sclerosis Societies 1985), which was developed by Kurtzke and Granger and is based on the PULSES (physical condition, upper limb function, lower limb function, sensory (verbal/hearing) functions, excretory functions, support factors (e.g. psychologic and financial)) profile and the Barthel Index. The scoring is based on interview and is determined according to the patient's actual level of function and not presumed abilities. Therefore, it may be affected by coexisting disease, which is an obvious limitation to its use in a clinical trial as a primary outcome. The ISS evaluates the following 16 items: stair climbing, ambulation, transfers, bowel function, bladder function, bathing, dressing, grooming, feeding, vision, speech and hearing, medical problems (either MS- or not MS-related), mood and thought disturbance, mentation, fatiguability, and sexual function. Each is scored from 0 (no dysfunction) to 4 (worst dysfunction); therefore, the maximum possible score is 64. There is obvious overlap with the FS, and many items are MS-non-specific. The scale has greater application as a device to monitor rehabilitation than as an outcome measure in clinical trials.

The environmental status scale (ESS) was developed by an international group chaired by E. Mellerup and T. Fog of Denmark to assess social dysfunction appropriate to one's cultural setting (International Federation of Multiple Sclerosis Societies 1985). It consists of seven items, each rated from 0 (no dysfunction) to 5 (greatest dysfunction). Again, the rating is based on performance. For example, someone capable of working, but who is unemployed, would be given the worst score (5) for actual work status if the evaluator deems that the "customary" role for that individual in their social background would be full-time employment. Other items rated are: financial/economic status, personal residence, personal assistance requirements, transportation, community services and social activities.

Few studies exist to assess impairment or handicap scales. Granger et al. (1990) evaluated a number of measurements of disability in handicap including the ISS and ESS in 24 patients. The investigators also evaluated the Functional Independence Measure scale (FIM) (Keith et al. 1987), the updated version of the older Barthel Index, which resulted from a national task force of the Academy of Physical Medicine and Rehabilitation and the American Congress of Rehabilitation Medicine, and the Brief Symptom Inventory (BSI) (Derogatis and Melisaratos 1983), a measure of psychologic distress. The FIM includes items for toileting and better distinguishes degrees of severity of bladder and bowel involvement. The FIM also separates transferring from bed or chair, bath or shower, and from a toilet. Theoretically, this improves precision and sensitivity compared with the ISS. There has been more extensive evaluation of the inter-rater agreement, redundancy and predictive value of the FIM than of the ISS, albeit not specifically for MS. Each of these measures and their component domains were evaluated as predictors of the help (minutes per day) required by MS patients and their self-expressed general life satisfaction. The FIM and ISS were each satisfactory in explaining approximately 75% of the variability among patients. A multiple regression analysis revealed that the predictors most likely to be associated with the need for help were transfers from the bath and shower (FIM), vision (ISS), and "walk or wheelchair" (FIM). With vision removed, multiple FIM items were predictive, including transfers from a chair or bed, memory, "walk or wheelchair", dressing the lower body, bladder management and eating. The items associated with general life satisfaction differed from those associated with the need for help, and included items from the BSI (inter-personal, sensitivity and hostility) and the ESS (transportation and social activity), as well as the FIM (toileting, dressing lower body and climbing stairs).

Cohen et al. (1993) found that the ability to accomplish ADL worsened exponentially once the EDSS exceeded 5. The predictive value of the EDSS on ADL was primarily due to its assessment of mobility. The EDSS did not adequately explain the variability in ADL between individuals.

Both the ISS and the ESS are tools that evaluate rehabilitation needs and progress, and increase the understanding of quality of life beyond the capability of the EDSS. Some prefer other scales such as the FIM because of greater sensitivity as determined in diseases other than MS. Psychologic inventories are essential adjuncts to understanding patient-perceived quality of life. Their subjective nature, unclear association with disease activity, measurement of disabilities and handicaps that are not necessarily directly attributable MS, and the use of an ordinal rating scheme, combine to render these scales unsuitable as primary outcome measures in the context of a clinical trial.

Quantitative Neuroperformance Testing

Quantitative evaluation of neurologic function (QENF) was proposed by Tourtellotte et al. (1965) as a battery of tests that can be timed and expressed as parametric data, often as a percentage of normal function. These measurements are not MS-specific but are designed to be objective measures sensitive to changes in function. The battery of tests includes the following: symbol digit modality test (cognitive), finger tapping, Purdue pegboard, foot tapping, standing/balance (two legs and one leg), tandem walking and simulated ADL (e.g. dressing, buttoning, zipping, tying a bow, cutting with knife, etc.). The testing is designed to be accomplished over approximately 1 hour by a trained technician at a consistent time of day.

Syndulko et al. (1993) have recently reviewed the experience at the UCLA/West Los Angeles VA group with the evaluation of this neuroperformance battery in patients enrolled at their centers in the USA cyclosporine study. They found that these tests were reproducible over multiple baseline examinations, and that changes over time correlated with changes on the EDSS and AI. They found that the neuroperformance tests were able to detect advantageous treatment effects at their center in favor of cyclosporine A, similar to those observed in the entire multicenter study, which used an EDSS-based primary outcome. In the same group of patients at their own center, they were unable to detect a treatment effect with EDSS or other standard clinical rating scales, which led the investigators to conclude that the QENF was more sensitive than EDSS. The magnitude of change and the difference between the placebo and active treatment groups were such that a smaller sample size would be necessary to detect an effect if the neuroperformance battery were used as the primary outcome measure rather than the EDSS. Learning effects were a problem for a relatively small number of subtests. (The authors did use parametric statistics to analyze treatment effect using EDSS and other clinical rating scale data, with which most would take issue.)

The proponents of this approach acknowledge the general lack of acceptance of neuroperformance testing. Conclusions based on this approach are conceptually difficult. It is unappealing to accept that a treatment is effective in altering the course of progressive MS because a single or composite neuroperformance score changes by a small, albeit statistically significant, amount. The issue of predictive criterion validity is especially important for these quantitative tests. However, given the need for more responsive and sensitive testing, this approach is promising, and, if confirmed as being feasible and predictive of future change, the neuroperformance battery may become an important and widely used assessment technique.

Noseworthy recently found that quantitative isometric strength assessment in a biomechanics laboratory was far more sensitive than assessment of two blinded neurologists in identifying muscle weakness in a pilot trial of IVIg to enhance recovery from recently acquired muscle weakness due to MS (Noseworthy et al. 1994). The reliability of isometric muscle testing was adequate with 73% and 80% reproducibility for markedly (≥50%) and mildly (<25%) weak muscle on repeated studies separated by at least 2 weeks. Of 432 muscles, with less than 50% power compared with normal isometric testing, two neurologists rated strength as normal in 41% and mildly reduced in 15%. The investigators concluded that the clinical neurologic examination underestimates the degree of MS-associated weakness, and that quantitative isometric testing might significantly enhance sensitivity with good reliability.

Goodkin et al. (1988) have assessed the use of the Box and Blocks and Nine-Hole Peg Tests as quantitative measures of upper extremity function. They investigated the frequency of impairment, the stability of the results over serial studies and the potential to use these tests as more sensitive measures that correlate with subjective deterioration in MS. The tests were administered by occupational therapists blinded to the neurologist's assessment of stability. Sixty to 90% of patients were impaired (scores <10% of age- and sex-matched normal controls). The tests showed deterioration of ≥10% in 15%–20% and ≥30% in 3%–4% of 68 MS patients who were apparently stable according to EDSS and P, Cll and V FS, but who had noted subjective deterioration in daily functional status.

Notably, a higher proportion of these individuals showed improvement than deterioration, raising the issue of whether the variability in this group is truly associated with their subjective worsening. Reproducibility was good for the controls who were assessed on several occasions at baseline, but substantially larger variation was encountered in patients who were followed over 6 months. Whether the greater variation was truly due to a change in function or to the greater interval between testing and retesting is uncertain. The authors conclude that these tests were more sensitive than the EDSS in detecting upper extremity function change. These upper extremity functional tests have been applied by Goodkin et al. (1995) in a randomized clinical trial of oral methotrexate in 60 ambulatory and chronically progressive MS patients. The most favorable results (i.e. the greatest difference in favor of treatment benefit) were seen in measures of upper extremity function, while no significant effect was detected in lower extremity function or ambulation.

Fatigue

Fatigue is a common disabling symptom in MS patients, and is poorly associated with other aspects of physical, cognitive or emotional impairment. In 32 consecutive patients with MS studied by Krupp et al. (1988) at the Albert Einstein Research and Training Center for MS, it predated other symptoms in 31% and was the most troublesome symptom in 28%. The Pearson correlation coefficient between EDSS and fatigue, as measured on a visual analog scale, was non-significant. The following factors distinguished MS-associated fatigue from fatigue in normal controls: prevents sustained physical functioning, aggravated by heat, interferes with responsibility, comes on easily, interferes with physical functioning, and causes frequent problems. Its severity was assessed with a visual analog scale. Patients were asked to place a mark on a 10 cm line ranging from "no fatigue" to "severe fatigue", appropriate to the point that best described their fatigue. Fatigue seems to be distinguishable from depression, but subjectivity and lack of association with other objective measurable dysfunction makes it a poor choice for a clinical trial primary outcome measure for progressive MS. However, its frequency and strong impact on quality of living make it an important secondary outcome measure. For clinical trials aimed at treatment of fatigue, a scale has been derived by Krupp et al. (1989), which requires that patients rate their fatigue from 1 to 7 (strongly disagree to strongly agree) on nine items that are able to distinguish fatigue in MS from that of normal subjects and from patients with systemic lupus erythematosus.

Conclusions

Clinical rating tools to assess outcome can be classified as follows:

1. Measures based on quantitation of the neurologic examination (e.g. the Scripps NRS);

2. Ordinal impairment scales (e.g. the EDSS and FS);
3. Disability and handicap scales that evaluate dysfunctions common in MS but not specific to MS-associated disabilities (e.g. ISS, ESS, FIM);
4. Quantitative neuroperformance scales (e.g. QENF of Tourtellotte, Nine-Hole Peg Tests, isometric strength testing);
5. Global rating scales, rated either by physician or patient (includes visual analog scales);
6. Hybrid scales (e.g. AI, which is a hybrid impairment scale and quantitative performance scale);
7. Self-rating scales sensitive to the emotional and functional impact on general health and quality of life.

The dilemma facing those who seek to develop a uniform rating battery of clinical outcome measures in MS is to develop sensitive, responsive measures that are reliable and clinically meaningful, yet are feasible and not redundant. Sensitivity has been repeatedly demonstrated to be inferior to MRI scanning, which often shows activity when MS is not clinically active. As long as clinical measures remain the affirmed primary outcome measures for Phase III clinical trials, they must be sufficiently sensitive and reliable to detect a clinically meaningful change over the short term of a 2–3-year clinical trial. Traditionally, clinically meaningful measures have been required to have intrinsic importance. However, given the generally slow progress of MS encountered in large groups of patients, even those recruited to clinical trials because of relatively rapid recent deterioration, the MS community must be prepared to consider outcome measures that may not be meaningful in their own right but reliably discriminate between stable and worsening disease and predict future worsening. Batteries of tests and rating scales, rather than single tests or scales, are necessary given the large number of relevant outcomes possible in progressive MS, which include neuropsychologic dysfunction (Chapter 6) along with traditional motor, sensory and sphincter dysfunction.

Both quantitative and qualitative assessments are of value. Quantitative assessments are intrinsically more sensitive, but changes on qualitative assessments are generally more meaningful clinically. Qualitative rating scales, such as the EDSS and FS, should be improved to increase precision and thereby improve intra- and inter-rater agreement. Certain FS scores should be updated to recognize current standards of assessment and treatment, especially those quantitating cognitive function and bladder dysfunction. Based on the experience of two decades of field testing of the EDSS in clinical trials, the choice of primary outcome measures should reflect the differing probabilities of worsening at the various levels. The theoretical and occasionally observed advantages of improved inter-rater agreement and sensitivity of the AI in assessing ambulation might encourage the development of hybrid quantitative neuroperformance and clinical rating scales. Quantitative testing needs to be studied further to develop a minimal feasible and non-redundant battery of tests. Prospective studies of predictive validity are necessary.

Neuropsychologic studies should be incorporated in clinical trials if their reliability and feasibility can be demonstrated. Fatigue assessment has great importance for assessing quality of life, given the major impact fatigue has on patient function. Because of the subjectivity inherent in quantitating fatigue and because multiple factors can aggravate fatigue, its assessment should be only a secondary outcome in clinical trials of progressive MS.

Disability and handicap are evaluated by interview through instruments not designed objectively to assess MS-specific dysfunction but patient performance. These instruments are of great importance in assessing the impact of MS, but the strong influence of psychologic and other processes not directly MS-related make them unsuitable for primary outcome measures in MS clinical trials.

References

Alexander L (1951) New concept of critical steps in course of chronic debilitating neurologic disease in evaluation of therapeutic response. Arch Neurol Psychiatry 66:253–271

Amato MP, Fratiglioni L, Groppi C, Siracusa G, Amaducci L (1988) Interrater reliability in assessing functional systems and disability on the Kurtzke Scale in multiple sclerosis. Arch Neurol 45:746–748

Arnold DL, Matthews PM, Francis G, O'Connor J, Antel JP (1992) Proton magnetic resonance spectroscopy for metabolic characterization of demyelinating plaques. Ann Neurol 31:235–241

Cohen RA, Kessler HR, Fischer M (1993) The extended disability status scale (EDSS) as a predictor of impairments of functional activities of daily living in multiple sclerosis. J Neurol Sci 115:132–135

Cook SD, Troiano R, Zito G et al. (1986) Effect of total lymphoid irradiation in chronic progressive multiple sclerosis. Lancet i:1405–1409

Derogatis LR, Melisaratos N (1983) The brief symptom inventory: an introductory report. Psychol Med 13:595–605

Ellison GW, Myers LW, Leake BD et al. (1994) Design strategies in multiple sclerosis clinical trials. Ann Neurol 36:S108–S112

Filippi M, Martinelli V, Sirabian G et al. (1993) Brain magnetic resonance imaging correlates of cognitive impairment in multiple sclerosis. J Neurol Sci 115(Suppl):S66–S73

Francis DA, Bain P, Swan AV, Hughes RAC (1991) An assessment of disability rating scales used in multiple sclerosis. Arch Neurol 48:299–301

Goodkin DE, Hertsgaard D, Seminary J (1988) Upper extremity function in multiple sclerosis: improving assessment sensitivity with Box-and-Block and Nine-Hole Peg tests. Arch Phys Med Rehabil 69:850–854

Goodkin DE, Bailly RC, Teetzen NL, Hertsgaard D, Beatty WW (1991) The efficacy of azathioprine in relapsing–remitting multiple sclerosis. Neurology 41:20–25

Goodkin DE, Cookfair D, Wende K et al. (1992) Inter- and intrarater scoring agreement using grades 1.0 to 3.5 of the Kurtzke Expanded Disability Status Scale (EDSS). Neurology 42:859–863

Goodkin DE, Rudick RA, Medendorp SV et al. (1995) Low dose (7.5 mg) oral methotrexate reduces the rate of progression in chronic progressive multiple sclerosis. Ann Neurol 37:30–40

Granger CV, Cotter AC, Hamilton BB, Fiedler RC, Hens MM (1990) Functional assessment scales: a study of persons with multiple sclerosis. Arch Phys Med Rehabil 71:870–874

Hauser SL, Dawson DM, Lehrich JR et al. (1983) Intensive immunosuppression in progressive multiple sclerosis. A randomized, three-arm study of high-dose intravenous cyclophosphamide, plasma exchange, and ACTH. N Engl J Med 308:173–180

IFNB Multiple Sclerosis Study Group (1993) Interferon beta-1b is effective in relapsing–remitting multiple sclerosis: 1. Clinical results of a multicenter randomized, double-blind placebo-controlled trial. Neurology 43:655–661

International Federation of Multiple Sclerosis Societies (1985) Minimal Record of Disability for multiple sclerosis. National Multiple Sclerosis Society, New York

Keith RA, Granger CV, Hamilton BB, Sherwin FS (1987) The functional independence measure: a new tool for rehabilitation. In: Eisenberg MG, Grzesiak RC (eds) Advances in clinical rehabilitation, vol. 1. Springer-Verlag, New York, pp 6–18

Krupp LB, Alvarez LA, LaRocca NG et al. (1988) Fatigue in multiple sclerosis. Arch Neurol 45:435–437

Krupp LB, LaRocca NG, Muir-Nash J, Steinberg AD (1989) The fatigue severity scale: application to

patients with multiple sclerosis and systemic lupus erythematosus. Arch Neurol 46:1121–1123
Kurtzke JF (1955) A new scale for evaluating disability in multiple sclerosis. Neurology 5:580–583
Kurtzke JF (1961) On the evaluation of disability in multiple sclerosis. Neurology 11:686–694
Kurtzke JF (1965) Further notes on disability evaluation in multiple sclerosis, with scale modifications. Neurology 15:654–661
Kurtzke JF (1983) Rating neurologic impairment in multiple sclerosis: an expanded disability status scale (EDSS). Neurology 33:1444–1452
Kurtzke JF (1989a) The disability status scale for multiple sclerosis: apologia pro DSS sua. Neurology 39:291–302
Kurtzke JF (1989b) Patterns of neurologic involvement in multiple sclerosis. Neurology 39:1235–1238
Kurtzke JF, Beebe GW, Nagler B et al. (1977) Studies on the natural history of multiple sclerosis: VIII. Early prognostic features of the later course of the illness. J Chronic Dis 30:819–830
McAlpine D, Compston N (1952) Some aspects of the natural history of disseminated sclerosis. Q J Med 21:135–167
Mumford CJ, Compston A (1993) Problems with rating scales for multiple sclerosis: a novel approach - the CAMBS score. J Neurol 240:209–215
Myers LS, Ellison GW, Leake BD (1993) Reliability of the disability status scale (DSS). Neurology 43(Suppl 2):A204
Noseworthy JH, Vandervoort MK, Wong CJ, Ebers GC and the Canadian Cooperative Multiple Sclerosis Study Group (1990) Interrater variability with the expanded disability status scale (EDSS) and functional systems (FS) in a multiple sclerosis clinical trial. Neurology 40:971–975
Noseworthy JH, Rodriguez M, Weinshenker BG et al. (1994) The assessment of muscle strength in an MS clinical trial. 10th Congress of European Committee for Treatment and Research in MS (ECTRIMS). Athens, Greece, November
Rao SM, Leo GJ, Haughton VM et al. (1989) Correlation of magnetic resonance in aging with neuropsychological testing. Neurology 39:161–166
Runmarker B, Andersson C, Oden A et al. (1994) Multivariate analysis of prognostic factors in multiple sclerosis. J Neurol 241:597–604
Sipe JC, Knobler RL, Braheny SL, Rice GPA, Panitch HS, Oldstone MBA (1984) A neurologic rating scale (NRS) for use in multiple sclerosis. Neurology 34:1368–1372
Syndulko K, Tourtellotte WW, Baumhefner RW et al. (1993) Neuroperformance evaluation of multiple sclerosis disease progression in a clinical trial: implications for neurological outcomes. J Neurol Rehabil 7:153–176
Tourtellotte WW, Haerer AF, Simpson JF, Kuzma JW, Sikorski J (1965) Quantitative clinical neurological testing: I. A study of a battery of tests designed to evaluate in part the neurologic function of patients with multiple sclerosis and its use in a therapeutic trial. Ann NY Acad Sci USA 122:480–505
Verdier-Taillefer MH, Zuber M, Lyon-Caen O et al. (1991) Observer disagreement in rating neurologic impairment in multiple sclerosis: Facts and consequences. Eur Neurol 31:117–119
Weinshenker BG (1995) The natural history of multiple sclerosis. Neurol Clin 13:119–146
Weinshenker BG, Gass B, Rice GPA et al. (1989) The natural history of multiple sclerosis: a geographically based study: 2. Predictive value of the early clinical course. Brain 112:1419–1428
Weinshenker BG, Rice GPA, Noseworthy JH et al. (1991) The natural history of multiple sclerosis: a geographically based study: 4. Applications to planning and interpretation of clinical therapeutic trials. Brain 114:1057–1067
Weinshenker BG, Issa M, Baskerville J (in press) Meta-analysis of the placebo-treated groups in clinical trials of progressive MS. Neurology
Wiebe S, Lee DH, Karlik SJ et al. (1992) Serial cranial and spinal cord magnetic resonance imaging in multiple sclerosis: clinical correlations and implications for classification of disease course. Ann Neurol 32:643–650
Willoughby EW, Paty DW (1988) Scales for rating impairment in multiple sclerosis: A critique. Neurology 38:1793–1798

6 Use of Neuropsychologic Outcome Measures in Multiple Sclerosis Clinical Trials: Current Status and Strategies for Improving Multiple Sclerosis Clinical Trial Design

Jill S. Fischer

Introduction

A number of significant advances in multiple sclerosis (MS) clinical research have occurred in the last decade. Within the past 3 years alone, positive outcomes have been reported in four clinical trials of therapeutic agents for relapsing–remitting MS (Durelli et al. 1994; IFNB Multiple Sclerosis Study Group 1993; Jacobs et al. 1996; Johnson et al. 1995) and two clinical trials in chronic progressive MS (Goodkin et al. 1995; Sipe et al. 1994). In addition, neuroimaging techniques have become increasingly refined, permitting the detection and quantitation of previously unrecognized cerebral lesions (see Chapter 8). Simultaneously, the widespread prevalence of MS-related cognitive impairment has been convincingly established (Fischer et al. 1994a; Rao 1990; Rao et al. 1991a).

In early 1994, the National Multiple Sclerosis Society, in conjunction with the National Institute of Neurological Disorders and Stroke and the International Federation of Multiple Sclerosis Societies, sponsored a workshop entitled "Outcomes assessment in multiple sclerosis clinical trials: a critical analysis". At this conference, the challenges of designing MS clinical trials were discussed, and the strengths and limitations of current clinical, imaging and laboratory-based measures were reviewed. In addition, the characteristics of an ideal MS clinical outcome measure were identified (Whitaker et al. 1995; see also Chapter 5). There was a strong consensus among conference participants that no existing clinical scale met these criteria; in addition, they agreed that current scales were inadequate in their assessment of cognitive function. A clinical outcome measure that assessed cognitive as well as physical impairment was strongly advocated, a rather remarkable development considering that the neuropsychologic manifestations of MS were barely mentioned at a similar workshop held in 1988 (Weiner and Paty 1989).

The purpose of this chapter is to:

1. Present the rationale for and potential limitations of including neuropsychologic measures in MS clinical trials;
2. Review recent experience using neuropsychologic measures to assess outcomes in both therapeutic and symptomatic trials;
3. Discuss conceptual and methodologic issues to consider when selecting and analyzing neuropsychologic measures in MS clinical trials.

The focus of this chapter will be primarily on the use of neuropsychologic measures as secondary outcome measures in Phase II and Phase III clinical trials in MS.

Advantages and Disadvantages of Using Neuropsychologic Measures in Multiple Sclerosis Clinical Trials

Rationale for Assessing Neuropsychologic Outcomes

There are several compelling reasons for using neuropsychologic measures to assess clinical outcomes in MS trials. First, cognitive impairment is clearly a common disease manifestation in MS: adjusted prevalence estimates derived from large-sample studies range from 43% for a community-based MS sample (Rao et al. 1991a) to 59% for a clinic-based sample (Heaton et al. 1985). Secondly, cognitive impairment is directly related to cerebral MS lesions: quantitated MS lesion burden on cranial magnetic resonance imaging (MRI) typically correlates more strongly with neuropsychologic test performance than it does with traditional clinical measures of neurologic function (Huber et al. 1992; Rao et al. 1989; Swirsky-Sacchetti et al. 1992). Furthermore, changes in neuropsychologic test performance over time reflect changes in underlying disease burden: neuropsychologic deterioration has been associated with significant increases in cerebral lesion burden over 1-year (Hohol et al. 1995) and 3-year intervals (S. M. Rao 1995, personal communication). Thirdly, MS-related cognitive impairment has important functional consequences: relative to cognitively intact patients of comparable physical disability, cognitively impaired MS patients are significantly less likely to be employed and to be involved in social activities, and are significantly more likely to need assistance with personal care and homemaking activities (Amato et al. 1995; Rao et al. 1989; Rao et al. 1991b).

Finally, contrary to the assumptions of many clinicians, the presence and degree of MS-related cognitive dysfunction is relatively independent of disease duration, disease course and physical disability (Fischer et al. 1994a). Neuropsychologic measures share only about 10%–15% variance with measures of physical disability, such as the Expanded Disability Status Scale (EDSS) (Kurtzke 1983), once the effects of confounding variables such as age and motor function are controlled (Beatty et al. 1990; Rao et al. 1991a; van den Burg et al. 1987). This tendency to overestimate the relationship between cognitive and physical impairment may in part explain why both neurologists' ratings (Fischer 1989; Peyser et al. 1980) and patients' perceptions of their cognitive function (Beatty and Monson 1991; Fischer 1989; Taylor 1990) often do not coincide with patients' objective neuropsychologic test performance.

Incorporating neuropsychologic assessment into MS clinical trials has a number of merits. Most importantly, objective neuropsychologic measures fulfill most of the criteria identified for an optimal MS clinical outcome measure (Table 6.1). Including neuropsychologic measures could also improve the design and conduct of a clinical trial. For example, neuropsychologic measures could be used to identify cognitively impaired patients who may be limited in their capacity to give informed consent or to follow a complicated treatment protocol. In such cases, a family member or other responsible individual could be enlisted to provide informed consent and assist with treatment compliance. If neuropsychologic status is expected to influence treatment response, patients could be stratified based on their neuropsychologic status at study entry, thereby increasing the sensitivity of the study design and reducing the likelihood of making a Type 2 error (i.e. failing to detect true treatment effects). In addition, neuropsychologic measures may be sensitive to subtle adverse effects that would otherwise be overlooked: this would be particularly important in Phase I trials of therapeutic agents such as interferon-alpha, which has been reported to have deleterious neuropsychologic effects in cancer patients (Meyers et al. 1991; Pavol et al. 1995; Poutianien et al. 1994).

Potential Drawbacks to Using Neuropsychologic Measures

Although neuropsychologic measures clearly have numerous advantages for MS clinical trials, they also have potential limitations that need to be considered. Some of these derive from our relatively primitive state of knowledge about MS-

Table 6.1. Comparison of features of neuropsychologic measures with criteria for optimal MS clinical outcome measure

Criterion for optimal MS outcome measure	Features of neuropsychologic measures
Sensitive	Recent studies suggest that neuropsychologic measures can detect change in MS patients over relatively brief periods, although information about the psychometric properties of many measures over time is limited.
Reliable	Neuropsychologic measures are administered and scored according to standardized procedures, producing objectively verifiable quantitative scores.
Valid	Neuropsychologic test performance is directly related to cerebral lesion burden on MRI, and cognitive impairment has a clear impact on a patient's daily functioning.
Multidimensional	Cognitive impairment does not correlate strongly with physical impairment in MS, making it a relatively independent dimension of the disease.
Widely applicable	Many neuropsychologic measures minimize sensory and motor demands, and, consequently, can be used with a broad range of MS patients.
Easy to administer	Many neuropsychologic measures are easy to administer; some are even automated.
Cost effective	Neuropsychologic measures can be administered by non-doctoral level personnel, given appropriate training and supervision.

related cognitive impairment. For example, although the pattern of MS-related cognitive impairment has been well established for MS patients as a group (e.g. Rao et al. 1991a), there is considerable heterogeneity across patients in terms of the nature and extent of cognitive impairment at any one point in time (Fischer 1988; Fischer and Rudick 1988; Fischer et al. 1992; Grossman et al. 1994; Rao et al. 1984). Furthermore, we know relatively little about the natural history of MS-related cognitive impairment or about the performance of specific neuropsychologic measures over time. Longitudinal studies of MS-related cognitive impairment have been few in number, and, due to methodologic limitations, most are of little assistance in selecting neuropsychologic outcome measures for MS clinical trials. An exception to this is the longitudinal study of Rao and his colleagues (Anderson et al. 1993; Bernardin et al. 1993), which is discussed later in this chapter.

Other potential limitations are not unique to the assessment of MS-related cognitive impairment, but rather, are endemic in the field of neuropsychology. For example, there is no universally accepted approach to neuropsychologic assessment, in MS or in any other patient population. Consequently, different investigators may prefer to use different measures of the same cognitive function. Fortunately, there is general agreement about the cognitive functions affected by MS and about the types of measures useful for assessing these (Peyser et al. 1990). Furthermore, as data about the psychometric properties of specific measures used in recent trials become available, consensus about the choice of specific measures is likely to emerge.

Restrictions in access to some neuropsychologic measures may pose an additional stumbling block. Many neuropsychologic tests are restricted to appropriately licensed professionals, usually psychologists, who have been trained in their administration, scoring and interpretation. Consequently, an appropriately trained professional needs to be involved in selecting measures and assuming responsibility for the use of restricted tests in the trial, or neuropsychologic measures that do not have these restrictions need to be used (e.g. measures developed in experimental, rather than clinical, contexts).

Some neuropsychologic measures may not lend themselves to use in clinical trials. Clearly, some tests that are useful in clinical settings or in studying specific neuropsychologic deficits may be too time-consuming or may require special equipment, limiting their applicability in most clinical trials. Other measures, such as those in which an element of novelty is critical, may not lend themselves to repeated administration. In addition, many neuropsychologic measures are susceptible to practice effects, regardless of the length of the intertest interval and despite the use of alternate forms (Anderson et al. 1993; Bever et al. 1995; Claus et al. 1991; Goldstein et al. 1991; McCaffrey et al. 1992). Practice effects do not preclude a measure from being sensitive to group differences in performance over time, however, as long as an appropriate control group is used (Bernardin et al. 1993).

Finally, the multidimensional nature of neuropsychologic assessment and the continuous nature of the scores generated by most neuropsychologic tests may be perceived as a limitation by many physicians, who are accustomed to thinking in terms of the presence or absence of pathology, rather than a continuum of performance. Although the absence of clear cut-offs for abnormal performance may complicate the interpretation of individual patient outcomes, the focus in controlled clinical trials is on performance of groups of patients, not individuals. In this context, continuous scores have definite advantages in terms of the variety of statistical approaches that can be taken. Integrating scores from multiple measures remains a challenge, both conceptually and statistically. Efforts are currently under way to use neuropsychologic data from recently completed trials to develop empirically based cut-offs for clinically significant change and to develop methods for aggregating performance across different measures.

In summary, MS-related cognitive impairment is an important clinical dimension of the disease by virtue of its prevalence and its functional significance. It is directly related to cerebral MS pathology, but relatively independent of physical impairment. Thus, the assessment of neuropsychologic outcomes complements the assessment of physical outcomes in MS clinical trials. Neuropsychologic measures fulfill most of the criteria identified for an optimal MS clinical outcome measure. Major drawbacks to their current use in assessing clinical trial outcomes are the heterogeneity inherent in neuropsychologic test performance (both cross-sectionally and longitudinally) and limitations in our knowledge about the evolution of MS-related cognitive impairment and the psychometric properties of specific measures over time. At this point in time, we cannot identify a single "best" measure for assessing neuropsychologic change in MS patients, and we cannot specify what constitutes clinically significant change. Analyses of neuropsychologic data from recently completed trials will soon provide an empirical basis for selecting measures to use in future MS clinical trials and specifying criteria for clinically significant change on these measures.

Natural History Studies Relevant to the Selection of Neuropsychologic Outcome Measures for Multiple Sclerosis Clinical Trials

Controlled natural history studies of MS-related cognitive dysfunction can provide invaluable information about the evolution of MS-related cognitive impairment, and also, potentially, about the psychometric properties of neuropsychologic measures. Unfortunately, only four controlled longitudinal studies have been carried out to date. Three of these used small clinic-based samples, and sampling restrictions limit their utility for planing clinical trials (Amato et al. 1995; Ivnik 1978; Jennekins-Schinkel et al. 1990). The community-based sample study by Rao and his colleagues (Bernardin et al. 1993) was larger, and consequently, may be a more valuable source of information about the development of MS-related cognitive impairment for investigators considering neuropsychologic outcome assessment in an MS clinical trial.

In this study, a comprehensive neuropsychologic battery was administered to a community sample of 100 MS patients and 100 healthy controls; the majority of these subjects (84 MS patients and 86 controls) were retested after a 3-year interval (Bernardin et al. 1993). The performance of the MS group deteriorated over this period relative to controls on nearly all of the measures administered, a difference that was statistically significant for approximately one-fourth of the measures administered ($P < 0.01$). This finding is particularly striking because practice effects were observed on nearly two-thirds of the measures administered (Anderson et al. 1993), including six of the seven measures on which statistically significant deterioration was observed. Statistically significant deterioration was not confined to a single cognitive domain, but rather, was evident on a range of neuropsychologic measures, including measures of verbal abilities and fluency, visuospatial abilities, calculation ability, information processing, recent memory and abstracting ability.

Not all patients deteriorated neuropsychologically over this 3-year period, however. Applying a stringent criterion for "significant" deterioration (<5th percentile of change scores for the control group), only about 20% of the MS patient group deteriorated significantly over this period (S. M. Rao 1995, personal communication). Thus, this study provides evidence of measurable deterioration in a range of cognitive functions in MS patients over a 3-year period, supporting the concept of assessing neuropsychologic change in MS trials. It also illustrates the heterogeneity of MS-related neuropsychologic change over time.

Multiple Sclerosis Clinical Trials Relevant to the Selection of Neuropsychologic Outcome Measures

As noted earlier, the prevalence and functional impact of MS-related cognitive dysfunction have only recently been appreciated. Consequently, it is not surprising that few MS clinical trials have incorporated neuropsychologic outcome measures. With the exception of the recently completed interferon-beta-1a (Jacobs et al. 1995) and copolymer 1 (Johnson et al. 1995) trials, neuropsychologic outcome measures have only been administered in small Phase II trials (Bever et al. 1994; Durelli et al. 1994; Fischer et al. 1994b; Smits et al. 1994) or at a subset of sites in larger multicenter trials (Multiple Sclerosis Study Group 1990; Pliskin et al. 1994). Furthermore, the neuropsychologic measures used in these trials have typically only covered a few cognitive domains. Despite these limitations, it is instructive to review the use of neuropsychologic measures in these clinical trials.

Therapeutic Trials Assessing Neuropsychologic Outcomes in Chronic–Progressive Multiple Sclerosis

The first controlled clinical trial known to have included neuropsychologic measures was the double-blind, placebo-controlled Phase III trial of cyclosporine. Cyclosporine (up to 10 mg/kg per day) significantly delayed time to becoming wheelchair bound for moderately disabled patients (EDSS = 3.0–7.0, inclusive) with chronic–progressive MS, but did not have a significant impact on two other primary outcome variables. Furthermore, substantial toxicity was observed (Multiple Sclerosis Study Group 1990). A comprehensive neuropsychologic battery was administered at a subset of the 12 sites in this study, but these neuropsychologic data were never extensively analyzed or presented (K. Syndulko 1995, personal communication). However, a measure of visual information processing, the Symbol-Digit Modalities Test (SDMT), was administered at all 12 sites as part of the Quantitative Examination of Neurologic Function (QENF) (Potvin and Tourtellotte 1985), and has been analyzed in conjunction with analyses of other QENF measures.

A total of 317 chronic–progressive MS patients (144 in the cyclosporine group and 173 in the placebo group) completed a single form of the SDMT at baseline and at 3-month intervals during the 2-year treatment phase (K. Syndulko, unpublished data). Significant practice effects were evident on the SDMT in both the cyclosporine and placebo groups ($P < 0.0001$), with performance improving almost 0.5 standard deviation (SD) due to repeated administration. The largest improvement in performance occurred between the first and second administrations, although stable performance was not achieved until the fifth administration (i.e. month 12). No significant differences in SDMT performance between the cyclosporine and placebo groups were observed as a function of treatment ($P = 0.73$ for the Treatment Group × Test Time interaction). Thus, this trial established that neuropsychologic measures can be administered study-wide in a multicenter trial, although no treatment effects were evident on this measure.

Neuropsychologic measures were also administered in a double-blind placebo-controlled Phase II trial of weekly low dose (7.5 mg) oral methotrexate (MTX). Like the cyclosporine trial, this trial involved moderately disabled patients (EDSS = 3.0–6.5, inclusive) with chronic–progressive MS (Goodkin et al. 1992; Goodkin et al. 1995; see also Chapter 12). MTX significantly delayed time to sustained progression of physical disability, as assessed by a composite outcome measure, in the 51 patients who completed the trial. A comprehensive neuropsychologic battery similar to the one proposed by Peyser and her colleagues (1990) was administered at baseline, after 1 year, and at the end of the 2-year treatment phase. Based on predetermined psychometric criteria for reliability and relative independence, five measures from the comprehensive battery were selected for the primary neuropsychologic outcome analysis. These included measures of confrontation naming (Boston Naming Test, 15-item version), visual construction (WAIS-R Block Design), auditory information processing (Paced Auditory Serial Addition Test, PASAT-2"), verbal recall (California Verbal Learning Test (CVLT), Long Delay Free Recall), and problem-solving flexibility (Wisconsin Card Sorting Test (WCST) Perseverative Responses). Details of the study design, other secondary outcome measures, and methods for selecting neuropsychologic measures for outcome analysis can be found in Chapter 12.

There were no statistically significant between-group differences in the baseline performance of the 40 patients (20 MTX, 20 placebo) who had complete data on these neuropsychologic outcome measures. The effect of MTX on neuropsychologic performance approached, but did not quite achieve, statistical significance ($P < 0.07$ for the treatment effect in a multivariate analysis of covariance of change scores, with age and education as covariates). With respect to performance on individual measures, the MTX group improved relative to the placebo group on all five measures, although, with the exception of the PASAT, the amount of change was generally modest (<0.33 SD for the MTX group, compared with a mean change of <0.15 SD for the placebo group). In contrast, the MTX group's performance improved nearly 1 SD on the PASAT, significantly more than that of the placebo group ($P = 0.002$), despite statistically significant practice effects ($P < 0.001$). Analysis of data from a subset of patients tested at 6-week intervals for the first 6 months of the trial indicated that the groups differed significantly in their PASAT performance after only 6 weeks of treatment, and that the treatment effect peaked in magnitude at 6 months to 1 year (see Chapter 12). Thus, this trial established that neuropsychologic measures can detect differential change between treatment conditions despite practice effects, and can do so at a very early point in the trial.

Therapeutic Trials Assessing Neuropsychologic Outcomes in Relapsing–Remitting Multiple Sclerosis

Four recently completed clinical trials with relapsing–remitting MS patients have also incorporated neuropsychologic outcome measures. One of these was the Phase II trial of high dose recombinant interferon alpha-2a (9×10^6 iu of rIFNα-2a), in which 20 patients (12 in the rIFNα-2a group and eight in the placebo group) with mild to moderate physical disability (EDSS = 0–6.0, inclusive) received intramuscular injections every other day for 6 months (Durelli et al. 1994; see also Chapter 11). Two memory measures (Wechsler Memory Scale (WMS) and Benton Visual Retention Test) and a measure of visual construction (Bender–Gestalt Test) were administered prior to treatment, at 3 months, and at the end of the 6-month treatment phase. Statistically significant treatment effects were observed on exacerbation rates, the presence of new or enlarging lesions on cerebral MRI, and cerebrospinal fluid CD4+ cell counts. The investigators reported that neuropsychologic test performance "did not show any change from baseline", but did not provide details of their statistical analyses. These results are encouraging, given the adverse neuropsychologic effects of high-dose IFN-α that have been observed in other patient populations (Meyers et al. 1991; Pavol et al. 1995; Poutianien et al. 1994). However, methodologic limitations of this study and the limited detail provided make it difficult to interpret the absence of treatment effects on neuropsychologic test performance.

Neuropsychologic measures were also administered to a subset of patients in the recent double-blind, placebo-controlled Phase III trial of beta-interferon (Betaseron®, IFN-β-1b) for mildly to moderately disabled patients (EDSS = 0–5.5, inclusive) with relapsing–remitting MS (IFNB Multiple Sclerosis Study Group 1993; see also Chapter 11). In the larger trial of 372 patients, the three treatment conditions (placebo, low dose IFN-β-1b (1.6×10^6 iu administered subcutaneously every other day), and high-dose IFN-β-1b (8×10^6 iu)) differed significantly on both primary outcome measures (exacerbation rate and proportion of exacerbation-free patients), as well as on secondary outcome measures such as unenhanced MRI activity (Paty et al. 1993). At the University of Chicago site, 30 patients (11 in the high dose IFNβ-1b group, ten in the low dose group, and nine in the placebo group) were administered a brief battery of neuropsychologic measures after 2 years on study, and again 25 months later (Pliskin et al. 1994). This battery included measures of visual information processing (Trails B, Stroop Test) and memory (WMS Logical Memory and Visual Reproduction subtests).

Statistically significant practice effects were evident on two neuropsychologic measures: the Stroop Test (Word Reading, $P < 0.03$) and WMS Visual Reproduction (Immediate Recall, $P < 0.001$). The performance of the three groups differed significantly over the study period on a measure of visual memory ($P < 0.03$ for the interaction between Treatment Condition and Test Time, in an analysis of variance of age corrected WMS Visual Reproduction Delayed Recall scores). This effect appeared to be dose related: the performance of the high dose IFNβ-1b group improved significantly over 2 years ($P < 0.003$), the low dose group's performance improved only modestly, and the placebo group's performance remained relatively stable. The performance of the high dose group also improved on a measure of information processing (Trails B), although the overall interaction effect did not achieve statistical significance. Unfortunately, a number of factors complicate the interpretation of these study results: the sample size was small, patients had already been on study for 2 years when they were first tested, and the groups differed in their initial performance levels on these measures. However, this study does suggest that neuropsychologic measures can detect differential change across treatment conditions in relapsing-remitting MS patients.

The results of neuropsychologic outcome analyses in two other Phase III trials are not yet available, but these trials deserve mention because neuropsychologic measures were implemented study-wide. One trial is the double-blind, placebo-controlled trial of copolymer 1 (Copaxone®, 20 mg, administered subcutaneously each day) in 251 mildly to moderately disabled patients (EDSS = 0–5.0, inclusive) with relapsing-remitting MS (Johnson et al. 1995; see also Chapter 13). Copolymer 1 significantly reduced the exacerbation rate (the primary endpoint) over the 2-year treatment phase, and also exerted statistically significant effects on several secondary outcome measures.

The Brief Repeatable Neuropsychological Battery (National MS Society Cognitive Functions Study Group 1990) was administered to all study participants at baseline and at 6-month intervals during the 2-year treatment phase; this battery consists of measures of verbal fluency (Word List Generation), information processing (PASAT and SDMT), and learning and memory (Buschke Selective Reminding Test (BSRT) and 10/36 Spatial Recall Test (10/36 SRT)). In addition, a more comprehensive battery of neuropsychologic measures was administered to patients at the University of Pennsylvania site, 19 of whom completed this battery at all five points in time (J. A. Cohen 1995, personal communication). Analysis of neuropsychologic data from this trial will not only elucidate the neuropsychologic effects of copolymer 1, but will also provide crucial information about the psychometric properties of the

Brief Repeatable Neuropsychological Battery in a large group of patients over time.

The recent double-blind placebo-controlled trial of interferon-beta-1a (Avonex®, 6×10^6 iu administered intramuscularly once a week) in 301 mildly-disabled patients (EDSS = 1–3.5) with relapsing-remitting MS also incorporated neuropsychologic tests as secondary outcome measures (Jacobs et al. 1994, 1996; see also Chapter 11). An extensive battery of clinical and experimental neuropsychologic measures was administered at baseline and at the end of the 2-year treatment phase to the first 276 patients enrolled in the study. In addition, a subset of this battery was administered at 6-month intervals during and after the treatment phase. A comprehensive battery was adopted in this trial for three reasons: to assess the neuropsychologic effects of IFN-β-1a on a broad range of cognitive functions; to identify the optimal set of neuropsychologic outcome measures through the application of statistical procedures that require large samples; and to develop empirically based methods for determining clinically-significant change on these measures. IFN-β-1a had a significant effect on the primary outcome variable, time to sustained progression of physical disability as assessed by the EDSS, as well as on several related secondary outcome variables, including exacerbation rate and the number and volume of enhancing lesions on MRI. Analysis of neuropsychologic data from this trial is currently under way.

Clinical Trials of Symptomatic Treatments Using Neuropsychologic Measures as Primary Outcome Measures

Neuropsychologic measures have served as primary outcome measures in several small-scale studies of treatments hypothesized to produce transient improvements in cognitive function in MS. These studies differ from trials of disease-modifying agents in that they use a within-subjects (i.e. crossover) design, which requires fewer subjects to achieve the same statistical power. In the first published study of a treatment for MS-related cognitive dysfunction (Leo and Rao 1988), four patients with definite MS, moderate physical disability (EDSS = 3.0–6.0, inclusive), and objectively established verbal memory impairment were enrolled in a 6-week double-blind, placebo-controlled cross-over study of intravenous physostigmine 1 mg. Despite the small sample size, the physostigmine significantly improved verbal memory, as assessed by the BSRT ($P < 0.05$ on paired t-tests of several BSRT variables), but not attention span (Digit Span). Examination of the performance of individual patients revealed that three of the four patients showed clear evidence of treatment effects.

The same investigator group also conducted an 8-week double-blind, placebo-controlled cross-over study of oral physostigmine (3 mg every 2 hours, for a total daily dose of 18 mg), using similar patients and an expanded set of outcome measures (Unverzagt et al. 1991). Consistent with the results of the intravenous physostigmine study, oral physostigmine significantly improved BSRT performance ($P < 0.05$ on a paired t-test of BSRT Consistent Long-Term Retrieval scores). However, it had an unanticipated adverse effect on information processing efficiency, as assessed by the PASAT-3" ($P < 0.05$, paired t-test). No statistically significant treatment effects were evident on other measures of memory (prose recall, 7/24 Spatial Recall Test, Serial Digit Learning) or information processing (complex reaction time, Sternberg Task, PASAT-2"). As in the prior study, only a subset of the eight patients who completed the study showed unequivocal treatment effects. Taken together, these studies provide evidence of the sensitivity of neuropsychologic measures to treatment effects in trials of short-acting symptomatic medications. They also illustrate the heterogeneity of treatment responses across patients, and the potential risks of misinterpreting treatment effects if only one measure of a specific cognitive function is administered.

Neuropsychologic measures also served as the primary outcome measure in a recent trial of 4-aminopyridine (4-AP), up to 10 mg four times a day. Based on subjective improvements in attention and memory reported by participants in a previous 4-AP trial (Polman et al. 1994), Smits and his colleagues (1994) enrolled 20 MS patients with a wide range of physical disability (EDSS = 2.5–8.0, inclusive) in a 4-week double-blind, placebo-controlled cross-over trial. A variant of the Brief Repeatable Neuropsychological Battery (substituting a Dutch verbal memory test for the BSRT) was administered twice prior to the treatment phase (2 weeks apart), at the cross-over (2 weeks later), and at the end of the 4-week treatment phase. There were trends for improved visual memory ($P < 0.06$, paired t-test of 10/36 SRT Delayed Recall) and information processing ($P < 0.09$, paired t-test of PASAT-2") with 4-AP, although these effects did not achieve statistical significance. Despite a number of methodologic factors that attenuated statistical power (e.g. small sample size, unanticipated baseline differences between groups, unanticipated carryover effects, heterogeneity of treatment response, and insensitive statistical analyses), the results of this study suggest that selected measures of information processing and visual memory can detect treatment effects.

Finally, in a similar trial, the Brief Repeatable Neuropsychological Battery was administered at baseline and every 4 weeks to 19 temperature-sensitive MS patients with a range of physical disability (EDSS = 3.0–8.0) participating in a 16-week trial of 3,4-diaminopyridine (DAP) 100 mg/day (Bever et al. 1994; Bever et al. in press). DAP produced significant improvements in both subjectively and objectively assessed physical disability ($P = 0.006$ and $P < 0.001$, respectively). The investigators reported that there were no statistically-significant treatment effects on the neuropsychologic outcome measures, but did not provide additional details of the statistical analyses. Rather, they emphasized the role that methodologic factors, such as the small sample size and the variability in neuropsychologic test performance observed both within and across patients, may have played in limiting their ability to detect any treatment effects.

To summarize, neuropsychologic outcome measures have detected treatment effects in several recent clinical trials of therapeutic and symptomatic medications for MS. Furthermore, there is suggestive evidence that they may be able to do so very early in a trial. Not all measures are equally sensitive; measures of information processing, and to a lesser extent visual memory, have shown the most promise. Clearly, the heterogeneity observed in neuropsychologic test performance both within and across patients, and the heterogeneity of treatment responses, make the detection of treatment effects challenging. Given methodologic variations across studies and inconsistencies in the results of some trials, it is premature at this time to recommend a specific neuropsychologic measure or set of measures for use in all MS trials. Data from the two recent multicenter trials discussed can be used to identify neuropsychologic measures with optimal psychometric properties for assessing MS trial outcomes, and to develop novel statistical approaches that address the heterogeneity inherent in neuropsychologic data.

Issues to Consider in Incorporating Neuropsychologic Measures into Multiple Sclerosis Clinical Trials

Some clinical investigators will decry the primitive state of knowledge about MS-related cognitive dysfunction, concluding that it is premature to assess neuropsychologic outcomes in MS clinical trials. More intrepid investigators may have been convinced that the advantages of assessing neuropsychologic outcomes in MS trials outweigh their limitations; the final section of this chapter is written for the latter group. This section covers a number of design and statistical considerations for investigators wishing to use neuropsychologic measures as secondary outcome measures in a randomized controlled clinical trial.

Defining the Question of Interest

What are the anticipated neuropsychologic effects of the experimental medication? Is it expected to slow the progression or development of MS-related cognitive impairment, to stabilize cognitive function at pretreatment levels, or to reverse cognitive impairment? At the present time, most experimental disease modifying agents are hypothesized to slow disease progression or dampen disease activity in some way, whereas symptomatic treatments are expected to improve a given symptom (e.g. a specific cognitive function). Ultimately, as disease modifying agents become more effective, it may be possible to arrest or even reverse MS-related cognitive impairment. The nature and direction of hypothesized treatment effects will have implications for both the choice of neuropsychologic outcome measures and the planning of statistical analyses.

Determining Which Patients to Assess

Should all patients entering a trial be monitored neuropsychologically, or only a subset of patients? Clearly, it is preferable to design the neuropsychologic outcome measures so that they can be administered along with other secondary outcome measures to all patients participating in a therapeutic trial. However, if it is impractical for some reason to administer the neuropsychologic measures to all patients in the trial, how should the investigator decide which patients to monitor during the trial?

One approach would be to monitor those patients who showed evidence of cognitive impairment on a set of neuropsychologic measures administered at baseline. While intuitively appealing, this approach has several drawbacks: it presumes that there are no adverse or beneficial neuropsychologic effects in patients who are cognitively intact at study entry; it requires normative data from a large group of age-, gender-, and education-matched healthy controls in order to establish appropriate criteria for cognitive impairment; and selecting patients based on their extreme neuropsychologic test scores runs the risk of capitalizing on statistical artifacts, such as regression to the mean (Hermann et al. 1991). Trials in which the experimental and control groups are not well matched neuropsychologically at the outset are particularly vulnerable to statistical biases such as these.

Consequently, if there are practical constraints on the number of clinical trial participants who can be monitored neuropsychologically, it is preferable to select these patients randomly or by site, rather than based on their initial cognitive status. Initial cognitive status could be used as a blocking factor to assign patients to treatments, however, in order to equate experimental and control groups neuropsychologically at study entry. As neuropsychologic measures gain broader acceptance, they may even be used to determine if patients meet "neuropsychologic inclusion criteria", much as the EDSS and exacerbation rates are used to identify patients meeting specific criteria for physical impairment and disease activity.

Selecting Appropriate Controls

It is important to distinguish between the type of control group needed to determine the presence and extent of cognitive impairment (i.e. neuropsychologic data from healthy controls), and the appropriate control group for MS therapeutic trials. In MS trials, one is asking the question, "How do neuropsychologic outcomes for MS patients who received the experimental treatment differ from those of MS patients who did not receive this treatment?" Consequently, the appropriate control group is not healthy controls, but rather, patients who are similar to those in the treatment group(s) at the study outset, but who receive placebo or "standard treatment". To evaluate neuropsychologic outcomes, patients in the experimental and control groups should be comparable both in terms of demographics (such as age, gender and education) and with respect to disease-related variables (including physical impairment and initial neuropsychologic status).

Selecting Neuropsychologic Outcome Measures: Single Versus Multiple Measures

Can a single measure be used to monitor neuropsychologic change in MS clinical trials, or are multiple measures necessary? The use of a single measure is certainly desirable from a statistical standpoint. However, as noted earlier, MS-related cognitive impairment is quite heterogeneous. For a single neuropsychologic outcome measure to be valid, it would need not only to be a measure of a cognitive function likely to change during the 2 or 3 years of a clinical trial, but also be predictive of concurrent or subsequent changes in other cognitive domains. No such measure has emerged from the clinical trials analyzed to date. Consequently, until additional information is available about the sequence of MS-related neuropsychologic changes and the psychometric properties of various neuropsychologic measures over time, it is advisable to include more than one neuropsychologic outcome measure.

The selection of a battery of neuropsychologic outcome measures can be grouped into focused and global approaches. In the focused approach, domain-specific measures from only one or two cognitive domains are chosen. This approach to neuropsychologic outcome selection has been used in MS trials, such as the recent copolymer 1 trial (Johnson et al. 1995), and in clinical trials in other diseases, such as the AZT trials for AIDS (Schmitt et al. 1988) and AIDS dementia complex (Sidtis et al. 1993). This approach is optimal if one expects an experimental treatment to affect only one specific cognitive domain, as in studies of symptomatic treatments for MS-related deficits in memory or information processing. It will also be the preferred approach in therapeutic trials if we learn that changes in one particular cognitive domain reliably predict either concurrent or subsequent changes in other domains in MS.

The global approach consists of domain-specific and multiply determined approaches. In the domain-specific approach, at least one measure of each major independent cognitive domain is selected. This was the approach taken in the methotrexate (Fischer et al. 1994b; Goodkin et al. 1992; see also Chapter 12) and interferon-β-1a (Jacobs et al. 1995; see also Chapter 11) trials in MS; it is also the approach adopted in the deprenyl and tocopherol (DATATOP) trial in Parkinson's disease (Kieburtz et al. 1994) and the Diabetes Complications and Control Trial (DCCT; Ryan et al. 1991). This approach to outcome measure selection is conceptually appealing, in that it allows one to determine if a therapeutic agent has a selective effect on a specific cognitive function or a global effect on several different functions. However, it can be time consuming. Furthermore, if the neuropsychologic effects of a therapeutic agent are subtle, or specific to only one or two cognitive domains, one runs the risk of making a Type 2 statistical error.

An alternative global approach is to select measures that each tap several different cognitive functions (i.e. are multiply determined), in the hope of producing a more parsimonious set of measures than the domain-specific approach. This approach was implicitly adopted in constructing the EDSS, in which the integrity of a number of partially overlapping functional systems is assessed. This method is relatively untested in the selection of neuropsychologic outcome measures for MS trials, although multiply determined measures of cognitive function, such as the Alzheimer's Disease Assessment Scale–Cognitive subscale and the Mini-Mental State Examination have been used to assess outcomes in clinical trials of tacrine in Alzheimer's disease (Davis et al. 1992). Unfortunately, this approach runs the risk of failing to detect change if MS-related neuropsychologic change is asynchronous across cognitive domains, or if an experimental treatment has dissimilar effects on different cognitive functions. Thus, until we know more about the sequence and synchrony of MS-related cognitive changes, the domain-specific approach is preferable.

Selecting Neuropsychologic Outcome Measures: Factors to Consider in Choosing Specific Measures

There are several additional factors to consider in selecting neuropsychologic outcome measures for use in MS clinical trials, many of which have been addressed by others and are only briefly mentioned here. For example, factors to consider in choosing neuropsychologic measures for cross-sectional studies of MS patients have been reviewed by Peyser and her colleagues (1990). Selecting neuropsychologic outcome measures for clinical trials with other patient populations has been discussed by Albert (1991) and by Ruff and Crouch (1991). Finally, Lezak (1995) is a rich source of information about specific neuropsychologic tests.

Clearly, there are a number of practical factors to consider in selecting specific neuropsychologic outcome measures for use in MS clinical trials. For example, efforts should be made to use measures that minimize sensory and motor demands unrelated to the function being assessed, so that these can be administered to all patients in a trial, even those who deteriorate over time. Similarly, one should select measures with minimal emotional demands, except when there is no other way to assess a particular cognitive function. Finally, measures that require minimal equipment and technical expertise are generally preferable, because they are likely not only to be more cost effective but also to yield more reliable data.

Psychometric factors must also be taken into account. Neuropsychologic outcome measures should be equally sensitive to positive and negative change, so that both beneficial and adverse effects can be assessed. Such measures should also produce a good range of scores and not be subject to "floor" and "ceiling" effects. If possible, efforts should be made to select neuropsychologic measures that yield scores that are normally distributed and lie on an interval scale of measurement.

While these practical and psychometric factors may seem obvious, two other considerations may not be so obvious to investigators accustomed to cross-sectional studies. The first of these pertains to the distinction between a measure's ability to discriminate between different groups and its ability to evaluate change over time (Guyatt et al. 1987). When neuropsychologic outcome measures have been included in MS clinical trials, these have typically been measures known to discriminate between MS patients and healthy controls, or between groups of MS patients (e.g. cognitively impaired and cognitively intact MS patients). Unfortunately, a measure's ability to detect differences between groups (its *discriminative* properties) may bear little relationship to its sensitivity to change over time (its *evaluative* properties). Furthermore, while the reliability of a measure (i.e. the reproducibility of scores on two different occasions) is important, it is no guarantee that a measure will be a good evaluative instrument. Guyatt and his colleagues have proposed a formula for conceptualizing a measure's "responsiveness", or sensitivity to change, which may be useful to apply to neuropsychologic measures being considered for use in MS clinical trials.

Secondly, much has been made of the dangers of practice effects on repeated neuropsychologic testing. This concern has been heightened by recent reports that many neuropsychologic measures are susceptible to practice effects, regardless of whether the intertest interval is brief (Claus et al. 1991; McCaffrey et al. 1992) or long (Anderson et al. 1993), or whether alternate forms were used (Goldstein et al. 1991; Anderson et al. 1993; Bever et al. 1995). Furthermore, the magnitude of practice effects may differ for different groups (e.g. patient groups versus controls) and even for different patients within a group (McCaffrey et al. 1992). However, recent work by Rao and his colleagues (Anderson et al. 1993; Bernardin et al. 1993) and results of recent MS clinical trials (e.g. Fischer et al. 1994b; see also Chapter 12) suggest that even measures susceptible to practice effects can detect differential change between groups over time. This work is encouraging, and highlights the importance of using an appropriate control group so that the significance of neuropsychologic changes in patients receiving experimental treatment(s) can be assessed.

Determining When to Administer Neuropsychologic Outcome Measures

The frequency with which neuropsychologic outcome measures are administered during a trial will depend in part on theoretical factors (such as the hypothesized action of an agent and anticipated time course of treatment effects) and in part on practical considerations (such as the length of the neuropsychologic battery and the budget available for assessment of secondary outcomes). Due to the weak correlation between physical and cognitive impairment in MS, equating groups on physical status at the outset of the trial does not guarantee that they will be comparable neuropsychologically. Consequently, neuropsychologic outcome measures must be administered prior to, as well as at the end of, the treatment phase, in order to establish the neuropsychologic equivalence of the groups at the outset of the trial and to evaluate treatment effects.

As noted earlier, there is often a great deal of variability in neuropsychologic test performance over time. Furthermore, neuropsychologic change in MS is typically a continous, rather than a discrete, process. In the light of this, it may be optimal to administer neuropsychologic outcome measures two or three times prior to the treatment phase and periodically throughout the trial. Administering neuropsychologic outcome measures at least twice prior to initiation of treatment enables the investigator to: estimate the measure's practice effects over brief periods (during which deterioration in the underlying condition would be unlikely); and establish a stable baseline prior to the treatment phase, thereby reducing error variance on subsequent testing and increasing the measure's sensitivity to treatment effects. Administering neuropsychologic outcome measures several times during the treatment phase permits the application of potentially more sensitive statistical techniques to separate practice effects and natural fluctuations in test performance from changes in the underlying cognitive function.

Obviously, it is neither practical nor advisable to administer a lengthy neuropsychologic battery repeatedly during a clinical trial. However, a comprehensive set of neuropsychologic measures could be administered at the outset of the trial and the end of the treatment phase, and a briefer subset of these measures could be administered repeatedly during the treatment phase. Selecting the optimal interval at which to administer this briefer battery is clearly a matter of judgment. Administering even a small set of neuropsychologic outcome measures every 6 weeks as was done in the MTX trial (Goodkin et al. 1992; see also Chapter 12) seems excessive, yet administering measures every 6 months as was done in the copolymer 1 and IFN-β-1a trials (Jacobs et al. 1995; Johnson et al. 1995; see also Chapters 11 and 13) may be too infrequent. Consequently, administering a subset of neuropsychologic outcome measures every 3 months, which is the interval at which neurologic examinations are performed in many trials, seems to be a reasonable compromise.

Planning Statistical Analyses of Neuropsychologic Outcomes

A detailed discussion of statistical issues and potential statistical approaches is well beyond the scope of this chapter; the reader is referred to Chapter 4 for this. There are two points regarding the selection of statistical procedures that deserve mention here, however.

One concerns the choice of statistical procedures when multiple neuropsychologic outcome measures are used. Performing multiple univariate statistical tests without adjusting the alpha level dramatically increases the probability of making Type 1 errors (i.e. concluding that the treatment has a significant effect when it does not). However, conventional procedures for adjusting the alpha level for the number of statistical tests performed (such as the Bonferroni procedure) are overly conservative. Consequently, they may inadvertently increase the probability of making a Type 2 error (i.e. falsely concluding that the treatment had no effect). Consequently, multivariate statistical procedures are generally preferable if their assumptions are met. In the future, it may be fruitful to develop novel techniques for simultaneously aggregating and analyzing changes in multiple outcome measures (e.g. profiling methods).

The other point concerns the impact that the primary question of interest has on the choice of statistical procedures. If all patients are followed for a fixed length of time, the investigator may be primarily interested in comparing the experimental and control groups in terms of mean change in performance over that period. In fact, the analysis of group differences in mean change using analysis of variance-based procedures has been the sole approach to the analysis of neuropsychologic outcome data in MS trials to date. While this approach to statistical analysis is necessary when there are relatively few subjects or only two observations on each subject, it can obscure important differences in the performance of subgroups of patients. Consequently, even in a small trial with few observations, it may be useful to use cluster analysis to identify subgroups of patients with different patterns of cognitive impairment at the trial outset in order to determine if they differ in terms of their neuropsychologic outcomes.

In addition, there are a number of other statistical approaches that can be used in trials with large samples and/or multiple observations on each subject. For example, techniques such as the "reliable change index" (Chelune et al. 1993; Jacobson and Truax 1991) could be applied to data from large trials such as the copolymer 1 (Johnson et al. 1995) or the interferon-beta-1a (Jacobs et al. 1996) trials to determine what constitutes "clinically significant change" on selected measures. Then, trials could be designed to determine if treatment groups differ in the length of time it takes to achieve that change, through the use of techniques such as survival analysis. Alternatively, investigators interested in the rate and pattern of change may want to include repeated assessment of neuropsychologic outcomes in order to take advantage of techniques such as slope analysis, which has been applied recently in HIV (Selnes et al. 1995; Stern et al. 1995a), or growth curve analysis, which has been applied in pediatric closed head injury (Francis et al. 1991), pediatric HIV (Fletcher at al. 1991) and Alzheimer's disease (Stern et al. 1995b).

Special Issues in Using Neuropsychologic Measures in Multicenter Clinical Trials

The use of neuropsychologic measures in multicenter trials brings with it several issues that may be unfamiliar to the investigator accustomed to single-center studies (Gracon et al. 1991). First, it is important that training should be centralized, and that there is ongoing supervision of study personnel administering neuropsychologic outcome measures in order to standardize administration and scoring of neuropsychologic measures, and keep measurement error to a minimum. This is best accomplished by involvement of a neuropsychologist coinvestigator, who can oversee the selection of neuropsychologic outcome measures prior to the trial, provide training in administration and scoring of the measures, and be responsible for quality control of the neuropsychologic data. If more than a few neuropsychologic measures are to be administered, it is preferable to have consulting neuropsychologists available at each site who can hire and supervise appropriate study personnel. Regardless of how many neuropsychologists are involved, administration and scoring of neuropsychologic outcome measures should always be reviewed at a central site. This neuropsychology co-ordinating center should be responsible for transcription of neuropsychologic data onto case report forms and providing timely feedback to sites about the accuracy of test administration and scoring.

Finally, the investigators should determine in advance of the trial whether, how and when neuropsychologic findings will be reported back to the patients enrolled in the study, and this should be spelled out on the consent form. Although the primary purpose of a clinical trial is to examine the performance of groups of patients, participants are often curious about their cognitive status after undergoing neuropsychologic testing. If normative data on the neuropsychologic outcome measures are available, neuropsychologic test results could be handled in the same manner as other laboratory data, with the treating physician being responsible for reporting abnormalities and making recommendations for further assessment to the study participant. In addition, once criteria for "clinically significant deterioration" are developed from analysis of existing data sets, study participants whose neuropsychologic performance deteriorated more than this amount could be referred to a clinical neuropsychologist for further assessment.

Conclusion

We have recently entered an exciting era in MS clinical trials, with a flurry of recent reports of positive trial outcomes. Despite this, we must not lose sight of the fact that our treatments and the measures that we use to gauge their effects are still imperfect. Clearly, any effective MS treatment will need to have an impact on cognitive as well as physical function, both of which are important to the patient. Neuropsychologic outcome measures offer a window through which to view previously invisible MS symptoms. Not only do they have many of the characteristics of an optimal MS outcome measure, but they have also demonstrated sensitivity to treatment effects in several recent trials. We are on the brink of being able to specify a parsimonious set of neuropsychologic tests to use as secondary outcome measures, based on data from recently completed multicenter trials. Ultimately, however, we must strive to develop not only more effective treatments for MS but also truly comprehensive outcome assessment methods that integrate assessment of physical and cognitive functions into a primary outcome measure.

Acknowledgements

I would like to thank Jeff Cohen, Lynn Grattan, Neil Pliskin, Steve Rao and Karl Syndulko for providing preprints and additional information about studies they have conducted. I am also grateful to Diane Cookfair and Roger Priore for helpful discussions about the statistical intricacies of analyzing neuropsychologic outcome data from MS clinical trials.

References

Albert MS (1991) Criteria for the choice of neuropsychological tests in clinical trials. In: Mohr E, Brouwers P (eds) Handbook of clinical trials: the neurobehavioral approach. Swets & Zeitlinger, Amsterdam, pp 131–139

Amato MP, Ponziani G, Pracucci G, Bracco L, Siracusa G, Amaducci L (1995) Cognitive impairment

in early-onset multiple sclerosis: pattern, predictors, and impact on everyday life in a 4-year follow-up. Arch Neurol 52:168–172
Anderson BL, Rao SM, Bernardin L, Luchetta T (1993) Long-term practice effects in neuropsychological testing. J Clin Exp Neuropsychol 15:61
Beatty W, Monson N (1991) Metamemory in multiple sclerosis. J Clin Exp Neuropsychol 13:309–327
Beatty W, Goodkin DE, Hertsgaard D, Monson N (1990) Clinical and demographic predictors of cognitive performance in multiple sclerosis: do diagnostic type, disease duration, and disability matter? Arch Neurol 47:305–308
Bernardin L, Rao SM, Luchetta TL et al. (1993) A prospective, long-term, longitudinal study of cognitive dysfunction in multiple sclerosis. J Clin Exp Neuropsychol 15:17
Bever CT, Panitch HS, Anderson PA et al. (1994) The efficacy and toxicity of oral 3,4-diaminopyridine in multiple sclerosis patients. Neurology 44 (Suppl 2):A374
Bever CT, Grattan L, Panitch HS, Johnson KP (1995) The brief repeatable battery of neuropsychological tests for multiple sclerosis: a preliminary serial study. Multiple Sclerosis 1:165–169
Chelune GJ, Naugle RI, Lüders H, Sedlak J, Awad IA (1993) Individual change after epilepsy surgery: practice effects and base-rate information. Neuropsychology 7:41–52
Claus JJ, Mohr E, Chase TN (1991) Clinical trials in dementia: learning effects with repeated testing. J Psychiatry Neurosci 16:2–5
Davis KL, Thal LJ, Gamzu ER et al. (1992) A double-blind, placebo-controlled multicenter study of tacrine for Alzheimer's disease. N Engl J Med 327:1253–1259
Durelli L, Bongioanni MR, Cavallo R et al. (1994) Chronic systemic high-dose recombinant interferon alfa-2a reduces exacerbation rate, MRI signs of disease activity, and lymphocyte interferon gamma production in relapsing-remitting multiple sclerosis. Neurology 44:406–413
Fischer JS (1988) Using the Wechsler Memory Scale-Revised to detect and characterize memory deficits in multiple sclerosis. Clin Neuropsychol 2:149–172
Fischer JS (1989) Objective memory testing in multiple sclerosis. In: Jensen K, Knudsen L, Stenager E, Grant I (eds) Mental disorders, cognitive deficits, and their treatment in multiple sclerosis. Libbey, London, pp 39–49 (Current problems in neurology, vol 10)
Fischer JS, Rudick RA (1988) Patterns of cognitive impairment in multiple sclerosis. Neurology 38(Suppl 1):A220
Fischer JS, Kawczak K, Daughtry MM, Schwetz KM, Rudick RA, Goodkin DE (1992) Unmasking subtypes of verbal memory impairment in multiple sclerosis. J Clin Exp Neuropsychol 14:32
Fischer JS, Foley FW, Aikens JE, Ericson GD, Rao SM, Shindell S (1994a) What do we *really* know about cognitive dysfunction, affective disorders, and stress in multiple sclerosis? A practitioner's guide. J Neurol Rehabil 8:151–164
Fischer JS, Goodkin DE, Rudick RA et al. (1994b) Low-dose (7.5 mg) oral methotrexate improves neuropsychological function in patients with chronic progressive multiple sclerosis. Ann Neurol 36:289
Fletcher JM, Francis DJ, Pequegnat W et al. (1991) Neurobehavioral outcomes in diseases of childhood: individual change models for pediatric human immunodeficiency viruses. Am Psychol 46:1267–1277
Francis DJ, Fletcher JM, Stuebing KK, Davidson KC, Thompson NM (1991) Analysis of change: modeling individual growth. J Consult Clin Psychol 59:27–37
Goldstein G and the DVA Cooperative Study Group on Anti-Hypertensive Agents (1991) Practice effect phenomena in a national hypertension study. Clin Neuropsychol 5:263
Goodkin DE, Rudick RA, VanderBrug Medendorp S et al. (1992) Low-dose (7.5 mg) oral methotrexate for chronic progressive multiple sclerosis: design of a randomized, placebo-controlled trial with sample size benefits from a composite outcome variable, including preliminary data on toxicity. Online J Curr Clin Trials Sep 25 (Doc No 19)
Goodkin DE, Rudick RA, VanderBrug Medendorp S et al. (1995) Low-dose (7.5 mg) oral methotrexate reduces the rate of progression in chronic progressive multiple sclerosis. Ann Neurol 37:30–40
Gracon SI, Gamzu ER, Mancini ADJ (1991) Multicenter clinical trials: design considerations, standardization and implication. In: Mohr E, Brouwers P (eds) Handbook of clinical trials: the neurobehavioral approach. Swets & Zeitlinger, Amsterdam, pp 275–291
Grossman M, Armstrong C, Onishi K et al. (1994) Patterns of cognitive impairment in relapsing-remitting and chronic progressive multiple sclerosis. Neuropsychiatry Neuropsychol Behav Neurol 7:194–210
Guyatt G, Walter S, Norman G (1987) Measuring change over time: assessing the usefulness of evaluative instruments. J Chron Dis 40:171–178
Heaton RK, Nelson LM, Thompson DS, Burks JS, Franklin GM (1985) Neuropsychological findings

in relapsing-remitting and chronic-progressive multiple sclerosis. J Consult Clin Psychol 53:103–110

Hermann BP, Wyler AR, VanderZwagg R et al. (1991) Predictors of neuropsychological change following anterior temporal lobectomy: role of regression toward the mean. J Epilepsy 4:139–148

Hohol MJ, Guttmann CRG, Orav EJ et al. (1995) Serial study of neuropsychological assessment and MRI analysis in multiple sclerosis. Neurology 45(Suppl 4):A233

Huber SJ, Bornstein RA, Rammohan KW, Christy JA, Chakeres DW, McGhee RB (1992) Magnetic resonance imaging correlates of neuropsychological impairment in multiple sclerosis. J Neuropsychiatry Clin Neurosci 4:152–158

IFNB Multiple Sclerosis Study Group (1993) Interferon beta-1b is effective in relapsing-remitting multiple sclerosis: I. Clinical results of a multicenter, randomized, double-blind, placebo-controlled trial. Neurology 43:655–661

Ivnik RJ (1978) Neuropsychological stability in multiple sclerosis. J Consult Clin Psychol 46:913–923

Jacobs LD, Cookfair DL, Rudick RA et al. (1995) A phase III trial of intramuscular recombinant interferon beta for exacerbating-remitting multiple sclerosis: design and conduct of study; baseline characteristics of patients. Multiple Sclerosis 1:118–135

Jacobs L, Cookfair D, Rudick R et al. (1996) Intramuscular interferon beta-1a for disease progression in relapsing multiple sclerosis. Ann Neurol 39:285–294

Jacobson JS, Truax P (1991) Clinical significance: a statistical approach to defining meaningful change in psychotherapy research. J Consult Clin Psychol 59:12–19

Jennekins-Schinkel A, Laboyrie PM, Lanser JBK, van der Velde EA (1990) Cognition in patients with multiple sclerosis: after four years. J Neurol Sci 99:229–247

Johnson KP, Brooks BR, Cohen JA et al. (1995) Copolymer 1 reduces relapse rate and improves disability in relapsing-remitting multiple sclerosis: results of a Phase III multicenter, double-blind, placebo-controlled trial. Neurology 45:1268–1276

Kieburtz K, McDermott M, Como P et al. (1994) The effect of deprenyl and tocopherol on cognitive performance in early untreated Parkinson's disease. Neurology 44:1756–1759

Kurtzke JF (1983) Rating neurological impairment in multiple sclerosis: an Expanded Disability Status Scale (EDSS). Neurology 33:1444–145[illegible]

Leo GJ, Rao SM (1988) Effects of intravenous physostigmine and lecithin on memory loss in multiple sclerosis: report of a pilot study. J Neurol Rehabil 2:123–129

Lezak MD (1995) Neuropsychological assessment, 3rd edn. Oxford University Press, New York

McCaffrey RJ, Ortega A, Orsillo SM, Nelles WB, Haase RF (1992) Practice effects in repeated neuropsychological assessments. Clin Neuropsychol 6:32–42

Meyers CA, Scheibel RS, Forman AD (1991) Persistent neurotoxicity of systemically administered interferon-alpha. Neurology 41:672–676

Multiple Sclerosis Study Group (1990) Efficacy and toxicity of cyclosporine in chronic progressive multiple sclerosis: a randomized, double-blinded, placebo-controlled clinical trial. Ann Neurol 27:591–605

National MS Society Cognitive Functions Study Group (1990) A manual for the Brief, Repeatable Battery of neuropsychological tests in multiple sclerosis. National MS Society, New York

Paty DW, Li DKB, UBC MS/MRI Study Group, IFNB Multiple Sclerosis Study Group (1993) Interferon beta-1b is effective in relapsing-remitting multiple sclerosis: II. MRI analysis results of a multicenter, randomized, double-blind, placebo-controlled trial. Neurology 43:662–667

Pavol MA, Meyers CA, Rexer JL, Valentine AD, Mattis PJ, Talpaz M (1995) Pattern of neurobehavioral deficits associated with interferon alfa therapy for leukemia. Neurology 45:947–950

Peyser JM, Edwards KR, Poser CM, Filskov SB (1980) Cognitive function in patients with multiple sclerosis. Arch Neurol 37:577–579

Peyser JM, Rao SM, LaRocca NG, Kaplan E (1990) Guidelines for neuropsychological research in multiple sclerosis. Arch Neurol 47:94–97

Pliskin NH, Towle VL, Hamer DP et al. (1994) The effects of interferon-beta on cognitive function in multiple sclerosis. In: Proceedings of the 119th annual meeting of the American Neurological Association. ANA, San Francisco, p 91

Polman CH, Bertelsmann FW, van Loenen AC, Koetsier JC (1994) 4-aminopyridine in the treatment of patients with multiple sclerosis: long-term efficacy and safety. Arch Neurol 51:292–296

Potvin AR, Tourtellotte WW (1985) Quantitative examination of neurologic function. CRC Press, Boca Raton

Poutiainen E, Hokkanen L, Niemi M-L, Färkkilä M (1994) Reversible cognitive decline during high-dose α-interferon treatment. Pharmacol Biochem Behav 47:901–905

Rao SM (1990) Neurobehavioral aspects of multiple sclerosis. Oxford University Press, New York

Rao SM, Hammeke TA, McQuillen MP, Khatri BO, Lloyd D (1984) Memory disturbance in chronic progressive multiple sclerosis. Arch Neurol 41:625–631

Rao SM, Leo GJ, Haughton VM, St. Aubin-Faubert P, Bernardin L (1989) Correlation of magnetic resonance imaging with neuropsychological testing in multiple sclerosis. Neurology 39:161–166

Rao SM, Leo GJ, Bernardin L, Unverzagt F (1991a) Cognitive dysfunction in multiple sclerosis: I. Frequency, patterns, and prediction. Neurology 41:685–691

Rao SM, Leo GJ, Ellington L, Nauertz T, Bernardin L, Unverzagt F (1991b) Cognitive dysfunction in multiple sclerosis: II. Impact on employment and social functioning. Neurology 41:692–696

Ruff RM, Crouch JA (1991) Neuropsychological test instruments in clinical trials. In: Mohr E, Brouwers P (eds) Handbook of clinical trials: the neurobehavioral approach. Swets & Zeitlinger, Amsterdam, pp 89–119

Ryan CM, Adams KM, Heaton RK, Grant I, Jacobson AM, DCCT Research Group (1991) Neurobehavioral assessment of medical patients in clinical trials: the DCCT experience. In: Mohr E, Brouwers P (eds) Handbook of clinical trials: the neurobehavioral approach. Swets & Zeitlinger, Amsterdam, pp 215–241

Schmitt FA, Bigley JW, McKinnis R et al. (1988) Neuropsychological outcome of zidovudine (AZT) treatment of patients with AIDS and AIDS-related complex. N Engl J Med 319:1573–1578

Selnes OA, Galai N, Bacellar H et al. (1995) Cognitive performance after progression to AIDS: A longitudinal study from the Multicenter AIDS Cohort Study. Neurology 45:267–275

Sidtis JJ, Gatsonis C, Price RW et al. (1993) Zidovudine treatment of the AIDS dementia complex: results of a placebo-controlled trial. Ann Neurol 33:343–349

Sipe JC, Romine JS, Koziol JA, McMillan R, Zyroff J, Beutler E (1994) Cladribine in treatment of chronic progressive multiple sclerosis. Lancet 344:9–13

Smits RCF, Emmen HH, Bertelsmann FW, Kulig BM, van Loenen AC, Polman CH (1994) The effects of 4-aminopyridine on cognitive function in patients with multiple sclerosis: a pilot study. Neurology 44:1701–1705

Stern Y, Liu X, Marder K et al. (1995a) Neuropsychological changes in a prospectively followed cohort of homosexual and bisexual men with and without HIV infection. Neurology 45:467–472

Stern Y, Liu XH, Tsai WY, Albert M, Brandt J (1995b) Growth curve models of the progression of Alzheimer's disease. Neurology 45(Suppl 4):A195

Swirsky-Sacchetti T, Mitchell DR, Seward J et al. (1992) Neuropsychological and structural brain lesions in multiple sclerosis: a regional analysis. Neurology 42:1291–1295

Taylor R (1990) Relationships between cognitive test performance and everyday cognitive difficulties in multiple sclerosis. Br J Clin Psychol 29:251–253

Unverzagt FW, Rao SM, Antuono P (1991) Oral physostigmine in the treatment of memory loss in multiple sclerosis. J Clin Exp Neuropsychol 13:74

van den Burg W, van Zomeren AH, Minderhoud JH, Prange AJA, Meijer NSA (1987) Cognitive impairment in patients with multiple sclerosis and mild physical disability. Arch Neurol 44:494–501

Weiner HL, Paty DW (1989) Diagnostic and therapeutic trials in multiple sclerosis: a new look. Neurology 39:972–976

Whitaker JN, McFarland HF, Rudge P, Reingold SC (1995) Outcomes assessment in multiple sclerosis clinical trials: a critical analysis. Multiple Sclerosis 1:37–47

7 "Quality of Life" Assessment in Multiple Sclerosis Clinical Trials: Current Status and Strategies for Improving Multiple Sclerosis Clinical Trial Design

Nicholas G. LaRocca, Paul G. Ritvo, Deborah M. Miller, Jill S. Fischer, Howard Andrews and Donald W. Paty

Health-Related Quality of Life

Sometime in the future, a multiple sclerosis (MS) patient comes to see the neurologist. Neurologist: "Well, your MRI looks great!" Patient: "That's wonderful doc, because my life is falling apart, I feel lousy and that medication you gave me made me sicker than my MS did". This situation is mirrored in clinical trials in which statistical imperatives dictate that outcomes be narrowly defined, often in terms of a single primary outcome measure. Although this strategy may help to avoid the type of error that occurs when so many outcomes are examined, it is problematic because a broad spectrum of other clinically relevant outcomes may be discounted.

The narrowly defined outcomes common to clinical trials run decidedly counter to the prevailing model of comprehensive care for MS. So firmly entrenched is this model that, in order to become a full member of the Consortium of Multiple Sclerosis Centers, a center must demonstrate that its care meets at least minimal criteria for comprehensiveness (Consortium of Multiple Sclerosis Center, 1994).

Clinical trials and comprehensive care centers could exist happily in differing orbits were it not for the fact that some patients pass through both. Putatively immunomodulatory agents are evaluated and approved based on narrow criteria, and are then introduced into the MS population with incomplete understanding of their real impact. Then these treatments are managed by providers committed to comprehensive care (i.e. co-ordinated attention to the whole person and his or her social context). Within the purview of comprehensive care, quality of life issues assume a significance barely hinted at in clinical trials undertaken thus far. Successful treatment with a given drug is contingent upon many issues beyond its direct effect on the disease. One of the key issues is whether the treatment, with its cost, side effects and benefits, improves quality of life for the patient.

Defining Quality of Life

In 1990 the National Institutes of Health (NIH) convened a workshop of 15 scholars to share their experience in health-related quality of life (HRQL) assessment (National Institutes of Health 1993). The goal of the conference was to explore the role of HRQL in NIH sponsored studies. A working definition emerged:

> Health-related quality of life is the value assigned to duration of life as modified by the impairments, functional states, perceptions, and social opportunities influenced by disease, injury, treatment, or policy (Patrick and Erickson 1993).

Thus HRQL is distinguished, somewhat, from the more general concept of "quality of life", which is seen as including:

> ...cultural, financial, political, temporal, and philosophical domains. Interaction occurs between dimensions of HRQL and other quality of life dimensions. Quality of life dimensions not directly affected by disease may affect a person's ability to cope with disease and respond to treatment. Disease or therapy can affect a person's perception or ability to enjoy dimensions of life other than those directly limited by disease *(National Institutes of Health 1993, p 2).*

The NIH conferees were sensitive to the need clearly to define the interface between HRQL and clinical trials. They thus said:

> HRQL can be conceptualized as a three-part model that includes (1) clinical status or biological functioning assessed by measures of disease pathology and organ system impairment; (2) disease-specific and treatment-specific symptoms and problems; and (3) generic health measures that focus on health concepts (including various aspects of functioning and general health perceptions) valued regardless of a person's age or health state *(National Institutes of Health 1993, p 1).*

Clinical trial endpoints have often emphasized outcomes in the first and second categories (e.g. survival time in cancer trials, Expanded Disability Status Scale (EDSS) in MS). In contrast, outcomes in the third category (e.g. general well-being) have been dealt with less directly.

Why Measure Quality of Life in a Clinical Trial?

If the basic purpose of a clinical trial is to slow or halt the progress of the disease, why should we assess HRQL? HRQL is an issue first of all because illness generally has an adverse impact on quality of life. If treatments effected perfect cures at reasonable cost and with no side effects, quality of life would probably be a peripheral concern. However, most treatments are only partially effective, are often expensive, and can have significant side effects.

Increasingly in clinical trials we not only ask how effective is a treatment, we also ask a number of other questions related to its cost benefit ratio and its utility. For example: Does the treatment restore, improve or at least stabilize quality of life? Does the treatment impair quality of life? Is the economic cost of the treatment high relative to the quality of life that can be achieved with the treatment? If neither complete cure nor imminent death are likely outcomes, what improvements can be achieved with respect to the patient's quality of life?

Such questions are not new. In 1947 the World Health Organization (WHO) adopted a broad definition of health as "a state of complete physical, mental, and social well-being, and not merely the absence of disease and infirmity" (World Health Organization 1947). As early as 1949, Karnofsky and Burchenal (1949) proposed expanding the criteria for evaluating success in cancer trials to include factors such as functional status, mood and general well-being. While mortality and morbidity are the traditionally measured parameters in clinical trials, they do not necessarily indicate how the patient feels subjectively or functions in everyday life. Yet these perceptions determine whether or not the patient considers the treatment a success (National Institutes of Health 1993). Thus the first reason to assess HRQL in clinical trials is to determine whether the treatment itself has a positive impact on quality of life.

Few treatments have no side effects and some (e.g. chemotherapeutic agents used in cancer) have severe negative consequences. Thus a second reason to measure HRQL in clinical trials is to assess the potential negative effects of the treatment on quality of life and balance this against the treatment's positive effects, if any.

Modern treatments are often very expensive over the long term. If an expensive treatment prolongs life but the quality of those extended years is poor, has our money been spent wisely? HRQL measurement can inform policy decisions concerning allocation of limited health care funds by quantifying what these buy in terms of quality of life. Therefore, a third reason to measure HRQL in clinical trials is to provide some basis for cost benefit and cost utility comparisons.

The NIH's interest in HRQL relates to the increasing relative prevalence of chronic illness (National Institutes of Health 1993). Many acute conditions have been eliminated or survival from them improved dramatically. The result is a greater emphasis on the management of chronic conditions, a costly enterprise and one that is difficult to evaluate. Traditional outcome measures, such as mortality or morbidity, have little relevance in chronic illness. Thus, a fourth reason to measure HRQL is to assess the course of chronic illness with a more meaningful set of parameters for determining the value of treatments for such disorders.

There has been an increasing emphasis in recent years on patient autonomy. Although assignment of treatment in a clinical trial is usually determined by a table of random numbers, in the real world, the decision is likely to be a joint one made by patient and physician. A fifth reason to include HRQL in clinical trials is therefore to obtain quantitative information on patient preferences and subjective perceptions that may have a powerful influence on real life treatment decisions.

In short, HRQL provides a comprehensive set of tools to compare the impacts of disease and to assess the relative merits of different treatments. HRQL includes the traditional measures used in clinical trials (e.g. biologic impairment), complementing them with methods that quantify the more subjective aspects of illness and its treatment. HRQL enables the physician, the patient and the policy maker to formulate informed decisions concerning medical care and allocation of limited resources.

Approaches to the Measurement of Health-Related Quality of Life

HRQL measures can be divided into two general types: generic and specific (Guyatt et al. 1993). Generic instruments can be used regardless of the nature of the medical condition and are thus useful for comparisons across conditions. Specific measures are specially tailored for a particular disease (e.g. MS), condition (e.g. speech disorders), or population (e.g. native Americans). Specific measures may be more sensitive to the nuances of a particular condition but render comparisons across conditions more difficult. We will discuss the strengths and weaknesses of both generic and specific measures and discuss at least one example of each.

Generic Instruments

Generic measures can be divided into two major classes: health profiles and utility measures (Guyatt et al. 1993). Health profiles have their roots in the psychometric tradition (e.g. intelligence tests) and consist of discrete scales that quantify the major dimensions of HRQL by means of patient self-report. In contrast, utility measures, grounded in econometrics and decision theory, elicit patients' preferences (i.e. utilities) for different health states. Comparisons of patient preferences for their current health state, obtained before and after treatment, yield values useful in summating treatment effects.

Health Profiles

Health profiles (also known as health surveys) are so named because they follow a "profile" approach to measurement based on psychometric theory. In this approach, each major dimension of HRQL is measured using several items for each dimension. A score is calculated for each dimension and these subscores can be displayed in the form of a profile. Examples of this approach include the Short Form from the Medical Outcomes Study (SF-36) (Ware and Sherbourne 1992), the Sickness Impact Profile (SIP) (Bergner et al. 1981), and the Nottingham Health Profile (Hunt et al. 1981). Health profiles assume that the impact of illness is multidimensional and thus permit the delineation of differential effects on different dimensions (Guyatt et al. 1993; Wiklund et al. 1990). Such multidimensional profiles also facilitate comparisons of the differential effects of various diseases on HRQL (Wiklund et al. 1990). However, assessment of so many dimensions in a reliable way can require a large number of items, making some profile approaches such as the SIP laborious for the patient to complete (Wiklund et al. 1990).

The SIP was one of the first HRQL instruments. It exists in different versions and has been modified and adapted by a number of researchers. The SIP consists of 136 items with a yes–no answer format. Subscales include ambulation, mobility, body care, movement, eating, work, home management, sleep, leisure, socialization, alertness, communication and emotions (Bergner et al.1981). Each item within a subscale is multiplied by an item-specific weight and then the items are summed into a subscale score. The SIP has been used in a wide variety of populations including MS surveys (Sanford and Petajan 1990).

The SIP comprehensively assesses a wide variety of health-related dimensions, making it suitable for in-depth studies of illness effects. Moreover, its widespread utilization in a variety of conditions encourages cross-condition comparisons. Thus, the usefulness of the SIP has been demonstrated in myriad studies addressing diverse questions. On the negative side, the SIP is quite long, which encourages many investigators to pick and choose among the subscales. In addition, some of the items are awkwardly worded. Some of the sections on physical dimensions of HRQL could probably be assessed more effectively by disease-specific measures. Despite these limitations, the breadth of the SIP and its wide use in a variety of conditions and populations make it an attractive instrument.

The SF-36 represents another example of a health profile. Consisting of 36 items organized into eight subscales, the SF-36 was derived from a much longer instrument developed for the Medical Outcomes Study (Ware and Sherbourne 1992; Ware et al. 1993). Most of these items were adapted from older instruments in which they had worked well psychometrically. Each item has a Likert-type format (multiple choices representing an ordinal gradation) with the items for each subscale summed without weighting into their respective scores. The subscales are physical, social and role functioning, mental health, general health perceptions, bodily pain, and vitality (Ware and Sherbourne 1992). The SF-36 was developed in order to provide a comprehensive and reliable measure of HRQL that could be used in situations where lengthy health surveys might not be practical (e.g. in national health surveys where a number of other instruments also have to be administered). The reliability of the SF-36 has been evaluated in a number of studies that were summarized by Ware (Ware et al. 1993). For all but one of the subscales, the median reliability coefficient was 0.80 or higher. The Social Functioning scale had a median reliability of 0.76. Thus all of the subscales of the SF-36 have reliabilities that exceed 0.70, the generally accepted standard necessary for group level analyses. The SF-36 has been used with thousands of individuals in the United States, Canada and the United Kingdom, and, in translated form, in many other countries. There thus exists a huge amount of data on the SF-36 against which new studies can be compared.

Utility Measures

While the profile measures described above are derived from psychometric theory (like IQ tests), utility measures are rooted in econometrics and decision theory (Guyatt et al. 1993). The decision theory in question was developed in the

1940s as a normative model for making individual decisions in the face of uncertainty (Torrance and Feeny 1989). When applied to health, utility measures elicit patients' preferences (i.e. utilities) for different health states, particularly current states. Comparisons of these preferences, pre- and post-treatment, yield single values summating treatment benefits as well as side effects. The term "utilities" refers to "...the numbers that represent the strength of the individual's preferences for particular outcomes when faced with uncertainty" (Torrance and Feeny 1989). Typically, HRQL is represented as a single number ranging from 0 (death) to 1 (full health). This number can be combined with life duration estimates to derive a quality adjusted life year (QALY) (i.e. QALY = numbers of years lived × the quality of life experienced per year). QALY comparisons provide a potentially useful means of understanding relative treatment benefit in both quantity and quality of life. The QALY metric can also be used to summate the course of a disease or treatment by estimating the time spent in each health state, multiplying it by the utility coefficient, and summing the total. When the utility coefficients are assigned by patient panels, the process conforms closely to the normative decision model. An example provided by Kaplan (1993) will serve to illustrate:

> ...suppose that a man dies of throat cancer at age 50 and he was expected to live to age 75. Survival analysis suggests that he lost 25 years of life. However, assume that there was a successful surgery that allowed the man to complete his life expectancy but with very significant impact upon his functioning and ability to communicate. Traditional survival analysis would indicate that the disease was cured since the life expectancy was the same as someone without the disease. However, analysis that takes quality of life into consideration would yield different results. Let's assume that the life after the surgery is scored as 0.5 on a 0.0 to 1.0 scale. The 25 years following surgery would be adjusted for this diminished quality to yield 12.5 quality adjusted years (25 years × 0.5 quality of life = 12.5 Quality Adjusted Life Years) *(pp 86–87)*.

This concept of QALY is closely identified with HRQL utility measures. QALY can be used in cost–utility analyses that seek to evaluate the allocation of health care resources by determining cost per QALY. The assumption is that health care should strive to achieve the lowest cost per QALY possible (Harris 1987). Carrying this concept a step further, it has even been suggested that limited health care resources might be "rationed" by allocating funds to those activities having the most favorable cost per QALY (Cubbon 1991; LaPuma and Lawlor 1990). QALY can also be useful in clinical decision making. For example, faced with two choices for treating MS, physician and patient might consider which gives the most QALY along with which carries the lowest cost per QALY (Harris 1987). While the concept of "rationing" remains controversial, it seems clear that QALY, along with similar methods, will play a role in setting health care priorities in the future.

Two of the best known HRQL utility measures will be used to illustrate this approach, the Quality of Well Being Scale (Kaplan and Anderson 1990) and Quality-Adjusted Time Without Symptoms and Toxicity (Q-TWiST) (Gelber et al. 1992).

The Quality of Well Being Scale (QWBS) is an outgrowth of the General Health Policy Model (GHPM). This model attempts to integrate information derived from a variety of health states in such a way as to have applicability across different providers and interventions (Kaplan and Anderson 1990). This model separates health status into distinct components, including life expectancy (mortality), functioning and symptoms (morbidity), preferences for functional states (utilities) and duration of various health states (prognosis) (Kaplan 1993). Unlike profile measures that conceptualize HRQL as a single point in time, the GHPM views it as a stochastic process extending over the life history of the individual (Schumacher et al. 1991).

The GHPM gave rise to the QWBS, which consists of lists of "health states" such as "in wheelchair, moved or controlled movement of wheelchair" (Kaplan 1993). These health states include three function scales: mobility, physical activity and social activity, as well as a scale for symptoms or problems. Each of these health states has been assigned a utility or weight by a panel of individuals thought to be representative of the target population. Scores for a single point in time are derived by adding together all the functional limitations and symptoms experienced by a given individual. Well years, or QALY, can be calculated by multiplying the utility for a given health state by the amount of time spent in that state and then adding all these together. This is best illustrated by example.

An individual with MS experiences the following health states with their respective utility coefficients: mobility – does not drive (–0.062), physical activity – able to propel own wheelchair (–0.060), social activity – unemployed but independent in most activities of daily living (–0.061), symptoms/problems – weakness (–0.299) and cognitive dysfunction (–0.340). The score for this individual for one day would be:

1 ("well" day) + (–0.062) + (–0.060) + (–0.061) + (–0.299) + (–0.340) = 0.178 (not so well day)

To simplify calculations, we will assume that this individual remains in each of these health states for 30 years and then dies suddenly from a myocardial infarction. This individual's well years (or QALY) would be: 30 × 0.178 = 5.34. The impact of intervention can be assessed using this formula. For example, if a new drug were found in clinical trials to eliminate his cognitive dysfunction, his QALY would rise to 15.54.

The QWBS combines information from a variety of HRQL dimensions into a single number and makes provision for expressing the result over the individual's life span. The scale is applicable across a wide variety of conditions and situations and allows for comparison of the cost per QALY for various health care initiatives. However, the single index does obscure information concerning variation among the different HRQL dimensions. The items in the scale cover a limited set of situations and there are some glaring omissions (e.g. depression). Moreover, in keeping with a normative decision model, utility weights are based on a representative panel with no provision for individual differences in preferences for various health states. As a result, the QWBS may be more useful for policy studies than for examining individual perceptions of disease and treatment. Using the QWBS over time in a changeable condition becomes complicated, since the health states have to be repeatedly assessed. Nevertheless, the QWBS provides a carefully conceived and developed approach to the assessment of HRQL that has proven useful in many research settings.

In clinical trials, a major issue is often the potentially negative impact of the treatment itself on quality of life. The Q-TWiST method evolved out of the desire to quantify this effect (Gelber et al. 1992; Gelber and Goldhirsch 1986). A common endpoint in cancer clinical trials has been survival time. However, as powerful chemotherapeutic agents were introduced that had toxic side effects, it was observed that in many cases patients were miserable during much of their survival time. Gelber and Goldhirsch (1986) introduced Time Without Symptoms and Toxicity (TWiST) as a new endpoint. This was a primitive attempt to partition survival time and consisted of simply subtracting the amount of time a patient experienced toxic side effects and the time following symptom relapse from survival time. In effect, this early system weighted time spent with toxic side effects or in relapse as zero. While time spent with toxic side effects can be miserable, it is worth something to most people. Thus Gelber et al. (1989) introduced Q-TWiST, which represents the time spent without symptoms or toxicity (weighted 1) plus time spent with toxic side effects and in relapse, with the two latter weighted somewhere between 0 and 1.

To illustrate Q-TWiST, consider an individual who is treated for breast cancer with chemotherapy and survives 5 years. Two of those years are spent free of either toxic side effects or symptom relapse and are thus assigned a utility coefficient of 1. Two years in total are spent with toxic side effects and 1 year is spent in symptom relapse prior to death; each are assigned a utility coefficient of 0.5. The 5 years of survival can be partitioned as follows:

$$2(\text{TWiST}) \times 1 + 2(\text{toxicity}) \times 0.5 + 1(\text{relapse}) \times 0.5 = 3.5 \text{ QALY}$$

A problem with this method has been that it was based on arbitrary utility weights. Extensions of the Q-TWiST method have emphasized threshold utility analysis, in which the outcome of a given treatment can be considered across a range of utility coefficients (Gelber et al. 1992) This has special application in individual clinical decision making, since it opens up the possibility of patients evaluating treatment alternatives based on individual preferences for various health states. However, in the absence of normative data on patient preferences, the utility coefficients used in the Q-TWiST remain arbitrary and theoretical. Gelber et al. (1992) have suggested that methods akin to profile approaches to HRQL may complement Q-TWiST and help to shed light on the issue of utility coefficients. Despite its mathematical elegance and intuitive appeal, Q-TWiST has not been very widely employed in cancer. In contrast to other methods such as the QWBS, it is difficult to utilize Q-TWiST across conditions. Q-TWiST is really an analytic method rather than a specific set of scale items. As such, it means something quite different in each of its applications. Q-TWiST is difficult to utilize in MS in its original form since it is hard to define survival endpoints and the health states are more numerous and more complex. However, some preliminary work is under way on an MS version of Q-TWiST and results have shown some promise (Schwartz et al. 1995).

Disease-Specific Instruments

In contrast to the broad focus of generic instruments, specific instruments attempt to concentrate more narrowly on quality of life issues particular to a single disease, symptom or group. This narrowing of focus does have certain advantages. Disease or symptom specific instruments may possess greater precision than the generics, rendering them more sensitive to small changes over time (Deyo and Centor 1986). For example, the Fatigue Impact Scale (Fisk et al. 1994), developed for use in MS, provides detailed information concerning the impact of MS fatigue on a variety of daily activities.

The list of specific HRQL instruments is nearly endless. One of the earliest to be developed was Karnofsky's index of performance status in cancer patients (Karnofsky et al. 1949). Others specific measures have been introduced for use in arthritis (Meenan et al. 1980), chronic obstructive pulmonary disease (Guyatt et al. 1987), chemotherapy in breast cancer (Levine et al. 1988), and many others. Such scales can be very specific indeed, such as the visual analog of voice quality for use in laryngeal cancer (Llewellyn-Thomas et al. 1984).

The disadvantage of such specific approaches is the inherent difficulty in comparing results to other conditions. Patrick and Bergner (1990) have suggested that the most desirable approach might be to use short, generic instruments in combination with disease-specific measures. An excellent example of this generic with specific approach was recently described by Vickrey et al. (1995a). The goal was to develop an improved method to measure outcome in surgery for intractable epilepsy. The common element in published reports of this type of surgery has been type and frequency of seizure, but with great variability in reporting this and other types of outcomes. The investigators constructed the 55-item Epilepsy Surgery Inventory (ESI-55) by combining 19 items of particular concern to epilepsy patients with the 36 items from the SF-36 (Ware and Sherbourne 1992), a generic HRQL instrument described earlier in this chapter. The ESI-55 contains 11 subscales that measure health perceptions, energy/fatigue, overall quality of life, social functioning, emotional well-being, cognitive functioning, role limitations due to emotional problems, role limitations due to memory problems, role limitations due to physical health problems, physical functioning, and pain. The ESI-55 was used to refine seizure-based outcome systems so that they more accurately reflect HRQL. The revised system divided seizure outcome during the past year into four broad categories: seizure-free; auras with or without one seizure; 2–12 seizures; and more than 12 seizures. Each of these four groups differed from all the others on at least two HRQL dimensions. The generic plus specific approach has generated increasing interest and is likely to become the standard in the future.

Strengths and Weaknesses of Quality of Life Measures

Table 7.1 summarizes some of the weaknesses and strengths of HRQL measures. In general it can be seen that adding HRQL measures can increase the cost and burden of clinical trials while generating data that may be complex and subtle in

Table 7.1. Weaknesses and strengths of health related quality of life measures

Weaknesses	Strengths
Measurement is time consuming, adding to cost and burden of trials	Utilize a comprehensive concept of health
Interpretation of data is complex and subject to differing interpretations	Capture positive aspects of health, not just absence of morbidity
Increase in the number of outcome measures complicates statistical analysis	Allow assessment of broad goals of treatment rather than just narrow goals of clinical trials
Multiple items are needed to assess "latent" variables that cannot be directly observed	Assess patient's perception of outcome (e.g. whether or not patient feels better)
Measurement process involves subjective value judgments	Help to separate physiology and function
Measurement is dependent on language and cognitive skills	Capture the possible negative effects of treatment
May be affected by factors unrelated to the disease or treatment	Can assess data correlated with health care costs
	Permit comparisons across conditions (e.g. MS versus epilepsy)

its interpretation. For example, what language a person speaks is irrelevant to the interpretation of an MRI scan. However, language and culture may be major factors to take into account in the measurement of depressive symptoms. On the plus side, HRQL measures help to broaden the focus of clinical trials and to anchor outcomes in terms of real life issues, such as whether or not a person feels well enough to perform daily activities. It is beyond the scope of this chapter to resolve the pros and cons of HRQL assessment in clinical trials. Instead, it is hoped that this presentation will help to stimulate thought, discussion, and research concerning this issue.

Multiple Sclerosis Quality of Life Inventory

The Multiple Sclerosis Quality of Life Inventory (MSQLI) is a project of the Consortium of Multiple Sclerosis Centers. Founded in 1985, the Consortium presently has more than 80 member centers in the United States and Canada. The mission of the Consortium includes fostering clinical research and the improvement of care for persons with MS. Toward these goals, the Consortium has always had an active interest in methodologies to evaluate the impact of MS and the effectiveness of treatments. In conjunction with the Albert Einstein College of Medicine, the Consortium held a Consensus Conference in 1991 on outcome measures in MS (Foley 1993). This conference was modeled on the prevailing practice of each professional discipline utilizing its own distinct methods.

Following this meeting, the Research Committee of the Consortium formed the Health Services Research Subcommittee (HSRS), charged with planning the Consortium's response to the need for a set of comprehensive measures, as had already been addressed in other conditions (Kaplan 1993; Kaplan and Anderson 1990; Schumacher et al. 1991).

Steps in the Development of the Multiple Sclerosis Quality of Life Inventory

The MSQLI was developed as a comprehensive assessment of quality of life among persons with MS. Based largely on a self-report format, the MSQLI was designed to be widely employed by both clinicians and researchers. The HSRS wanted the MSQLI to be sensitive to differences between patient groups at a single point in time as well as changes in individual patients over time. The MSQLI was thus intended to be an assessment of the impact of MS on quality of life as well as the value of treatments in ameliorating such changes.

Review and Discussion

The HSRS held a number of meetings and conference calls to establish the theoretical rationale for the MSQLI, discuss candidate measures and review the literature. As a result of these discussions, it was decided to adopt the WHO's classification of impairment, disability and handicap as the theoretical framework for the MSQLI (World Health Organization 1980). The WHO classification had been adopted earlier as the basis for the first set of measures to achieve international consensus for use in MS, the Minimal Record of Disability (Haber and LaRocca 1985). As far as the HSRS could determine, this was the first time that the WHO's classification had been integrated in this way with the quality of life construct. Utilizing the WHO schema, quality of life may be thought of as physical, psychologic and social well-being. As utilized in the MSQLI, the quality of life construct, in the context of health experience, has several components:

1. Impairment is any loss or abnormality of physiologic or anatomic structure or function that is based on objective assessment.
2. Disability is any restriction or lack (resulting from impairment) of ability to perform an activity in the manner or within the range considered normal for a human being. Disability is the subjectively perceived impact of impairment by the individual who experiences that impairment.
3. Handicap is a disadvantage for a given individual, resulting from an impairment or disability that limits or prevents the fulfillment of a role that is normal for that individual.

Using these definitions as a guide, the HSRS assembled a set of candidate measures that could be subject to independent review.

Content Validation

The goal of content validation was to ensure that the MSQLI covered all relevant domains in sufficient but not excessive detail. Secondarily, it was designed to evaluate the clarity and acceptability of each item in the MSQLI. The HSRS compared the set of candidate measures to those in existing MS and generic quality of life research to determine if anything had been overlooked. However, the most important part of this step was a comprehensive review of the MSQLI by three panels: neurologists, allied health care professionals and consumers. As a result of these reviews, a number of changes were made in the MSQLI, particularly in the domains of objective physical measures, bladder and bowel problems, caregiving, sexual functioning and others.

Advisory Committee Review

Based upon the results of the content validation, the HSRS revised the MSQLI and applied to the National Multiple Sclerosis Society (NMSS) for funding to begin field testing of the instrument. This application was successful and in November, 1993, the HSRS met with an expert advisory committee assembled by the NMSS to review the research plan and make recommendations. The members of this committee included Chris Bever, Robert Kaplan, Sarah Minden and John Ware. Based upon the results of this meeting, a number of changes were made in the content of the MSQLI and in the research plan.

Field Testing

Field testing of the MSQLI had a number of objectives:

1. To evaluate the reliability of the component measures;
2. To identify redundancy in the MSQLI and eliminate unnecessary items;
3. To explore the empirically-defined dimensions of quality of life in MS;
4. To compare the usefulness of generic quality of life scales with MS-specific measures;
5. To compare the MSQLI results for defined groups such as high versus low neurologically impaired patients;
6. To assess the practicality of the MSQLI in actual clinical settings.

The field testing of the MSQLI began in late 1994 at four sites: the Mellen Center in Cleveland, Ohio, St Michael's Hospital in Toronto, Ontario, the Dalhousie MS Center in Halifax, Nova Scotia, and St Agnes Hospital in White Plains, New York. The sample for the field test consists of 300 patients with clinically definite MS. All subjects are seen by a neurologist who rates the objective physical impairment measures and by an interviewer who completes the remainder of the MSQLI. Those patients who are capable of doing so, answer the questions by circling answers on the printed questionnaires. Patients with visual or motor problems that preclude the above method, are read the questions by the interviewer. The entire procedure takes approximately 3 hours and is done in one session if possible.

Data Analysis

Analysis of the MSQLI will focus on the reliability of the individual measures, redundancy of items, and validity of scales. Reliability of analysis will assess internal consistency of scales and cohesiveness of individual items. Factor analysis will be used to explore the distinct dimensions of HRQL in MS. In addition, factor analysis and other multivariate methods will be used to evaluate redundancy of items and scales within the MSQLI with a view toward shortening it. The final step will be to compare the quality of life of various dichotomously-defined groups of subjects. For example, one such analysis might compare quality of life for subjects with mild versus severe neurologic impairment. A question of particular interest will be whether the MS-specific instruments add substantially to the information available from generic measures such as the SF-36.

Components of the Multiple Sclerosis Quality of Life Inventory

Space limitations do not permit a complete description of each part of the MSQLI. The specific measures are listed in Tables 7.2–7.4, along with information on the source for each. These are organized according to the WHO concept of health. With the exception of the 9-Hole Peg Test, all the objective measures of neurologic impairment are rated by a neurologist. The remaining parts of the MSQLI are administered by a specially trained interviewer.

Table 7.2. MSQLI impairment measures

Objective measures of neurologic impairment:
Date of onset and diagnosis
Kurtzke's Functional Systems and EDSS (Kurtzke 1983)
Visual acuity
Ambulation Index (Hauser et al. 1983)
Nine Hole Peg Test (Goodkin et al. 1988)
Objective Measures of cognitive impairment:
Hopkins Verbal Learning Test (Brandt 1991)
Symbol Digits Modalities Test (Smith 1973)
Paced Auditory Serial Addition Test (Gronwell 1977)
Brief Test of Attention (Schretlen and Bobholz 1992)

Table 7.3. MSQLI disability measures

Self-assessment of perceived disability
Physical Functioning dimensions of the Sickness Impact Profile (Bergner et al. 1981)
Fatigue Inventory, based on items from the Medical Outcomes Study (Fisk et al. 1994; Stewart et al. 1992)
Sensory and Pain Inventory, based on items from the Medical Outcomes Study and the work of Archibald et al. (1994)
Sexual Functioning and Satisfaction Questionnaire, adapted from Schover and Jensen (1987)
Bowel and Bladder Questionnaire, constructed by the HSRS, along with the SIP Bowel and Bladder Subscale (Bergner et al. 1981)
Perceived (cognitive) Deficits Questionnaire (Sullivan et al. 1990)
Mental Health Inventory, 18-item version (Davies et al. 1988; Veit and Ware 1983)
Social Support Questionnaire (Sherbourne and Stewart 1991)
Revised UCLA Loneliness-Companionship Scale (Russell et al. 1980)
Health Status Questionnaire SF-36 (Ware and Sherbourne 1992)
MS Symptom Distress Survey, constructed by the HSRS
Impact of Visual Impairment, constructed by the HSRS

Table 7.4. MSQLI handicap measures

Self-assessment of social handicap
Social Interaction Subscale of the SIP
Work Role Subscale of the SIP
Home Management Subscale of the SIP
Recreation and Pastimes Subscale of the SIP
Income and Financial Inquiry, constructed by the HSRS
Satisfaction with Care Questionnaire, constructed by the HSRS
Housing and Transportation Questionnaire, constructed by the HSRS

Other Approaches to the Measurement of Quality of Life in Multiple Sclerosis

The MSQLI is only one of many possible approaches to HRQL measurement in MS. At present, several research groups have studies under way in this field. Thomas Choi has been investigating the combined use of generic and MS-specific measures (T. Choi et al. unpublished observations). Carolyn Schwartz has adapted the Q-TWiST method for use in MS and is currently evaluating it at a number of sites in the USA (Schwartz et al. 1995). Barbara Vickrey has developed and tested an MS quality of life measure similar to the ESI-55, named the MSQOL-54 (Vickrey et al. 1995b). Results from these and other studies will be available soon and will enable investigators to make an informed decision concerning the use of HRQL measures in MS.

Future Directions

Investigators and sponsors planning definitive efficacy trials should consider broadening the outcome assessment beyond measures of disease pathologies. Specifically, measurement of the actual impact of an intervention calls for:

1. MS-specific and condition-specific measures (e.g. the Fatigue Impact Scale);
2. One or more generic profile measures (e.g. the SF-36);
3. A generic utility measure (e.g. the Q-TWiST).

These recommendations closely follow the suggestions made at the NIH Workshop on Quality of Life Assessment in 1990. Incorporating HRQL will help to make clinical trials vastly more informative and, at the same time, will address the impact of the intervention and disease in the person as a whole.

References

Archibald CJ, McGrath T, Ritvo PG, Fisk JD, Murray TJ (1994) Pain in multiple sclerosis: prevelance, severity, and impact on mental health. Pain 58:89–93

Bergner M, Bobbitt RA, Carter WB, Gilson BS (1981) The Sickness Impact Profile: development and final revision of a health status measure. Med Care 19:787–805

Brandt J (1991) The Hopkins Verbal Learning Test: development of a new memory test with six equivalent forms. Clin Neuropsychol 5:125–142

Consortium of Multiple Sclerosis Centers (1994) Charter and bylaws. Consortium of Multiple Sclerosis Centers, Teaneck, NJ

Cubbon J (1991) The principle of QALY maximisation as the basis for allocating health care resources. J Med Ethics 17:181–184

Deyo RA, Centor RM (1986) Assessing the responsiveness of functional scales to clinical change: an analogy to diagnostic test performance. J Chron Dis 39:897–906

Davies AR, Sherbourne CD, Peterson JR, Ware JE (1988) Scoring manual: adult health status and patient satisfaction measures used in RAND's Health Insurance Experiment, N-2190-HHS. The RAND Corporation, Santa Monica, CA

Fisk JD, Pontefract A, Ritvo PG, Archibald CJ, Murray TJ (1994) The impact of fatigue on patients with multiple sclerosis. Can J Neurol Sci 21:9–14

Foley FW (1993) Foreword: Comprehensive evaluation of outcome of care in multiple sclerosis. J Neurol Rehabil 7:85–86

Gelber RD, Goldhirsch A (1986) A new endpoint for the measurement of adjuvant therapy in postmenopausal women with operable breast cancer. J Clin Oncol 4:1772–1779

Gelber RD, Goldhirsch A, Simes RJ, Glasziou P, Castiglione M (1989) Integration of quality-of-life issues into clinical trials of breast cancer. In: Cavalli F (ed) Endocrine therapy of breast cancer III. Springer, Heidelberg, pp 27–36

Gelber RD, Lenderking WR, Cotton DJ et al. (1992) Quality-of-life evaluation in a clinical trial of zidovudine therapy in patients with mildly symptomatic HIV infection. Ann Intern Med 116:961–966

Goodkin DE, Hertsgaard D, Seminary J (1988) Upper extremity function in multiple sclerosis: improving assessment sensitivity with Box and Block and Nine Hole Peg Tests. Arch Phys Med Rehabil 69:850–854

Gronwell DMA (1977) Paced auditory serial-addition task: a measure of recovery from concussion. Percept Mot Skills 44:367–373

Guyatt GH, Townsend M, Berman LB, Pugsley SO (1987) Quality of life in patients with chronic airflow limitation. Br J Dis Chest 81:45–54

Guyatt GH, Feeney DH, Patrick DL (1993) Measuring health-related quality of life. Ann Intern Med 118:622–629

Haber A, LaRocca NG (1985) Minimal Record of Disability in multiple sclerosis. National Multiple Sclerosis Society, New York

Harris J (1987) QALYfying the value of life. J Med Ethics 13:117–123

Hauser SL, Dawson DM, Lehrich JR et al. (1983) Intensive immunosuppression in progressive multiple sclerosis: a randomized three-arm study of high dose intravenous cyclophosphamide, plasma exchange, and ACTH. N Engl J Med 308:173–180

Hunt SM, McKenna SP, Williams J (1981) Reliability of a population survey tool for measuring perceived health problems: a study of patients with coxarthrosis. J Epidemiol Community Health 35:297–300

Kaplan RM (1993) Quality of life assessment for cost/utility studies in cancer. Cancer Treat Rev 19 (Suppl A):85–96

Kaplan RM, Anderson JP (1990) The general health policy model: an integrated approach. In: Spilker B (ed) Quality of life assessments in clinical trials. Raven Press, New York, pp 131–149

Karnofsky DA, Burchenal JH (1949) Clinical evaluation of chemotherapeutic agents in cancer. In: McLeod CM (ed) Evaluation of chemotherapeutic agents. Columbia University Press, New York, 191–205

Karnofsky DA, Abelmann WH, Craver LF, Burchenal JH (1949) The use of the nitrogen mustards in the palliative treatment of carcinoma. Cancer 20:634–656

Kurtzke JF (1983) Rating neurological impairment in multiple sclerosis: an expanded disability status scale (EDSS). Neurology 33:1444–1452

LaPuma J, Lawlor EF (1990) Quality-adjusted life-years. JAMA 263:2917–2921

Levine MN, Guyatt GH, Gent M et al. (1988) Quality of life in stage II breast cancer: an instrument for clinical trials. J Clin Oncol 6:1798–1810

Llewellyn-Thomas HA, Sutherland HJ, Hogg SA et al. (1984) Linear-analogue self assessment of voice quality in laryngeal cancer. J Chron Dis 73:917–924

Meenan RF, Gertman PM, Mason JH (1980) Measuring health status in arthritis: the arthritis impact measurement scale. Arthritis Rheum 23:146–152

National Institutes of Health (1993) Quality of life assessment: practice, problems, and promise (NIH Publication no. 93-3505). US Department of Health and Human Services, Washington, DC

Patrick DL, Bergner M (1990) Measurement of health status in the 1990s. Ann Rev Public Health

11:165–183

Patrick DL, Erickson P (1993) Health status and health policy: quality of life in health care evaluation and resource allocation. Oxford University Press, New York

Russell D, Peplau LA, Cutrona CE (1980) The revised UCLA loneliness scale: concurrent and discriminant validity evidence. J Pers Soc Psychol 39:472–480

Sanford ME, Petajan JH (1990) Effects of multiple sclerosis on daily living. In: Rao SM (ed) Neurobehavioral aspects of mulitple sclerosis. Oxford University Press, New York, pp 251–265

Schretlen D, Bobholz JH (1992) Standardization and initial validation of a brief test of executive attentional ability. J Clin Exp Neuropsychol 14:65(abstract)

Schumacher M, Olschewski M, Schulgen G (1991) Assessment of quality of life in clinical trials. Stat Med 10:1915–1930

Schwartz CE, Cole BF, Gelber RD (1995) Measuring patient-centered outcomes in neurologic disease: extending the Q-TWiST methodology. Arch Neurol 52:754–762

Schover LR, Jensen SB (1988) Sexuality and chronic illness: a comprehensive approach. Guilford Press, New York

Sherbourne CD, Stewart AL (1991) The MOS Social Support Survey. Soc Sci Med 32:705–714

Smith A (1973) Symbol Digit Modalities Test manual. Western Psychological Services, Los Angeles, CA

Stewart AL, Hayes RD, Ware JE (1992) Health perceptions, energy, fatigue, and health distress measures. In: Stewart AL, Ware JE (eds) Measuring functioning and well being. Duke University Press, Durham, NC, pp 143–172

Sullivan MJL, Edgley K, Dehoux E (1990) A survey of multiple sclerosis. Part 1: perceived cognitive problems and compensatory strategy use. Can J Rehabil 4:99–105

Torrance GW, Feeny D (1989) Utilities and quality-adjusted life years. Int J Technol Assess Health Care 5:559–575

Veit CT, Ware JE (1983) The structure of psychological distress and well-being in general populations. J Consult Clin Psychol 51:730–732

Vickrey BG, Hays RD, Engel J et al. (1995a) Outcome assessment for epilepsy surgery: the impact of measuring health-related quality of life. Ann Neurol 37:158–166

Vickrey BG, Hays RD, Harooni R, Myers LW, Ellison GW (1995b) A health-related quality of life measure for multiple sclerosis. Qual Life Res 4:187–206

Ware JE, Sherbourne CD (1992) The MOS 36-item Short Form Health Survey (SF-36). Med Care 30:473–481

Ware JE, Snow KK, Kosinski M, Gandek B (1993) SF-36 Health Survey: manual and interpretation guide. The Health Institute, New England Medical Center, Boston, MA

Wiklund I, Dimenas E, Wahl M (1990) Factors of importance when evaluating quality of life in clinical trials. Control Clin Trials 11:169–179

World Health Organization (1947) The constitution of the World Health Organization. WHO, Geneva, Chron 1:29

World Health Organization (1980) International Classification of Impairments, Disabilities, and Handicaps. WHO, Geneva

8 Magnetic Resonance Imaging: Current Status and Strategies for Improving Multiple Sclerosis Clinical Trial Design

Robert I. Grossman

Introduction

Magnetic resonance (MR) has clearly evolved into the primary modality for the paraclinical evaluation of patients with multiple sclerosis (MS). The value of MR in controlled clinical trials and studies of natural history lies in its ability to detect sensitively the extent and evolution of lesion burden in the central nervous system. It has been demonstrated that MR is more sensitive than the clinical examination in both the detection and extent of progression of cerebral disease (Baum et al. 1990; Grossman et al. 1986; Isaac et al. 1988). In one study, subclinical evolution of lesions was observed by MR in 56% of clinically stable patients (Truyen et al. 1991). Investigators have reported a disparity between degree of disability and lesion burden (Huber et al. 1988; Mauch et al. 1988). One reason for this disparity is that clinical disability measurements are difficult to quantitate and inaccurately reflect disease burden (Noseworthy et al. 1990). This has contributed to the widespread acceptance of MR as a surrogate marker of therapeutic efficacy in clinical trials (IFNB Multiple Sclerosis Study Group 1993). McDonald et al. have suggested that MR is presently positioned to: screen putative therapies and determine which modify the evolution of disease; and serve as a supplementary marker of disease activity in Phase III studies in which disability is the primary outcome measure (McDonald et al. 1994).

This chapter will focus on a variety of MR techniques that have proven, or may in the future prove, useful in monitoring disease-related activity in MS clinical trials or studies of the natural history of MR lesions. Brief descriptions are provided so that the strengths and limitations of the proposed methodologies can be understood by the non-physicist. The approach that will prove most worthy to the understanding of MS will involve an open-minded researcher, one who will incorporate as many techniques as possible in his/her examination, acknowledging the constraints of time and patient tolerance. One must recognize that each technique provides a slightly different piece of the very complex puzzle. Magnetization transfer (MT), 1H magnetic resonance spectroscopy (1H MRS), T2 lesion volume, enhanced lesion number, etc., all furnish information that could potentially indicate the benefit of a therapeutic regimen. However, since it is not possible to use every technique in every study, MR probes must be applied prudently to analyze the results of treatment. We shall begin with important imaging principles that impact on protocols for MS clinical trials.

Imaging Principles

Effect of Partial Volume Blurring on Lesion Characterization

This section is based on work by Chung and colleagues (Chung et al. (1995).

Lesion detection is a complex function. It is primarily related to the contrast-to-noise ratio (CNR) that reflects the relative signal (brightness) intensity differences between the region of interest and the background. If a lesion fills the entire voxel, its detectability is related primarily to the contrast of the abnormality. However, the smaller the abnormality, the higher the CNR necessary for detection. In this situation, the percentage of the voxel filled by the lesion and the inherent contrast of the lesion determine its detectability (Plate 8.1). This is important since the variability of volumetric measurement increases as tissue contrast decreases.

A general imaging principle is that signal-to-noise ratio (SNR) (the mean intensity within a region of interest (signal) divided by the the standard deviation in the background containing only noise) scales linearly with image voxel size. The larger the voxel, the greater the SNR, and the smaller the slice thickness, the lower the SNR. Another generalization is that, all other things being equal, signal intensity increases with field strength. To obtain comparable signal-to-noise to a 1.5 Tesla magnet (standard high field magnet) on magnets of field strength below 1.5 Tesla, at similar imaging times, requires an increase in voxel size. Resolution, on the other hand, increases at the expense of both the SNR and image acquisition time.

Partial volume blurring is the result of imaging slices that are larger than the lesion you are trying to detect, but thin slices have lower SNR because of their decreased voxel size. It has been demonstrated that for small, low contrast abnormalities such as MS lesions the detection rate is greater for thin slices, even with a gap, than for thick, contiguous slices (Bradley and Glenn 1987).

Slice Thickness and Lesion Volume

Using a computerized volumetric technique Mitchell et al. studied an MS phantom with both 5 mm and 3 mm slices and reported an absolute error of 0.21 cm^3 for the former versus 0.15 cm^3 for the latter (Mitchell et al. 1994). This is the result of partial volume effects on accuracy. They also observed that, as lesion volume increases, the relative error in lesion volume measurement decreases (accuracy increases as lesions become larger). Precision, defined by the standard deviation of the volume measurements divided by the actual volume, was also noted to improve with increasing lesion volume. Finally, thinner sections produced better precision in measurement of smaller lesion volumes. The bottom line is that thinner is better. The trade-off in the past was time; however, with fast spin echo imaging this is less of a problem.

Conventional Spin Echo Imaging

The conventional spin echo pulse sequence has been used, in the past, for most clinical trials. It is a robust methodology where one line of k-space (raw data – see section on Fast Spin Echo) is acquired per time to repetition (TR) interval. Here, scan time for conventional two-dimensional Fourier transform imaging is given by the following equation:

Scan time = TR interval × number of phase encodings × number of excitations (NEX)

There are important relationships that are the foundation for imaging protocols (Tables 8.1 and 8.2). Many imaging trade-offs are based on this equation. Doubling the phase encoding (from 128 to 256) decreases the signal-to-noise by a factor of two because the voxel size is halved but increases resolution by a factor of two. In addition, increasing the phase encoding steps to 256 increases the signal-to-noise by $\sqrt{2}$ because the acquisition time is doubled. The net effect is a decrease in the signal-to-noise by $\sqrt{2}/2$ or 0.71. Increasing the number of excitations (or averages) increases the signal-to-noise, but also the examination time. If the field of view is doubled, the voxel size is quadrupled (doubled in two dimensions of the matrix, resulting in poorer resolution) and the signal-to-noise doubles. Reducing the field of view or increasing the number of phase-encoding steps (matrix) effectively increases the number of pixels the lesion spans, thus reducing the loss of contrast through blurring.

Table 8.1. How to increase signal-to-noise

Increase excitations
Decrease TE
Use surface coils
Increase field of view
Decrease matrix size
Sample full echo
Reduce bandwidth
Thicker slices
Higher field strength

Table 8.2. Dependence of signal-to-noise on scan parameters

√NEX
√frequency encoding steps
√phase encoding steps
√1/√bandwidth
Pixel area
Slice thickness

To reduce the slice thickness by half decreases the signal-to-noise by half. To maintain the same signal-to-noise in this case requires doubling of the imaging time. Because of the time constraints regarding thinner slice thicknesses, this technique has been replaced in many centers by fast spin echo imaging.

The receiver bandwidth refers to the range of frequencies that are sampled in the frequency-encoded dimension and is proportional to the number of points sampled over time. The greater the range of frequencies sampled, the less the signal-to-noise obtainable at any one frequency. Therefore, as bandwidth increases signal-to-noise decreases by a factor of the square root of the reciprocal of the bandwidth ($\sqrt{1/\text{bandwith}}$) Decreasing the bandwidth to increase the signal-to-noise decreases the resolution. Increasing the field strength of the magnet generally increases the signal-to-noise (all other things being equal).

Fast Spin Echo Imaging

The principles of this technique are covered in many technical articles beyond the scope of this chapter (Hennig and Friedburg 1988; Hennig et al. 1986; Listerud et al. 1992; Melki et al. 1991). However, there is a minimal amount of knowledge of the physical principles required to understand the relevance of this pulse sequence with respect to MS. K-space is where the raw data of spatially-encoded MR signals, collected during the application of the frequency-encoding gradient, are placed. Each point in k-space contributes to the entire image. In conventional spin echo images, one "line" of k-space is encoded per TR interval. One line of k-space is acquired per echo, and for each line of k-space the phase-encoding gradient amplitude is incremented. The central lines of k-space are responsible for the majority of signal in the image, whereas the outer lines of k-space are responsible for the spatial resolution. In conventional spin echo MR, phase-encoding would be repeated 128 or 256 (size of the matrix, i.e. number of phase encodings) times per TR interval to fill k-space. This results in significant time being required to complete the scan, taking approximately 9–12 minutes for a conventional T2-weighted scan. With fast spin echo (FSE) imaging, the phase-encoding gradient is incremented from two to 16 or more times per TR interval. Multiple different phase encodings are performed per TR and multiple echoes per TR are acquired. Thus, instead of one line of k-space per TR interval, from two to 16 or more lines of k-space per TR are encoded. Therefore, if we performed a scan with a 256 matrix and had 16 phase-encoding steps per TR, we would only need 16 repetitions (256/16 rather than 256 repetitions). The number of echoes applied per TR is called the echo train length and the time between each echo is called the echo space.

The acquisition of multiple lines of k-space per TR has some very important effects. Since all the echoes during a TR interval contribute to the signal instead of an echo time (TE) we have the combination of these echoes termed an effective TE. Here the effective TE is determined by which echo has the lowest phase-encoding gradient (central line of k-space). Although the image may look similar to a proton density or T-2 weighted image there are contributions from other echoes in the image. The variation of TE throughout the scan can theoretically produce signal loss because of broadening of the point spread function with blurring and of contrast for small lesions (Constable and Gore 1992). Reduction in echo loss spacing and echo train length can decrease this problem because this minimizes the discontinuities in T2 attenuation. Blurring is also maximal for short effective TE sequences because there are the greatest changes in signal (in the beginning of the T2 decay curve), i.e. maximal discontinuity (steepest portion of the T2 decay curve) and this is encoded in central k-space (lowest order spatial frequencies). Furthermore, the late echoes, placed at the periphery of k-space, have the greatest signal loss (i.e. from the flattest portion of the T2 decay curve) but the outer region of k-space is also responsible for resolution. Hence, there is some loss of resolution, which may also relate to marginal lesion blur (Norbash et al. 1992). Conversely, for a long TE image, central k-space is composed of late echos and the high spatial frequencies contain early echoes producing edge enhancement (Norbash et al. 1992). For MS, in most cases, we want to obtain dual echo images with both short and long effective TEs so that cerebrospinal fluid (CSF) is dark and the lesion is bright (short TE), and the CSF and the lesion are both bright (long TE). This is useful in many computer quantitation programs. To obtain a short effective TE image, short echo train lengths are recommended (Constable and Gore 1992). The above arguments were tested and FSE and conventional spin echo images produced quantitatively equivalent images with respect to the detection of high intensity lesions (Norbash et al. 1992).

Another less important issue in MS patients is the reduction in detecting magnetic susceptibility differences (i.e. hemorrhagic lesions). This is the result of multiple 180° refocusing pulses reducing signal loss from diffusion.

There are, however, two important advantages for the FSE sequence that are relevant to MS. The first involves the ability to produce thinner contiguous imaging sections with high signal-to-noise and contrast-to-noise in times comparable to thicker section spin echo images. This is important because thinner sections decrease volume averaging. This problem limits the accuracy of lesion determinations. The second benefit of FSE images is the magnetization transfer effect from the multiple 180° pulses per slice. This may increase the conspicuity between lesions with myelin loss and normal brain. Thus, the FSE sequence appears to be a better choice than spin echo imaging for lesion quantitation studies.

Fluid-Attenuated Inversion Recovery Imaging

The fluid-attenuated inversion recovery (FLAIR) technique is a recently introduced pulse sequence that yields heavily T2-weighted images in which CSF is nulled (De Coene et al. 1992). The technique couples an inversion pulse with a long inversion time (TI) to a long echo time (TE) readout. FLAIR images have the ability to increase the conspicuity of lesions that are at the interface between the brain and the CSF. Cortical/subcortical lesions are generally difficult to visualize with conventional spin echo imaging because of the lack of conspicuity between high intensity cortex and high intensity CSF. This is also true for periventricular lesions and adjacent brain (Figure 8.1). This methodology is

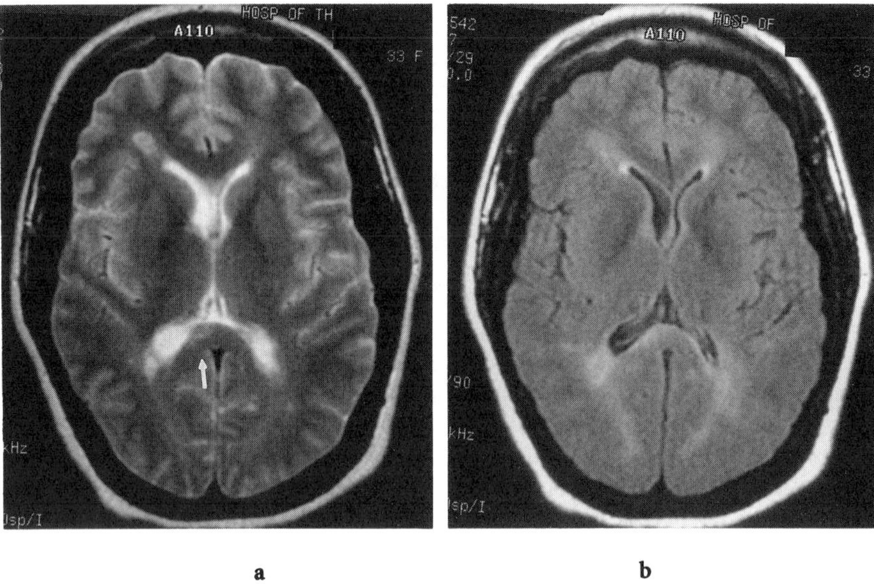

Figure 8.1. FLAIR images. (a) T2-weighted fast spin echo image demonstrating periventricular high intensity lesions. Note the subtle high intensity in the splenium of the corpus callosum (arrow). (b) FLAIR image revealing greater conspicuity of lesions in the periventricular region and in the splenium of the corpus callosum.

potentially useful for MS, as it increases the number of lesions visualized (De Coene et al. 1993; White et al. 1992). However, as initially reported, this technique required long imaging times (13 minutes as originally reported) because of the long TIs and repetition times (TRs) to null CSF and produce T2-weighted images. To speed up this process the inverting pulse can be combined with an FSE pulse sequence, termed fast FLAIR, and can perform 36 slices of 5 mm thickness in just over 5 minutes (Rydberg et al. 1994). This sequence demonstrated improved lesion detectability, lesion conspicuity and lesion to CSF contrast compared with conventional spin echo imaging (Rydberg et al. 1994). Is this technique the ideal for MS lesions? The answer is yes and no! The positive aspects of the technique are enumerated above. Additionally, when using an FSE sequence, there is the additonal magnetization transfer effect.

This methodology has particular utility in single studies to investigate the presence of MS lesions. Fast FLAIR imaging would be useful for studies determining whether or not patients presenting with optic neuritis or brainstem lesions have additional asymptomatic lesions. It adds sensitivity when compared with conventional spin echo images in determining the lesion load a patient may possess.

The major drawback of the technique involves its use in lesion quantitation programs. Unfortunately, there are regions of the brain that are normal, but present as high intensity areas on FLAIR images. These include the posterior limb of the internal capsule and cerebellar white matter, as well as in the parietopontine tract. The high signal from the white matter is the result of less attenuation of signal from unmyelinated or sparsely myelinated fibers (secondary to susceptibility differences produced by myelin) to a greater extent than one or more long T2 components associated with unmyelinated or sparsely myelinated fibers (Hajnal et al. 1992). A computer program for lesion quantitation could not easily separate out those normal high intensity regions from lesions. That is not to say a set of rules could not be written for such a program to exclude these regions, but the complications of such an approach detract from its easy implementation. The bottom line is that at this time FLAIR appears to be a very sensitive pulse sequence for MS but it would be difficult to implement for volumetric quantitation.

The evolution of pulse sequences and imaging methodology indicates the relativity of the term normal "appearing white matter". As our knowledge progresses, this notion needs to be refined, since it is dependent on our techniques. Clearly, when performing a longitudinal study, all pulse sequences need to be fixed. Apples must be compared with apples. Equally important is the goal of the study. Thus, if one were interested in having the most sensitive method for MS lesion detection to determine which patient would enter a prospective treatment protocol based upon number of lesions, then a FLAIR sequence might be quite useful. If, on the other hand, the goal was to assess the efficacy of a particular treatment protocol as it affects lesion volume, then one would more likely choose an FSE pulse sequence without FLAIR because of the high intensity normal brain that presents a complicated computer volumetric problem.

Techniques to Increase Lesion Specificity and Lesion Quantitation

We have just described the relationships of imaging parameters and have focused on the strengths and weaknesses of certain common pulse sequences. We will now focus on the methods that help to refine our knowledge and increase our specificity with respect to MS. This is the most exciting part of research in MS. With the increasing sophistication of our probes, the possibility of better understanding of the disease process is improved.

Enhancement in Multiple Sclerosis

The concept of the blood-brain barrier (BBB) dates back to the nineteenth century, when the noted bacteriologist, Paul Ehrlich observed that intravenous dyes stained all the organs of an animal except the brain. The BBB is responsible for the lack of significant enhancement in the normal brain parenchyma following contrast injection. Alterations of the BBB result in parenchymal contrast enhancement. This is a non-specific phenomenon. Any alteration of the BBB, such as inflammation, infection or trauma, can render intraparenchymal tissue susceptible to contrast enhancement. Factors determining the degree of enhancement include the intravascular concentration of contrast, the interval between injection and imaging, the delivery of the contrast material to the region of the brain and the permeability of the lesion area, as well as the particulars related to imaging sequence (e.g. use of a preparatory magnetization transfer pulse, the pulse sequence used to detect enhancement, etc.), (Kermode et al. 1990; Larsson and Tofts 1992).

MS lesions enhance following injection of contrast media because of a transient abnormality in the BBB produced by a perivenous inflammatory process. On MR, enhancement is traditionally and best observed on the so-called T1-weighted (short TR) image. From serial MR studies we have learned that MS lesions are dynamic, but both active and inactive (non-enhancing) lesions may change over time (Grossman et al. 1988). Histopathologically active lesions, characterized by the degree of macrophage infiltration, have been correlated with contrast enhancement (Katz et al. 1990; Nesbit et al. 1991). In approximately 78% of MS patients with acute relapses it was noted that gadolinium (Gd) enhancement of specific lesions disappeared within 3–5 weeks and no enhancement was observed of any lesion for more than 6 months (Miller et al. 1988). It has also been suggested that Gd enhancement may precede high intensity changes on T2-weighted images (Kermode et al. 1988, 1990). Thus, enhancement, one marker of a particular abnormality (the BBB) that is transiently abnormal in MS patients, is widely accepted as a surrogate measure of disease activity.

Enhancement has been observed to be more sensitive in detecting disease-related "activity" than changes in lesion size on T2-weighted images and may, when combined with quantitative T2 measures, increase the statistical power of a study (Miller et al. 1993). Does the absence of enhancement suggest inactivity? The answer is definitely not! Lesions may appear or change in size without enhancement (Grossman et al. 1986; Wong et al. 1994). Additionally, there appear to be differences in the patterns of enhancement between groups of clinically classified MS patients (benign and early relapsing–remitting MS) (Thompson et al. 1992). In early relapsing–remitting MS, the majority of new lesions demonstrated enhancement, whereas only one-third of new lesions in the benign group enhanced (Thompson et al. 1992). Chronically progressive patients subdivided into primary progressive and secondary progressive groups were reported to have different enhancement patterns (Thompson et al. 1991). Over a 6-month interval, those patients with primary progressive disease displayed enhancement in 5% of new lesions, whereas secondary progressive patients displayed enhancement in 87% of their new lesions. These results suggested a difference in the inflammatory nature of the lesions and were thought to be important in the selection of patients and the monitoring of disease activity in therapeutic trials.

Clearly, enhancement is a transient phenomenon, and cannot describe the full biologic activity of the disease process in MS. Conceptually, the range of histopathologic disease activity is much greater than can be attributed directly to alterations of the BBB. The precise relationship of the BBB abnormality and the disease course is not well understood. It has been regarded as a primary problem by some investigators, but may also be viewed as an epiphenomen

(Miller et al. 1988). There is no doubt that it is important to quantitate enhancement (Frank et al. 1994). Both the number of enhancing lesions and the enhanced volume can be reliably monitored (Simon et al. 1995). There are some lesions (particularly in the cortex) that may only be detected with contrast (Barkhof et al. 1991). What has not been established is the predictive validity of imaging changes as they relate to traditional clinically-based outcome measures. If one could prove that a particular therapy can suppress enhancement on a long-term basis and that this suppression can translate into a measurable clinical outcome effect, then measurements of enhancement could be proffered as a cost-effective measure of response to therapy. Recent work suggests the high incidence and relative stability of measurements of enhancement, suggesting that therapeutic effects can be detected by an annual MR scan (Simon et al. 1995). There are data that reveal a trend between enhancement and clinical disease but this has not been correlated with long-term prognosis (Smith et al. 1993). Newly enhancing lesions may occur without clinical worsening (Capra et al. 1992; Harris et al. 1991). Steroids can clearly suppress the BBB abnormalities in MS and decrease the number of enhancing lesions. Indeed, it has been reported that, after treatment with methylprednisolone, there was a dissociation between the number of enhancing lesions and the number of lesions on T2-weighted images (Barkhof et al. 1991), yet few would argue that steroids favorably influence the long-term outcome of MS (Compston 1988; Menken 1989). The debate is not whether to monitor enhancement; it is one visible marker that should be studied. Rather, the question is in what context should the results be interpreted and, more importantly, what other markers should be studied?

Concept of Disease Activity

Disease-related activity, as measured by MR, is a complex issue. New lesions, Gd enhancement and enlarging lesions have all been cited as potential measures of lesion activity (Goodkin et al. 1992). Pitfalls are associated with each of these measures and their derivatives, including total T2-weighted and enhanced lesion number and volume (area).

Reliable measurement of lesion size can be compromised by measurement error. This is particularly problematic for lesions smaller than 0.6 cm^2 in which the coefficient of variation of measurement may be as high as 23% (Goodkin et al. 1992). The detection of a new lesion is based upon the assumption that the lesion was not present on a previous MR. This necessitates that the precise location be evaluated on serial images. Attempting to fix head position by perpendicular scout images does not prevent subtle changes in brain position. To do serial comparisons in a scientific manner demands a reliable registration program. Eyeballing two MRs performed at different times is fine for clinical work, but is neither reliable nor reproducible for use in scientific investigation. This is also the case when assessing lesion enlargement. Unless a validated registration program is utilized, small positional changes can produce results that are attributable to measurement error instead of biologic activity. Lesions can "grow" or "shrink" because the observer is viewing a slightly different region caused by minimal differences in scan plane. Therefore, the assessment of comparison images must be performed using such a registration program.

Measurement of enhancement is another activity marker that is associated with several potential confounding variables. Enhancement is a time-dependent phenomenon (Grossman et al. 1986). The first issue is that images performed at different times will have different enhanced volumes. This can be best appreciated in patients who have had both axial and coronal images. When the coronal images are performed after the axial images in the same patient, there may be a difference in the enhancement in a particular lesion based upon the time interval.

Secondly, a precise pulse sequence is required and, optimally, should be standardized. Not all T1-weighted sequences are the same or result in the same degree of enhancement. A goal in a multicenter trial must be that all scanners use the same or similar equipment.

Thirdly, the dose of drug to be used in the study must be considered. As one increases the Gd contrast dose from 0.1 mmol/kg to 0.5 mmol/kg, there is an increased quantity of enhancement detected. Abnormalities of the BBB are not an all or none response, but rather are a graded phenomenon. Total contrast load influences the degree and number of detected enhancing lesions. This variable must be decided and standardized before any study commences. Yet, the optimal dose for a study could be a very controversial decision. The higher the contrast dose the greater the sensitivity (i.e. degree of enhancement, number of lesions detected, and volume of enhanced lesion), and the greater the cost for this higher contrast dose. In addition, with respect to natural history, the two doses may produce different results in terms of duration of enhancement, detection of lesions and volume of enhanced lesion.

The fourth issue is the implementation of an off-resonance saturation pulse (magnetization transfer pulse) (Elster et al. 1994; Finelli et al. 1994; Mathews et al. 1994). At any contrast agent dose, imposition of a magnetization transfer pulse will be similar to increasing the contrast agent dose. Thus, an enhanced T1-weighted magnetization transfer image using a Gd dose of 0.1 mmol/kg will produce an effect almost comparable with giving 0.3 mmol/kg. It goes without saying that pulse sequence protocols must be the same, but how should they initially be constituted? Should post-Gd images be done with standard dose, double dose or triple dose, or with magnetization transfer technique or without? As we increase the sensitivity of such studies, we increase the costs and may decrease the number of centers that can participate because of hardware and software requirements to perform these studies.

The advantage of using enhancement as a marker of lesion activity is that, by one definition, anything that enhances is considered active. It is not necessary to consider the more difficult issue of whether a lesion has changed in size (Miller et al. 1993). The technique used to count the enhanced lesion must be reproducible. Automated programs to do this have had limited success because normal small blood vessels and structures such as the infundibulum, pituitary, cavernous sinuses and choroid plexus, all demonstrate enhancement. Manual lesion counting is subject to inter-reader variability. The best alternative is probably a semiautomated program which detects all the regions of enhancement and then lets the reader reject non-lesions.

In summary, disease activity data must be viewed in the context of the particular techniques utilized. Protocols should be evaluated not only by their inherent ability to detect lesion activity but also by their practical application in the context of multicenter clinical trials. It is useless to have different centers using dissimilar equipment or protocols and then pool the results with respect to activity. Measurement of enhancement is not a simple straightforward calculation. Likewise, the longitudinal comparison of lesions requires the requisite registration program. Without it, minor changes in head positioning can lead to invalid conclusions regarding activity or drug effects.

Quantitation of Lesion Burden in Multiple Sclerosis Patients

At first approximation, quantitative information is the essence of contemporary MR studies on MS. MR is uniquely positioned to image the entire brain and, using various techniques, separate normal from abnormal tissue. The issue of disease burden has been addressed by a number of investigators using a variety of different approaches. These include manual tracing of individual lesions, pixel value thresholding, histogram, linear combination, and multispectral classification or feature map partitioning techniques (Cline et al. 1990; Isaac et al. 1988; Jackson et al. 1993; Vannier et al. 1985). Two important generalizations regarding these approaches are that the more automated the technique, the lower the intra- and inter-reader variability, and the less time-consuming the process (Kikinis et al. 1992)

Certain techniques, such as grading lesion size by diameter, have proven to be too imprecise to have a place in a modern drug trial (Ormerod et al. 1987). A manual outlining technique was used in the interferon beta-1b trial (IFNB Multiple Sclerosis Study Group 1993). This trial demonstrated the power of MR to detect a treatment effect more convincingly than conventional clinically-based outcome measures. With a highly experienced individual, the intra-reader variability for determining the presence of lesions was 6%. However, the success of manual methods overall is very low because of the high inter-rater variability. Furthermore, systematic errors (for example, in this study where a 10% reduction in lesion load was found after 3 years in both treated and untreated patients) with manual methods raise significant questions concerning its reliability in clinical trials (McDonald et al. 1994).

Another issue is the stability of measurements over the long term. Evolution of a particular imaging technique or computer program presents a dilemma to the researcher. It is wonderful to make progress with such developments; however, data collected using an earlier method may be discordant. The best way to handle these issues is to adopt state-of-the-art methodology at the beginning of a study. This philosophy generally enables studies of relatively long durations that generate robust data. An alternative approach, when significant progress compels modification of methodology, is to provide a "congruence test". Old and new data must be reconciled before changes in methodology in any longitudinal study can be implemented. Furthermore, one should assume that even the slightest modification in methodology (even a change in TE from 30 ms to 20 ms) will affect results. A major technical shift, such as changes in slice width from 5 mm to 3 mm, or in pulse sequences from spin echo to FSE, will have measurable effects on data. Thus, strict adherence to imaging protocols must be guaranteed throughout the duration of the study.

Quantitative data must be reproducible. The reproducibility of the measurements are more important than their accuracy. After all, the major issues are the change from baseline measurements and the impact that a therapeutic intervention has on this change. Data must be able to be reproduced by more than one individual. All results should be subjected to rigid internal and external audits.

The use of 2-dimensional histogram analysis has been advocated as a quantitative methodology (Kikinis et al. 1992; Kohn et al. 1991). Here, the intensity on a histogram is proportional to the number of voxels with the identical intensity on proton density and T2-weighted images (Plate 8.2). The histogram provides a number of clusters, which theoretically should correspond to a distinct feature of imaged tissue (i.e. CSF, normal brain, lesion). Unfortunately, this is not invariably the case due to radiofrequency inhomogeneity, partial volume effects and other problems. However, such techniques designed to classify these clusters, using statistical methodology, can produce very good results (Mitchell et al. 1994).

Another method of segmentation of component tissue regions and lesions in MR images based upon a new theory and recently developed algorithms offers an alternative approach (Udupa and Samarasekera 1995; Udupa et al. 1994). The theory is based upon manipulation of "fuzzy connected components". An object such as the white matter region is considered to be a fuzzily connected entity, wherein every pair of voxels has a "strength of connectivity" with which it is associated. This "strength" is a global property, which determines how voxels "hang together" in a fuzzy way to form an object. The power of this new method compared with other segmentation methods comes from considering an object as a fuzzily defined, as well as a fuzzily connected, entity. For volume computation, the fractional (fuzzy) membership of voxels in tissue regions is taken into account.

This method allows for the analysis of a gradation of strengths of connectedness. In the context of MS lesions, this means that a strong fuzzy component includes mainly the core of the lesion, which will be associated with a weaker fuzzy component that extends into the periphery of the lesion. This is a more natural, realistic and accurate description of the lesion than the descriptions based on hard decisions. In a longitudinal analysis, this method allows us to scrutinize the various graded components rather than treating a lesion as a homogeneous lump. Plates 8.3a and 8.3b show the proton density and T2 images of an MS patient. Plates 8.3c–e show the "fuzzy connectivity scenes" for white matter (Plate 8.3c), gray matter (Plate 8.3d), and the ventricle (Plate 8.3e). Here, brighter values mean greater "strength of connectivity" and "hanging togetherness" for the particular material. Plate 8.3f shows the lesions detected for the first time instant superimposed on the image in Plate 8.3b. This method requires less than 1 minute per patient of operator time. It is highly reproducible, with a maximum inter- and intraoperator variability of 1.5%.

In a study of one chronic-progressive MS patient, Mitchell et al. observed considerable change in individual lesions and lesion volume over an 18-month period (Mitchell et al. 1994). This variation has also been observed by other groups (Harris et al. 1991; Isaac et al. 1988; Kappos et al. 1988; Koopmans et al. 1989; Miller et al. 1991; Thompson et al. 1990). The variation of MS lesion volume must be appreciated lest it confound interpretation of a therapeutic study. Lesion volume is clearly dynamic; thus, long-term studies are necessary to determine a true therapeutic effect.

It must also be stressed that quantitation of lesion volume does not provide a full measure of individual lesion activity. MS lesions fluctuate, with individual lesions increasing, decreasing or disappearing (Grossman et al. 1988; Harris et al. 1991; Miller et al. 1993). Lesions can display various patterns of contrast enhancement with or without changes in size (Harris et al. 1991; Miller et al. 1993). In this context, the sum of lesion activity may result in little overall net volume change over a long duration. Methodology must also seek to increase sensitivity to the contribution of individual lesions to total lesion volume and to provide new measures of individual lesion activity.

Measurement of T1 and T2 Relaxation Times

Measurement of relaxation times has been proposed as a method for increasing the sensitivity and specificity of MR (Wehrli et al. 1984). This methodology involves a computer analysis of a set of saturation recovery or inversion recovery (T1 and proton density) and multiple spin echo images (T2) to determine T1, proton density and T2 values for regions of interest (Carr–Purcell–Meiboom–Gill sequence) (Wehrli et al. 1985). Using this technique, the T2 relaxation times are markedly abnormal in MS lesions (Lacomis et al. 1986; Larsson et al. 1988; Wehrli et al. 1985). Testing the reproducibility of T2 relaxation measurements revealed a variance of up to 4% between consecutive scans, 7% across the field of view, and up to 10% longitudinally. Interinstrument variation was up to 10% (Breger et al. 1986). Another group achieved a standard deviation of 3% in T1 and T2 relaxation times (Miller et al. 1989). These variability measures are below the range variation associated with pathologic processes. However, other groups have argued that relaxation times are unable to differentiate various pathologic processes (Bottomley et al. 1987). Errors in calculated T2 relaxation times have been the result of unwanted echoes due to tip-angle imperfections at the edges of slices (Crawley and Henkelman 1987). Other sources of error include partial volume effects, the presence of flow or diffusion variations caused by magnet and radiofrequency inhomogeneity, rephasing gradient adjustment after slice selection, eddy currents and coil loading (Breger et al. 1986; Miller et al. 1989).

Calculated relaxation times have demonstrated abnormalities in normal appearing white matter (NAWM) in MS (Miller et al. 1989; Ormerod et al. 1987). It has been argued that disease burden may be better addressed if it were based on relaxation times rather than high signal on conventional T2-weighted images, because of the increased sensitivity of relaxation time measurements when compared with direct interpretation of images (Haughton et al. 1992).

In summary, calculation of relaxation times has provided increased sensitivity compared with conventional MR with respect to NAWM and lesion load. However, the reproducibility has never been tested in a large study. As noted above, there are many difficulties that investigators need to address if multicenter data are to be gathered using this methodology.

Multiexponential T2 Relaxation Analysis

Another method utilized for increasing the specificity of high intensity abnormalities in MS is analysis of the T2 decay curve (Figure 8.2). This requires multiparametric fitting of the T2 decay curve and has been proposed as a method to characterize tissue (Gersonde et al. 1985). The technique applies multiple (128, 256, etc.) 180° pulses per TR interval and produces 128 (or more) T2 images. (Carr-Purcell-Meiboom-Gill-CPMG pulse train). The T2 decay curve of each pixel can be then constructed. This curve is made up of 128 (or more) points from each 128 (or more) echo images. Such multiparametric curve fitting is thought to reflect the relative molecular compartmentalization of the protons. (i.e. water with edema, inflammation, gliosis, axonal loss and demyelination) (Mulkern et al. 1989; Rumbach et al. 1991).

Without addressing the mathematical argument regarding this analysis, one can appreciate that there are many mathematical functions that may describe the

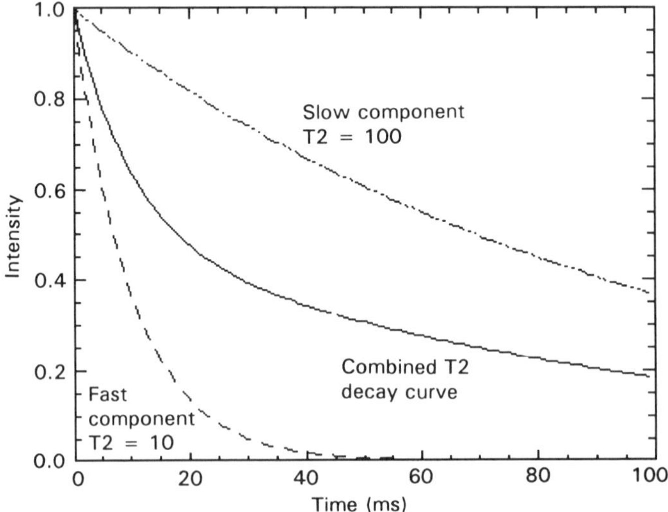

Figure 8.2. Multiexponential T2 relaxation. A hypothetical system consisting of two "compartments" having different T2 relaxation times. The upper curve depicts the relaxation of the "slow T2 relaxation" compartment while the lowest curve depicts the relaxation of the "fast T2 compartment". The combined curve (solid line) represents the observed T2 decay of this system.

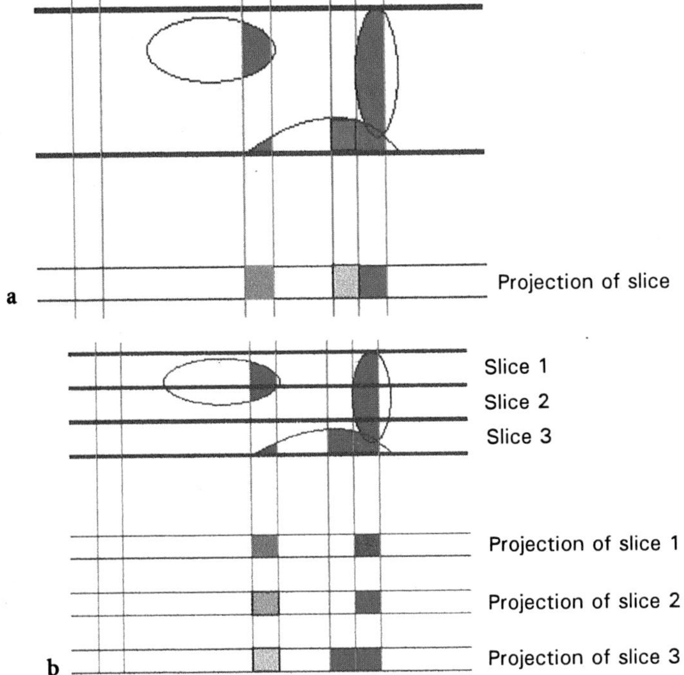

Plate 8.1. Partial volume effects. **a** With a thick slice, a structure that does not extend through the entire slice is detected at reduced intensity, compared with a structure (or combination of structures) that does extend through the slice. Here, the slice contains three structures, and the pixel boundaries (in red) define regions that are filled to greater or lesser extents by the structures. The resultant intensity (projection of slice) represents the extent to which the structure fills the sensitive area. **b** If the slab is divided into three slices, the ability to discriminate between fine structures (resolution) is enhanced.

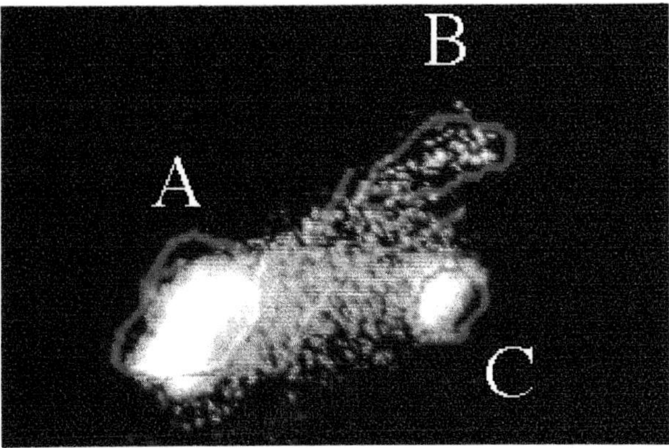

Plate 8.2. Two-dimensional histogram. The x-axis represents the intensity of each pixel on the proton-weighted image, while the y-axis represents the intensity of the pixel on the T2-weighted image. Using statistical methods, the computer has found three clusters (circles). Cluster B has high intensity on proton density and T2-weighted images, and represents those pixels corresponding to the MS lesions, while cluster A has lower intensity on T2-weighted images and represents brain. Cluster C corresponds to CSF, lower in intensity than lesion on proton density and high intensity on T2-weighted images.

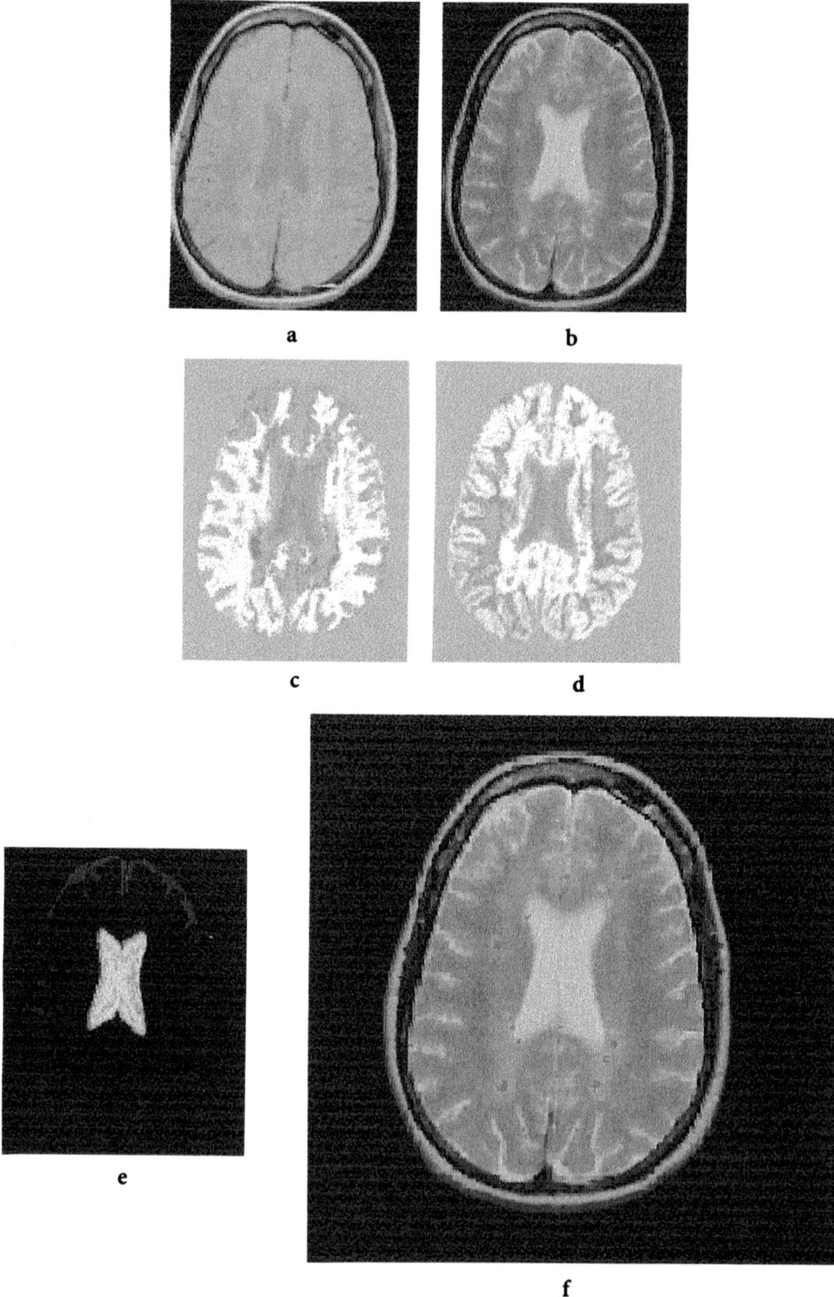

Plate 8.3. Fuzzy connectivity. a Proton density weighted image in an MS patient; b T2-weighted image at the same level in this patient; c–e Fuzzy "connectivity scenes" for white matter (c), gray matter (d) and ventricle (e). Here, brighter values mean greater "strength of connectivity" and "hanging togetherness" for the particular material. f Shows the lesion (red) detected by this method superimposed on the image in (b).

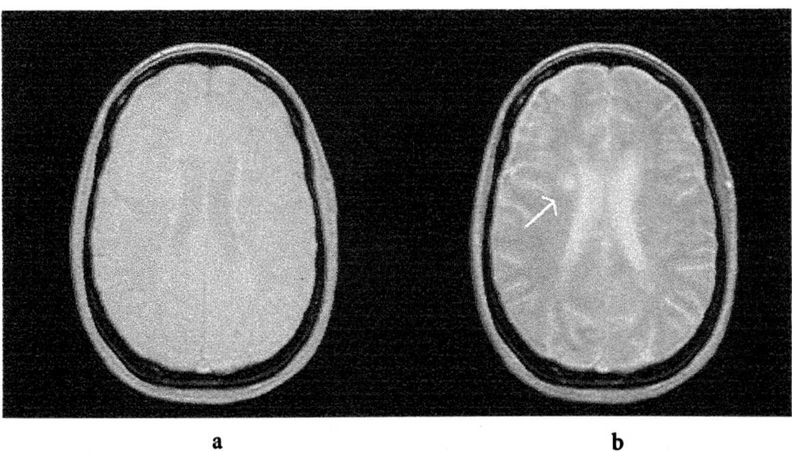

a b

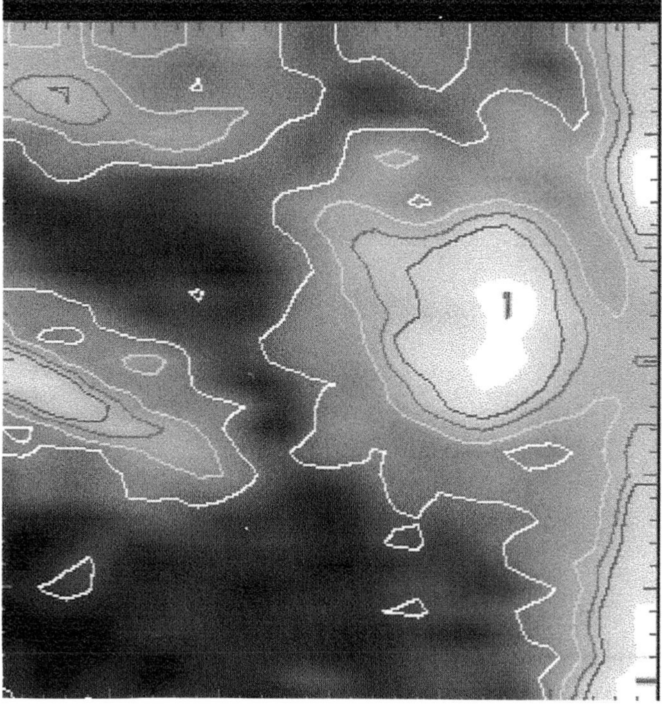

c

Plate 8.4. MTR map. MR images from a patient with MS: **a** Proton density weighted image; **b** MT weighted image: a large MS lesion is apparent on the right side adjacent to the lateral ventricle (arrow); **c** Detail of this lesion with contours of MTR (at 5% intervals).

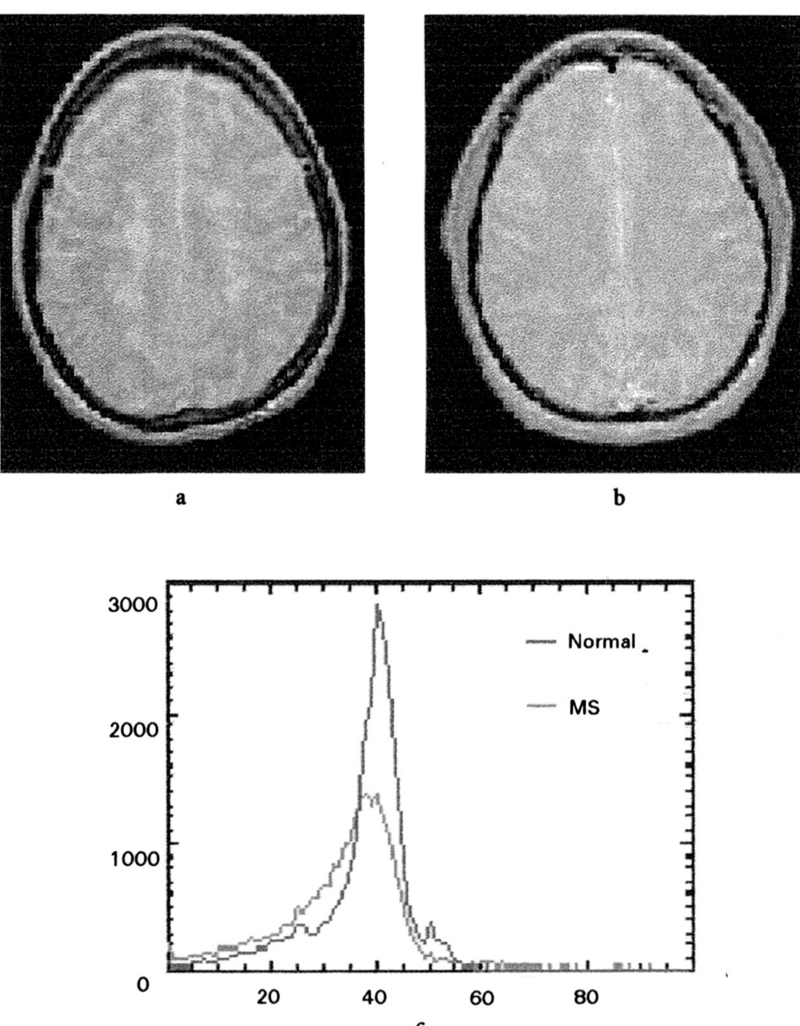

Plate 8.5. MTR histogram analysis of single brain slices in normal brain and MS: a and b are axial images with MT contrast obtained from similar locations in a patient with clinically diagnosed MS (a) and in a normal control (b). Histograms demonstrating the distribution of MTR appear in c: the MS curve is flatter and shifted to the left, consistent with overall reduced MTR and a reduced volume of tissue with normal MTR.

T2 decay curve. It may be fitted to a monoexponential, biexponential, triexponential function, etc. Statistical analysis can then determine which function best fits the particular T2 decay curve. Thus, various regions of high intensity that appear similar on a T2-weighted image may have different exponential components when studied by this technique. On a pixel by pixel basis, a particular pixel can be assigned by its relaxation time. By performing region of interest (ROI) measurements we can derive mean T2 relaxation values for particular ROIs. The T2 decay curve of normal white matter appears best to fit a monoexponential curve, whereas that of visible lesions best fits a biexponential curve.(Larsson et al. 1988). The short and long relaxation times can then be quantitated by histogram analysis. The final step, currently being investigated, is to determine if there is correlation between individual patterns of relaxation times and histopathology. Many reports have correlated various long T2 relaxation times with particular histopathology (≥300–500 ms vasogenic edema; <300 ms gliotic lesions) (Armspach et al. 1993; Rumbach et al. 1991). Such analysis can also be performed in NAWM, and has been reported to be slightly abnormal (Armspach et al. 1991).

Magnetization Transfer Techniques

Neither MR imaging alone nor with Gd is specific with respect to the pathologic substrate of the MS lesion (edema, demyelination, gliosis). A new MR imaging technique, magnetization transfer (MT) imaging, has been proposed to specify the in vivo water content and its relationship to either macromolecules or membranes of tissues and to generate a novel form of image contrast (Wolff and Balaban 1989). MT contrast is based mostly on the cross-relaxation between the immobile protons (on macromolecules such as protons in myelin membranes) and the free protons (bulk water) of tissues. MT contrast is introduced by application of an off-resonance radiofrequency (RF) pulse of sufficient power to saturate the energy level of populations of protons in immobile water. Exchange of this saturated magnetization with free water thus affects the signal intensity observed on a subsequent MR image. MT can characterize multiple sclerosis lesions so that new plaques, with mostly edema and low grade demyelination, may be distinguished from chronic, highly demyelinated or gliotic lesions (high free water states). It can detect abnormalities attributable to microscopic lesions in NAWM, as imaged by conventional MR.

MT techniques represent a means of expanding the measured parameters in an MR examination beyond proton density, T1 and T2, through exploitation of the interaction of macromolecular components with components in the aqueous phase. Derived from the chemical exchange model and modified Bloch equations of McConnell, which led to the use of the double resonance technique to investigate multicomponent chemical exchange systems, MT imaging was demonstrated in vivo by Wolff and Balaban in 1989. In their study, MT contrast was achieved through the continuous application of an RF field at a frequency several kHz removed from the resonance frequency of water. This RF irradiation was designed preferentially to saturate (i.e. hold the magnetization at or near zero) the proton spins associated with macromolecules while having little direct effect on water protons. The transfer of magnetization into the water proton pool through exchange was observed as a signal intensity decrease leading to relative hypointensity on a magnetic resonance image. The experiments of Balaban, as well as subsequent studies, confirmed that the decrease of image intensity accompanying the application of MT preparation pulses was reproducible and tissue specific, suggesting that MT provided a novel form of contrast in an MR image (Dousset et al. 1992; McGowan and Leigh 1994; McGowan et al. 1994a, b; Outwater et al. 1992).

Selective saturation is possible, due to the very short T2 (and large T1/T2 ratio) associated with the solid-like macromolecular protons. Although complete selective saturation cannot be accomplished, proper selection of experimental parameters can minimize the effect of the MT irradiation on the water protons (called the direct effect) while providing significant saturation of the macromolecular proton spins. The differential effect of off-resonance irradiation on image intensity is dependent on the relaxation parameters of both proton pools (macromolecular pool and free water proton pool) as well as the exchange rate for transfer of magnetization.

In addition to the continuous irradiation MT method, two alternative approaches have been proposed and demonstrated. Pulsed off-resonance MT is achieved through modification of a gradient-echo pulse sequence to include off-resonance RF pulses in each TR period (Dousset et al. 1992; McGowan et al. 1994a; Outwater et al. 1992). A steady-state MT effect is quickly established, as is predicted by theory and confirmed by observation (McGowan 1993). This MT method is easily incorporated into a clinical MR examination, requiring no additional hardware components, and has been found to be quite robust.

MT contrast may also be produced by so-called on-resonance saturation methods. These techniques are reminiscent of the selective saturation inversion technique of Edzes and Samulski, in which a pulse is given at the proton resonance frequency over a time period that is long compared with the T2 of the macromolecular (or bound) spins and short with respect to the T2 of the water protons (Edzes and Samulski 1977, 1978). In this way, the water proton spins may be inverted (as in the Edzes and Samulski experiment) or returned to their equilibrium position while the bound spins experience saturation. The exchange of magnetization between the macromolecular and water proton spins is observed once again as a change in the water proton signal (Hu et al. 1992). The results with this technique are apparently similar to those of the off-resonance technique, which is not unexpected as a series of on-resonance pulses transforms into the frequency domain as off-resonance irradiation. Pulsed, on-resonance MT has been applied in clinical research by several investigators (Hu et al. 1992; Pike et al. 1992; Yeung and Aisen 1992). Like the off-resonance pulsed technique, it may be implemented on many MR scanners without the use of additional hardware, but it places more stringent demands on the precision with which the RF pulses are given, as well as the main magnetic field (B_0) homogeneity, than does the off-resonance method.

Contrast in the MT image is a complicated function of the relaxation and exchange properties of the environments that influence the behavior of the protons, and therefore may be difficult to interpret. However, it is generally true that tissue appears hypointense with respect to fluid and fluid-filled spaces on MT. It has also been observed that MT contrast is similar in some cases to T2-weighted contrast, suggesting a possible link between T2 relaxation and the exchange of transverse magnetization (McGowan 1993). Thus, quantitative MT may be useful in the investigation of pathology that results in observed changes in T2.

A quantitative measure of the MT effect is obtained by acquiring two sets of MR images, one with MT saturation pulses, the other a control image without saturation pulses, but with otherwise identical acquisition parameters. This enables the calculation of the effect of the MT saturation, known as the magnetization transfer ratio (MTR), in a region of interest through the use of the following equation:

$$\mathrm{MTR} = \frac{M_0 - M_s}{M_0} \tag{1}$$

where M_0 represents the average pixel intensity in the region when the saturation pulses are off, and M_S the corresponding intensity with MT saturation. Thus, MTR represents the fractional signal loss due to the complete or partial saturation of the bound proton pool, and ranges from near zero in blood and CSF to 50% or more in tissue that contains a high proportion of poorly mobile macromolecules, such as muscle.

When the calculation described by Equation (1) is carried out on a pixel-by-pixel basis, an MTR map results, as illustrated in Plate 8.4, which shows images from the brain of a patient with multiple sclerosis. Specific MTR values calculated in regions of interest are shown on the MTR map (Plate 8.4c).

MTR has been found to be highly reproducible in studies of normal and diseased tissue, although the measured MTR is dependent upon the experimental parameters imposed. MTR may be correlated with the extent of tissue abnormality in MS lesions, offering the potential of increased sensitivity and specificity for MR studies of white matter disease or monitoring therapeutic effects in clinical trials.

As in Plate 8.5, we can perform histogram analysis of a single slice (or the whole brain) and appreciate the extent of volumetric MTR abnormality in the brain. This could be a powerful methodology for determining the efficacy of a potential treatment for MS.

Magnetic Resonance Occult Lesion

A discrepancy exists between visible (T2-weighted) lesion volumes and measurements of functional disability. This can in part be attributed to poorly characterized spinal cord disease. The pathophysiologic heterogeneity of lesions that all appear the same (high intensity) on conventional T2-weighted images may also contribute to the reported discrepancy between T2 lesion volume and disability.

In this case, certain lesions (demyelination and axonal loss) may produce significant disability, whereas inflammatory changes may be less incapacitating (Miller et al. 1996). Other factors include weak quantitation techniques and short follow-up intervals (Miller at al. 1996). Another underappreciated component is the presence of invisible or occult lesions in the NAWM, as defined by conventional MR. Neuropathologists have commonly observed microscopic regions of disease resembling acute inflammatory lesions in patients with definite MS (Raine 1991). Indeed, up to 72% of macroscopically NAWM in MS patients has been demonstrated to be abnormal on histologic study (Allen and McKeown 1979), and there is growing MR evidence that confirms the existence of a significant quantity of magnetic resonance occult lesions (MROLs) (Brainin et al. 1989; Dousset et al. 1992; Haughton et al. 1992). In a recent report, MROLs (as measured by abnormal T1 and/or T2 relaxation times) constituted approximately 50% of the total detected lesion load per slice, which appeared to vary widely from patient to patient (Barbosa et al. 1994). This feature of MS is presently less appreciated and clearly not detected by conventional MR imaging. There also exists a small group of patients with no apparent lesion burden as judged by MR, although categorized as clinically definite MS (Filippi et al. 1994; Miller et al. 1987).

MT offers the most robust methodology for quantitating MROL. It has recently been reported that white matter in nine healthy volunteers had an average calculated MTR value of 42.93 ± 0.73%, ranging from 41.62 to 44.50, while the NAWM in the 23 patients with MS had an average calculated MTR value of 40.13 ± 1.5% and ranged from 36.31 to 42.09. When analyzed statistically, the difference in average MTR between normals and MS patients was significant with $P < 0.0001$ (Loevner et al. 1994).

In addition to being a possible explanation for the poor correlations between volumetric analysis and clinical measurements, changes in MROLs may also be an important factor to monitor during therapeutic drug trials. If MS lesions arise from MROLs, then therapeutic efficacy studies should also be targeted at assessing the effect of drugs on this component of MS lesions. There is no question that MROLs are important to quantitate. This new information will be additive to standard T2 disease burden measurements and provide a more accurate measurement of true lesion burden currently not obtained with conventional MR.

Proton Magnetic Resonance Spectroscopy in Multiple Sclerosis

Another technique that may provide biochemical information about MS lesions is proton magnetic resonance spectroscopy (1H MRS) (Figure 8.3). This probe enables the investigator to characterize the biochemical constituents of individual lesions and their evaluation, or interrogate large regions of the brain for biochemical abnormalities. There has been considerable progress with regard to the smallest voxel volumes that can be interrogated by 1H MRS, so that volumes of less than 1 cm^3 are easily attainable. Unfortunately, there remain differences in the data reported in the literature. This may be the result of the heterogeneous nature of the disease or the fact that the spectral data have been acquired with different pulse sequences, localization methods and echo delays.

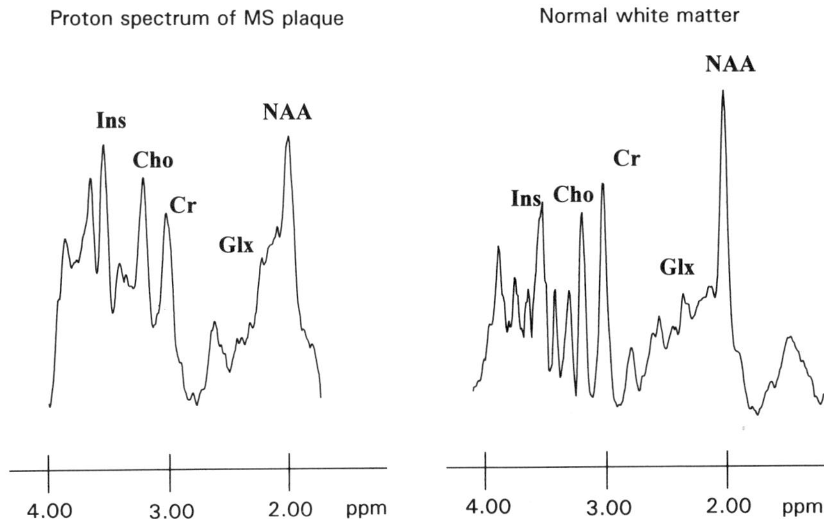

Figure 8.3. ^{1}H spectroscopy. A representative proton spectrum from an MS plaque and comparision with normal white matter. There are increases in the Ins and Cho peaks, and a decrease in the NAA peak compared with the normal white matter. Ins: inositol; Cho: choline; Cr: creatine; Glx: glutamine, glutamate, GABA; NAA: *N*-acetyl aspartate.

Narayana et al. used ^{1}H MRS to study MS lesions and found resonances consistent with the presence of cholesterol and/or fatty acids in some lesions (Narayana et al. 1991). Some of these resonances disappeared after 2 weeks, perhaps indicating that demyelination could be monitored based on changing levels of cholesterol and/or fatty acids. Narayana later studied patients with lesions that enhanced after injection of Gd-DTPA, and observed prominent resonances in the 0.5–2.0 ppm region in six of nine enhancing lesions (Narayana et al. 1992). They speculated that these resonances arose in lipids and other myelin breakdown products. In their cohort of enhancing lesions, there was no significant decrease in *N*-acetyl asparate (NAA), a putative marker of neuronal structural integrity.

Arnold et al. examined seven patients with MS and noted that in three patients with moderate to severe chronic disability, the NAA/creatine (Cr) ratio was lower (1.6–2.0) than observed in normals (2.4–2.9) (Arnold et al. 1990). In three of four patients with minimal or no disability, the NAA/Cr ratio was normal. No lipid resonances (putative markers of acute myelin breakdown) were observed in any of the patients studied. The authors attributed the decrease in the NAA/Cr ratio to cumulative irreversible neuronal damage rather than a response to acute inflammation. Based on these results, the authors suggested that: in hyperacute plaques, the NAA/Cr ratios would be unchanged; demyelinating plaques would exhibit increased choline (Cho)/Cr ratio, since choline is a putative marker of myelin breakdown; and subacute to chronic plaques would have decreased NAA/Cr ratios. The same authors employed MRS in a longitudinal study with examinations performed every 6 months (Arnold et al. 1994). Initially the NAA/Cr ratio was lower than normal in the MS patients as compared with controls. This ratio decreased in subsequent studies but neither the MR lesion volume nor the disability scores changed significantly. The changes in NAA/Cr between successive 6-month intervals showed a significant correlation with lesion volume in the relapsing patients. Van Hecke et al. noted a significant reduction in NAA relative to normals (Van Hecke et al. 1991). Larsson et al. reported that resonances corresponding to free lipids were observed as early as day 10 and as late as 1 year after occurrence of the plaques (Larsson et al. 1991). The relative concentration of NAA was significantly lower in patients than in controls, and the relative concentration of Cho was significantly higher in patients than in controls. The authors suggested that these differences were most pronounced in older plaques. MR spectroscopic demonstration of elevations in Cho/Cr and lipid marker peaks in an MS plaque probably reflects disintegration of myelin, and a decreased NAA/Cho ratio may be related either to gliosis or to axonal degeneration, which sometimes occurs in longstanding MS.

Husted et al. used both 1H and 31P (phosphorous) MRS and reported that the metabolite ratio NAA/Cr and the total ^{31}P peak integrals were significantly reduced compared with controls (Husted et al. 1994). In addition, in MS lesions NAA/Cho and phosphodiesters/total ^{31}P were significantly reduced compared with controls, and in MS NAWM imaged with conventional MR there was a trend for NAA/Cho to be reduced compared with controls. In the NAWM of patients with MS, the total Cr and phosphocreatine (PCr) were significantly increased compared with controls, as detected with both 1H (total Cr peak integrals) and ^{31}P (PCr/total ^{31}P) MRS. These results suggest reduced neuronal density and altered phospholipid metabolites in white matter lesions in MS.

Grossman et al. demonstrated decreased levels of NAA, but no correlation was found between NAA concentration and degree of enhancement with Gd-DTPA (Grossman et al. 1992). Extra peaks were observed between 2.1 ppm and 2.6 ppm, ranging in concentration from 10 to 50 mm protons. This region corresponds to areas of known amino acid resonance, including GABA and glutamate. As these peaks were observed in five of seven enhancing lesions and an enhancement is thought to correlate with lesion activity, the authors termed these peaks, "marker peaks", representing possible markers of demyelination.

What can be seen from the preceding review of MRS reports on MS is that there is a great deal of diversity regarding the findings in MS. As a probe of individual lesions 1H MRS has the potential to yield very interesting information. For instance, lesions interrogated before and after a particular therapeutic regimen can provide infomation on the biochemical changes that the drug can produce and may furnish the earliest evidence regarding efficacy. It is also true that NAA can suggest early evidence of neuronal loss, and perhaps irreversibility of lesions. MRS must be combined with lesion registration for precise longitudinal data. MRS has clear promise, offering biochemical insights not obtainable by any other method.

Spinal Cord Lesions in Multiple Sclerosis

There have been a number of reports in which MR has been utilized to examine lesions in the spinal cords of patients with MS (Maravilla et al. 1984; Miller et al. 1987; Nilsson et al. 1987; Thomas et al. 1993; Turano et al. 1991; Uldry et al. 1993; Wiebe et al. 1992). Many investigators attribute the lack of correlation between the Kurtzke Expanded Disability Status Scale (EDSS) and quantitative lesion burden to spinal cord diseases (Honig and Sheremata 1989; McDonald 1992). One recent study reported a lack of correlation between cord lesions and disability but did observe a relationship between cord atrophy and disability (Kidd et al. 1993). This excellent work did not, however, use a computerized volumetric program, a problem which the authors acknowledge might have provided a more reliable assessment of spinal cord lesion load. Others have reported good correspondence between spinal cord lesions and the presence of motor tract signs (Papadopoulos et al. 1994). However, there has been no longitudinal study correlating spinal cord lesion burden with clinical measurements (including Kurtzke EDSS) and/or brain lesion burden. Spinal cord lesion quantitation is important because: it represents a proportion of tissue affected by MS but presently not taken into account with brain lesion burden measurements; it may be a major factor in disability in some MS patients; a disproportionately small number of lesions can produce a profound effect; and, in some cases, only the spinal cord may be affected in patients with MS.

The Bottom Line

MR is critical to the understanding of MS. In the present era, any therapeutic assessment should optimally present MR data. No one MR protocol will provide all the answers. There will be drugs that have utility demonstrated with any one or a combination of techniques described in this chapter. Protocol development should focus on preliminary experimental data suggesting the role a particular drug or drugs may play. If a drug produces remyelination, then 1H and MT might be extremely useful markers. If a technique is noted to stabilize the BBB, then enhancement and T2 lesion burden might be important markers. As stated earlier, the greater the number of MR probes utilized the higher the probability of detecting an effect. A recent Task Force of the US National MS Society concluded that monthly T2-weighted and enhanced MR could potentially serve as a primary endpoint for short trials of new agents; however, the primary endpoint in a definitive trial is still clinical outcome (Miller et al. 1996).

It goes without saying that imaging protocols must be rigidly followed. Reliable quantitation techniques will have low intra- and inter-reader variability, providing precise results and enabling internal and external auditing.

MR ushered in a new and exciting era with dramatic improvement in detection of MS lesions in the brain and spinal cord. Researchers have moved from the descriptive qualitative aspects of MR to more robust quantitative techniques. These methodologies promise to recognize therapeutic effects more rapidly, and (when performed in well controlled studies) for less costs than those completed in the past. Advances in drug therapy combined with modern MR and state-of-the-art computer programs generate an optimistic vision for future controlled clinical trials in MS.

References

Allen I and McKeown S (1979) A histological histochemical and biochemical study of the macroscopically normal white matter in multiple sclerosis. J Neurol Sci 41:81–91

Armspach J P, Gounot D, Rumbach L et al. (1991) In vivo determination of multiexponential T2 relaxation in the brain of patients with multiple sclerosis. Magn Reson Imaging 9:107–113

Armspach JP, Gounot D, Namer IJ et al. (1993) Quantitative cerebral magnetic resonance imaging during ACTH treatment of multiple sclerosis. Magn Reson Imaging, 11:1147–1153

Arnold DL, Matthews PM, Francis G et al. (1990) Proton magnetic resonance spectroscopy of human brain in vivo in the evaluation of multiple sclerosis: assessment of the load of disease. Magn Reson Med 14:154–159

Arnold DL, Riess GT, Matthews PM et al. (1994) Use of proton magnetic resonance spectroscopy for monitoring disease progression in multiple sclerosis. Ann Neurol 36:76–82

Barbosa S, Blumhardt LD, Roberts N et al. (1994) Magnetic resonance relaxation time mapping in multiple sclerosis: normal appearing white matter and the invisible lesion load. Magn Reson Imaging 12:33–42

Barkhof F, Hommes OR, Scheltens P et al. (1991) Quantitative MRI changes in gadolinium-DTPA enhancement after high-dose intravenous methylprednisolone in multiple sclerosis. Neurology 41:1219–1222

Baum K, Nehrig C, Schorner W et al. (1990) Long-term follow-up of MS: disease activity detected clinically and by MRI. Acta Neurol Scand 82:191–196

Bottomley PA, Hardy CJ, Argersinger RE et al. (1987) A review of 1H nuclear magnetic resonance in pathology: are T1 and T2 diagnostic? Med Phys 14:425–448

Bradley WG, Glenn BJ (1987) The effect of variation in slice thickness and interslice gap on MR lesion detection. AJNR Am J Neuroradiol 8:1057–1062

Brainin M, Reisner T, Neuhold A et al. (1989) Involvement of apparently normal white brain substance in the disease process of multiple sclerosis [Ger]. Nervenarzt 60:159–162

Breger R, Wehrli F, Charles H et al. (1986) Reproducibility of relaxation and spin-density parameters in phantoms and the human brain measured by MR imaging at 1.5 T. Magn Reson Med 3:649–662

Capra R, Marciano N, Vignolo L A et al. (1992) Gadolinium-pentetic acid magnetic resonance imaging in patients with relapsing remitting multiple sclerosis. Arch Neurol 49:687–689

Chung H-W, Wehrli F, Williams J et al. (1995) Quantitative analysis of trabecular microstructure by 400 Mhz nuclear magnetic resonance imaging. J Bone Miner Res 10:803–811

Cline HE, Lorensen WE, Kikinis R et al. (1990) Three-dimensional segmentation of MR images of the head using probability and connectivity. J Comput Assist Tomogr 14:1037–1045

Compston A (1988) Methylprednisolone and multiple sclerosis. Arch Neurol 45:669–670

Constable R, Gore J (1992) The loss of small objects in variable TE imaging: implications for FSE, RARE, and EPI. Mag Reson Med 28:9–24

Crawley A, Henkelman R (1987) Errors in T2 estimation using multislice multiple-echo imaging. Magn Reson Med 4:34–47

De Coene B, Hajnal JV, Gatehouse P et al. (1992) MR of the brain using fluid-attenuated inversion recovery (FLAIR) pulse sequences. AJNR Am J Neuroradiol 13:1555–1564

De Coene B, Hajnal JV, Pennock JM et al. (1993) MRI of the brain stem using fluid attenuated inversion recovery pulse sequences. Neuroradiology 35:327–331

Dousset V, Grossman RI, Ramer KN et al. (1992) Experimental allergic encephalomyelitis and multiple sclerosis: lesion characterization with magnetization transfer imaging [published erratum appears in Radiology 1992;183:878]. Radiology 182:483–491

Edzes HT, Samulski ET (1977) Cross relaxation and spin diffusion in the proton NMR of hydrated collagen. Nature 265:521–523

Edzes HT, Samulski ET (1978) The measurement of cross-relaxation effects in the proton NMR spin-lattice relaxation of water in biological systems: hydrated collagen and muscle. J Magn

Reson 31:207–229

Elster A, King J, Matthews V et al. (1994) Cranial tissues: appearance at gadolinium-enhanced and nonenhanced MR imaging with magnetization transfer contrast. Radiology 190:541–546

Filippi M, Horsfield MA, Morrissey S P et al. (1994) Quantitative brain MRI lesion load predicts the course of clinically isolated syndromes suggestive of multiple sclerosis. Neurology 44:635–641

Finelli D, Hurst GC, Gullapali RP, Bellon EM (1994) Improved contrast of enhancing brain lesions on postgadolinium, T1-weighted spin-echo images with use of magnetization transfer. Radiology 190:553–559

Forsen S, Hoffman R (1963a) A new method for the study of moderately rapid chemical exchange rates employing nuclear magnetic double resonance. Acta Chem Scand 17:1787–1788

Forsen S, Hoffman R (1963b) Study of moderately rapid chemical exchange reactions by means of nuclear magnetic double resonance. J Chem Phys 39:2892–2901

Forsen S, Hoffman R (1964) Exchange rates by nuclear magnetic multiple resonance: III. Exchange reactions in systems with several nonequivalent sites. J Chem Phys 40:1189–1196

Frank JA, Stone LA, Smith ME et al. (1994) Serial contrast-enhanced magnetic resonance imaging in patients with early relapsing-remitting multiple sclerosis: implication for treatment trials. Ann Neurol 36:S86–S90

Gersonde K, Tolxdorff T. Felsberg L (1985) Identification and characterization of tissues by T2-selective whole-body proton NMR imaging. Magn Reson Med 2:390–401

Goodkin DE, Ross JS, Medendorp SV et al. (1992) Magnetic resonance imaging lesion enlargement in multiple sclerosis. disease-related activity, chance occurrence, or measurement artifact? Arch Neurol 49:261–263

Grossman RI, Gonzales-Scarano F, Atlas SW et al. (1986) Multiple sclerosis: gadolinium enhancement in MR imaging. Radiology 161:721–725

Grossman RI, Braffman BH, Brorson JR et al. (1988) Multiple sclerosis: serial study of gadolinium-enhanced MR imaging. Radiology 169:117–122

Grossman RI, Lenkinski RE, Ramer KN et al. (1992) MR proton spectroscopy in multiple sclerosis. AJNR Am J Neuroradiol 13:1535–1543

Hajnal J, De Coene B, Lewis P et al. (1992) High signal regions in normal white matter shown by heavily T2-weighted CSF nulled IR sequences. J Comput Assist Tomogr 16:506–513

Harris JO, Frank JA, Patronas N et al. (1991) Serial gadolinium-enhanced magnetic resonance imaging scans in patients with early, relapsing-remitting multiple sclerosis: implications for clinical trials and natural history. Ann Neurol 29:548–555

Haughton VM, Yetkin FZ, Rao SM et al. (1992) Quantitative MR in the diagnosis of multiple sclerosis. Magn Reson Med 26:71–78

Hennig J, Friedburg H (1988) Clinical applications and methodological developments of RARE technique. Magn Reson Imaging 6:391–395

Hennig J, Nauerth A, Friedburg H (1986) RARE imaging: a fast imaging method for clinical MR. Magn Reson Med 78:823–833

Honig LS, Sheremata WA (1989) Magnetic resonance imaging of spinal cord lesions in multiple sclerosis. J Neurol Neurosurg Psychiatry 52:459–466

Hu BS, Conolly SM, Wright GA et al. (1992) Pulsed saturation transfer contrast. Magn Reson Med 26:231–240

Huber SJ, Paulson GW, Chakeres D et al. (1988) Magnetic resonance imaging and clinical correlations in multiple sclerosis. J Neurol Sci 86:1–12

Husted CA, Goodin DS, Hugg JW et al. (1994) Biochemical alterations in multiple sclerosis lesions and normal-appearing white matter detected by in vivo 31P and 1H spectroscopic imaging. Ann Neurol 36:157–165

IFNB Multiple Sclerosis Study Group (1993) Interferon beta-1b is effective in relapsing-remitting multiple sclerosis: I. Clinical results of a multicenter, randomized, double-blind, placebo-controlled trial. Neurology 43:655–661

Isaac C, Li DK, Genton M et al. (1988) Multiple sclerosis: a serial study using MRI in relapsing patients. Neurology 38:1511–1515

Jackson EF, Narayana PA, Wolinsky JS et al. (1993) Accuracy and reproducibility in volumetric analysis of multiple sclerosis lesions. J Comput Assist Tomogr 17:200–205

Kappos L, Stadt D, Ratzka M et al. (1988) Magnetic resonance imaging in the evaluation of treatment in multiple sclerosis. Neuroradiology 30:299–302

Katz D, Taubenberger J, Raine C et al. (1990) Gadolinium-enhancing lesions on magnetic resonance imaging: neuropathological findings. Ann Neurol 28:243

Kermode AG, Tofts PS, MacManus DG et al. (1988) Early lesion of multiple sclerosis [letter]. Lancet ii:1203–1204

Kermode AG, Tofts PS, Thompson AJ et al. (1990) Heterogeneity of blood-brain barrier changes in multiple sclerosis: an MRI study with gadolinium-DTPA enhancement. Neurology 40:229–235

Kidd D, Thorpe JW, Thompson AJ et al. (1993) Spinal cord MRI using multiarray coils and fast spin echo: II. Findings in multiple sclerosis. Neurology 43:2632–2637

Kikinis R, Shenton M, Jolesz F et al. (1992) Routine quantitative MRI-based analysis of brain and fluid spaces. J Magn Reson Imaging 2:619–629

Kohn M, Tanna N, Herman G (1991) Analysis of brain and cerebrospinal fluid volumes with MR imaging. Radiology 178:115–122

Koopmans RA, Li DK, Oger JJ et al. (1989) Chronic progressive multiple sclerosis: serial magnetic resonance brain imaging over six months. Ann Neurol 26:248–256

Lacomis D, Oabakken M, Gross G (1986) Spin lattice relaxation (T1) times of cerebral white matter in multiple sclerosis. Magn Reson Med 3:194–202

Larsson H, Tofts P (1992) Measurement of blood-brain barrier permeability using dynamic Gd-DTPA scanning – a comparison of methods. Magn Resone Med 24:174–176

Larsson HB, Frederiksen J, Kjaer L et al. (1988) In vivo determination of T1 and T2 in the brain of patients with severe but stable multiple sclerosis. Magn Reson Med 7:43–55

Larsson HB, Christiansen P, Jensen M et al. (1991) Localized in vivo proton spectroscopy in the brain of patients with multiple sclerosis. Magn Reson Med 22:23–31

Listerud J, Einstein S, Outwater E et al. (1992) First principles of fast spin echo. Magn Reson Q 8:199–244

Loevner LA, Grossman RI, Lexa FJ et al. (1995) Microscopic disease in normal-appearing white matter on conventional MR images in patients with multiple sclerosis: assessment with magnetization-transfer measurements. Radiology 196:511–515

Maravilla KR, Weinreb C, Suss R et al. (1984) Magnetic resonance demonstration of multiple sclerosis plaques in the cervical cord. AJNR Am J Neuroradiol 5:685–689

Mathews VP, King JC, Elster AD et al. (1994) Cerebral infaction: effects of dose and magnetization transfer saturation at gadolinium-enhanced MR imaging. Radiology 190:547–552

Mauch E, Schroth G, Kornhuber HH et al. (1988) Importance of cranial magnetic resonance imaging in diagnosis of multiple sclerosis without supraspinal signs [letter]. Lancet i:822–823

McConnell HM (1958) Reaction rates by nuclear magnetic resonance. J Chem Phys 28:430–431

McDonald W, Miller D, Thompson A (1994) Are magnetic resonance findings predictive of clinical outcome in therapeutic trials in multiple sclerosis? The dilemma of interferon-β. Ann Neurol 36:14–18

McDonald WI (1992) Multiple sclerosis: diagnostic optimism [editorial]. Br Med J 304:1259–1260

McGowan JC (1993) Characterization of biological tissue with magnetization transfer. University of Pennsylvania, Philadelphia, PA

McGowan JC, Leigh J (1994) Selective saturation in magnetization transfer experiments. Mag Resn Med 32:517–522

McGowan JC, Schnall MD, Leigh JS (1994a) Magnetization transfer imaging with pulsed off-resonance saturation: contrast variation with saturation duty cycle. J Magn Reson 4:79–82

McGowan JC, Schotland J, Leigh J (1994b) Oscillations, stability, and equilibrium in magnetic exchange networks. J Magn Reson [A] 108:201–205

Melki P, Mulkern R, Panych L et al. (1991) Comparing the FAISE method with conventional dual-echo sequences. J Magn Reson Imaging 1:319–326

Menken M (1989) Consensus and controversy in neurologic practice. The case of steroid treatment in multiple sclerosis. Arch Neurol 46:322

Miller DH, McDonald WI, Blumhardt LD et al. (1987) Magnetic resonance imaging in isolated noncompressive spinal cord syndromes. Ann Neurol 22:714–723

Miller DH, Rudge P, Johnson G et al (1988) Serial gadolinium enhanced magnetic resonance imaging in multiple sclerosis. Brain 111:927–939

Miller DH, Johnson G, Tofts PS et al. (1989) Precise relaxation time measurements of normal-appearing white matter in inflammatory central nervous system disease. Magn Reson Med 11:331–336

Miller DH, Barkhof F, Berry I et al. (1991) Magnetic resonance imaging in monitoring the treatment of multiple sclerosis: concerted action guidelines. J Neurol Neurosurg Psychiatry 54:683–688

Miller DH, Barkhof F, Nauta JJ (1993) Gadolinium enhancement increases the sensitivity of MRI in detecting disease activity in multiple sclerosis. Brain 116:1077–1094

Miller DH, Albert PS, Barkhof F et al. (1996) Guidelines for the use of magnetic resonance techniques in monitoring the treatment of multiple sclerosis. Neurology (in press)

Mitchell JR, Karlik SJ, Lee DH et al. (1994) Computer-assisted identification and quantification of multiple sclerosis lesions in MR imaging volumes in the brain. J Magn Reson Imaging 4:197–208

Mulkern R, Bleier A, Adzamli I et al. (1989) Two-site exchange revisited: a new method for extracting exchange parameters in biological systems. Biophys. J 55:221–232

Narayana PA, Johnston D, Flamig DP (1991) In vivo proton magnetic resonance spectroscopy studies of human brain. Magn Reson Imaging 9:303–308

Narayana PA, Wolinsky JS, Jackson EF et al (1992) Proton MR spectroscopy of gadolinium-enhanced multiple sclerosis plaques. J Magn Reson Imaging 2:263–270

Nesbit GM, Forbes GS, Scheithauer BW et al. (1991) Multiple sclerosis: histopathologic and MR and/or CT correlation in 37 cases at biopsy and three cases at autopsy. Radiology 180:467–474

Nilsson O, Larsson EM, Holtas S (1987) Myelopathy patients studied with magnetic resonance for multiple sclerosis plaques. Acta Neurol Scand 76:272–277

Norbash A, Glover G, Enzmann D (1992) Intracerebral lesion contrast with spin-echo and fast spin-echo pulse sequences. Radiology 185:661–665

Noseworthy J, Van der Voort M, Wong C et al. (1990) Interrater variability with the expanded disability status scale (EDSS) and functional systems (FS) in a multiple sclerosis clinical trial. Neurology 40:971–975

Ormerod IE, Miller DH, McDonald WI et al. (1987) The role of NMR imaging in the assessment of multiple sclerosis and isolated neurological lesions. A quantitative study. Brain 110:53–76

Outwater E, Schnall MD, Braitman LE et al. (1992) Magnetization transfer of hepatic lesions: evaluation of a novel contrast technique in the abdomen. Radiology 182:535–540

Papadopoulos A, Gatzonis S, Gouliamos A et al. (1994) Correlation between spinal cord MRI and clinical features in patients with demyelinating disease. Neuroradiology 36:130–133

Pike GB, Hu BS, Glover GY et al. (1992) Magnetization transfer time-of-flight magnetic resonance angiography. Mag Reson Med 25:372–379

Raine CS (1991) Demyelinating diseases. In: Davis RL, Robertson DM (eds) Textbook of neuropathology. Baltimore, Williams & Wilkins, 535–620

Rumbach L, Armspach JP, Gounot D et al. (1991) Nuclear magnetic resonance T2 relaxation times in multiple sclerosis. J Neurol Sci 104:176–181

Rydberg JN, Hammond CA, Grimm RC et al. (1994) Initial clinical experience in MR imaging of the brain with a fast fluid-attenuated inversion-recovery pulse sequence. Radiology 193:173–180

Simon JH, Jacobs J, Cookfair R et al. (1995) The natural history of MS based on an annual MR snapshot: results from the MSCRG study of intramuscular recombinant interferon beta-1a. Neurology 45(Suppl 4):A418

Smith ME, Stone LA, Albert PS et al. (1993) Clinical worsening in multiple sclerosis is associated with increased frequency and area of gadopentetate dimeglumine-enhancing magnetic resonance imaging lesions. Ann Neurol 33:480–489

Thomas DJ, Pennock JM, Hajnal JV et al. (1993) Magnetic resonance imaging of spinal cord in multiple sclerosis by fluid-attenuated inversion recovery. Lancet 341:593–594

Thompson AJ, Kermode AG, MacManus DG et al. (1990) Patterns of disease activity in multiple sclerosis: clinical and magnetic resonance imaging study. Br Med J 300:631–634

Thompson AJ, Kermode AG, Wicks D et al. (1991) Major differences in the dynamics of primary and secondary progressive multiple sclerosis. Ann Neurol 29:53–62

Thompson AJ, Miller D, Youl B et al. (1992) Serial gadolinium-enhanced MRI in relapsing/remitting multiple sclerosis of varying disease duration. Neurology 42:60–63

Truyen L, Gheuens J, Parizel PM et al. (1991) Long term follow-up of multiple sclerosis by standardized, non-contrast-enhanced magnetic resonance imaging. J Neurol Sci 106:35–40

Turano G, Jones SJ, Miller DH et al. (1991) Correlation of SEP abnormalities with brain and cervical cord MRI in multiple sclerosis. Brain 114:663–681

Udupa JK, Samarasekera S (1995) Fuzzy connectedness and object definition. SPIE Proc 2431:2–11

Udupa JK, Samarasekera S, Venugopal K et al. (1994) Fuzzy objects and their boundaries. SPIE Proc 2359:50–58

Uldry PA, Regli F, Uske A (1993) Magnetic resonance imaging in patients with multiple sclerosis and spinal cord involvement: 28 cases. J Neurol 240;41–45

Van Hecke P, Marchal G, Johannik K et al. (1991) Human brain proton localized NMR spectroscopy in multiple sclerosis. Magn Reson Med 18:199–206

Vannier M, Butterfield R, Jordan D et al. (1985) Multispectral analysis of magnetic resonance images. Radiology 154:221–224

Wehrli F, MacFall J, Glover G et al. (1984) The dependence of nuclear magnetic resonance (NMR) image contrast on intrinsic and pulse sequence timing parameters. Magn Reson Imaging 2:3–16

Wehrli F, Breger R, MacFall J et al. (1985) Quantification of contrast in clinical MR brain imaging at high magnetic field. Invest Radiol 20:360–369

White S, Hajnal J, Young I et al. (1992) Use of fluid-attentuated inversion-recovery pulse sequences

for imaging the spinal cord. Magn Reson Med 28;153–162
Wiebe S, Lee DH, Karlik SJ et al. (1992) Serial cranial and spinal cord magnetic resonance imaging in multiple sclerosis. Ann Neurol 32: 643–650
Wolff SD, Balaban RS (1989) Magnetization transfer contrast (MTC) and tissue water proton relaxation in vivo. Magn Reson Med 10:135–144
Wong KT, Grossman RI, Kapouless I, Cohen J (1994) Multiple sclerosis lesion activity: more than just enhancement. Proceedings of the 80th Scientific Assembly and Annual Meeting of the Radiological Society of North America, 319
Yeung HN, Aisen AM (1992) Magnetization transfer contrast with periodic pulsed saturation. Radiology 183:209–214

9 Magnetic Resonance Imaging of Patients with Isolated Idiopathic Optic Neuritis, Brainstem Syndromes and Myelopathy

David H. Miller

Background

In about 90% of patients with multiple sclerosis (MS), the initial clinical event is an acute and usually reversible monosymptomatic episode of central nervous system dysfunction (Matthews 1990). In most instances, the symptoms and signs indicate the presence of a lesion in either the spinal cord (about 50% of cases), optic nerves (25%) or brainstem (15%). However, not all patients presenting with such syndromes go on to develop further neurologic events disseminated in time and space that allow the diagnosis of MS (Poser et al. 1983). Indeed, such syndromes can sometimes be a manifestation of the monophasic demyelinating disorder, acute disseminated encephalomyelitis (ADEM), or they may be due to a focal structural lesion for which there is an effective treatment.

It follows that the two major clinical requirements when assessing patients with clinically isolated syndromes are to make the correct diagnosis, and, when it is concluded that the syndrome is due to inflammatory demyelination, to assign prognosis for the future development of MS and, in particular, disability. In the last decade, magnetic resonance imaging (MRI) has made a vital contribution in both of these areas. Because of the lack of bone hardening artifact, a high sensitivity to soft tissue pathology, and an ability to obtain images in multiple planes, MRI has largely replaced myelography and CT scanning as the investigation of choice in the diagnosis of spinal cord and brainstem disorders (Thompson and Miller 1992). Using fat-suppressed sequences and gadolinium enhancement, it also makes an important contribution in the investigation of patients with optic neuropathies (Gass et al. 1995; Lee et al. 1991a).

Most of this chapter concerns those patients with acute clinically isolated syndromes in whom inflammatory demyelination is suspected and an alternative cause has not been identified by MRI and other appropriate investigations. It will review brain MRI findings at presentation and their predictive value for future progression to clinically definite MS and disability. This review will be placed in the context of the appropriate clinical syndrome and other laboratory investigations that have been used to assist with diagnosis and prognosis. There will be a short discussion on MRI of the acute symptomatic lesion and the chapter concludes with a section on chronic progressive myelopathy.

The Acute Clinical Syndromes and Risk for Development of Multiple Sclerosis

Optic Neuritis

Optic neuritis is the most distinctive and homogeneous of all clinically isolated syndromes due to demyelinating disease. It is therefore not surprising that it has been most carefully documented with respect to the risk of subsequent conversion to MS, and the contribution of MRI and other laboratory features in assigning prognosis. Compared with isolated spinal cord or brainstem syndromes, historical data prior to MRI is likely to have more diagnostic reliability in optic neuritis, since the clinical manifestations are more specific for demyelination. Several prospective long term clinical follow-up studies have reported that 30%–70% of adults presenting with acute unilateral optic neuritis will develop MS, with rather higher figures apparent in the United Kingdom than in the United States (Bradley and Whitty 1968; Cohen et al. 1979; Francis et al. 1987; Landy 1983; Perkin and Rose 1979; Rizzo and Lessell 1988; Sandberg-Wollheim et al. 1990). Bilateral simultaneous optic neuritis, which in adult life is relatively uncommon, probably carries a lower risk of developing MS (Morrissey et al. 1995; Parkin et al. 1984), although this group of patients has not been studied as often as those with acute unilateral optic neuritis. Other (non-demyelinating) causes are more likely to be found in patients with a bilateral simultaneous optic neuropathy, most notably Leber's hereditary optic neuropathy, which was identified by mitochondrial DNA analysis in 4/23 (17%) patients in a recent series (Morrissey et al. 1995). The risk for MS developing after an episode of optic neuritis in childhood, at which age it is usually bilateral and simultaneous, is low; it was reported in only 1/17 patients in one series (Parkin et al. 1984).

Acute Isolated Syndromes of the Spinal Cord or Brainstem

Until recently, there was very little follow-up data available on patients presenting with an acute isolated syndrome of the spinal cord or brainstem. Lipton and Teasdall (1973) reported that only one of 29 patients presenting with a complete transverse myelitis subsequently developed MS over more than 5 years of follow-up. However, a complete transverse myelitis is unusual in MS, whereas partial cord syndromes occur very frequently. The prognosis for MS following an acute partial spinal cord syndrome or brainstem syndrome has been more difficult to define than in the case of optic neuritis. This difficulty arises because the clinical syndromes are more heterogeneous, and have a wider differential diagnosis than acute optic neuritis. With the improved diagnostic precision of MRI, it has been recently possible to identify those cohorts with these syndromes in which demyelination is considered likely and other structural lesions can be excluded confidently. In such a cohort, Morrissey et al. (1993) have described the rate of conversion to MS after a mean follow-up of 5 years. MS had developed in 24/44 (56%) patients who presented with optic neuritis (mean follow-up 66 months), 8/17 (47%) with a brainstem syndrome (mean follow-up 70 months), and 11/28 (39%) with a spinal cord syndrome (mean follow-up 56 months). Allowing for slight differences in the length of follow-up, it appears that the overall risk for developing MS is similar for all three syndromes.

When patients present with a single episode of suspected demyelination, questions regarding prognosis are inevitable. Unfortunately, clinical features of the early stages of MS are of relatively little prognostic value. A number of studies agree that presentation with optic neuritis or purely sensory symptoms are favourable features (McAlpine 1964; Poser et al. 1982), while initial weakness or ataxia is less favorable (Phadke 1987; Visscher et al. 1984; Thompson et al. 1986). Nevertheless, the predictive value of such features is weak and of little value in counselling individual patients. Rather more predictive is the patient's disability status 5 years after the onset of symptoms (Kurtzke 1977; Miller et al. 1992), but this observation is hardly surprising since once a substantial disability is established it is unlikely to resolve. What is most needed is a reliable predictor of outcome *before* disability develops. Not only would this be of value in counselling patients, it would also enable the appropriate selection of patients for trials of new therapies at the earliest stages of the illness.

The Predictive Value of Laboratory Markers

In the absence of useful clinical prognostic indicators, attention has turned to potential laboratory markers. The human leukocyte antigens (HLA) and cerebrospinal fluid (CSF) parameters have been the most intensively studied. Patients with optic neuritis or other clinically isolated syndromes who are HLA DR2-positive, are more likely to progress to clinically definite MS within 5 years (Compston et al. 1978, Morrissey et al. 1993), but the relative risk is modest. Thus, Morrissey et al. (1993) reported progression to MS in 65% who were DR2-positive and 36% of DR2-negative individuals. Furthermore, with longer follow-up, the increased risk disappears (Francis et al. 1987; Sandberg-Wollheim et al. 1990).

Numerous reports have established that the presence of CSF oligoclonal IgG bands at presentation with suspected MS (seen in about 50% of patients) confers an increased risk of progression to definite disease over the next few years (Lee et al. 1991b; Moulin et al. 1983; Nikolskelainen et al. 1981; Sandberg-Wollheim et al. 1990); one study found that oligoclonal IgM bands are even more predictive than IgG bands (Sharief et al. 1991). Nevertheless the predictive value of oligoclonal bands is moderate rather than marked (e.g. one large study with a mean follow-up of 34 months reported conversion to clinically definite MS in 24% of those who had oligoclonal IgG bands at presentation and 9% who did not (Moulin et al. 1983)), and the invasive nature of lumbar puncture makes it unattractive as a routine investigation in many patients with mild, early symptoms, particularly now that MRI is widely used.

Conventional T2-Weighted Brain Magnetic Resonance Imaging and the Risk for Multiple Sclerosis

Many groups have reported brain MRI findings at presentation with isolated syndromes suggestive of MS. Acute unilateral optic neuritis has been most extensively studied. There is a consistent agreement that about 50%–70% of individuals with acute unilateral optic neuritis demonstrate clinically silent cerebral white matter lesions (Frederiksen et al. 1991; Jacobs et al. 1986; Martinelli et al. 1991; Ormerod et al. 1986a,; Stadt et al. 1990). The lesions are usually multiple and their appearances indistinguishable from those of established MS (Figure 9.1). Excluding those in whom MRI has revealed an alternative diagnosis, a similar proportion of patients presenting with acute isolated partial syndromes of the spinal cord and brainstem also manifest cerebral white matter lesions (Ford et al. 1992; Ormerod et al. 1986b; Miller et al. 1987a).

The presence of such lesions does not allow an immediate diagnosis of MS, since the criteria of dissemination in time is not yet fulfilled; it is conceivable that some of these patients have ADEM. Indeed, the MRI appearances of ADEM and MS may be indistinguishable (Kesselring et al. 1990). However, in adult life, ADEM is rare and MS is common, so it is likely that the lesions are most often due to MS. The critical question is whether the MRI abnormalities predict future clinical events.

A number of follow-up studies, ranging from 1 to 5 years, have consistently reported a higher rate of progression to MS in those with MRI abnormalities at presentation compared with those with a normal scan (Table 9.1). The earliest report was after a mean follow-up of 12 months in 53 patients presenting with

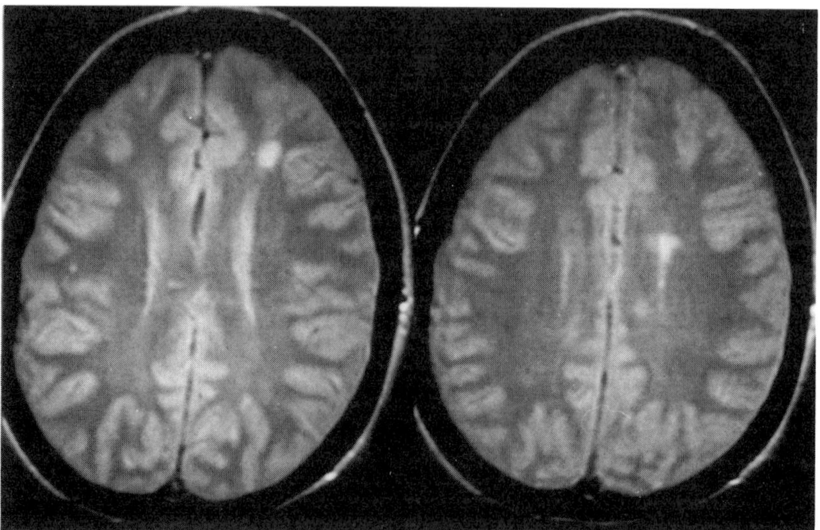

Figure 9.1. T2-weighted brain MRI in a patient with a clinically isolated acute spinal cord syndrome reveals multiple cerebral white matter lesions characteristic of demyelination.

Table 9.1. Clinical isolated syndromes: brain MRI at presentation and risk for MS

Study	Duration of follow-up (months)	Progression to MS[a]	
		Abnormal MRI (%)	Normal MRI (%)
Martinelli et al. 1991	32	7/21 (33)	0/22 (0)
Frederiksen et al. 1991	11	7/31 (23)	0/19 (0)
Lee et al. 1991b[b]	24	52/118 (44)	3/66 (5)
Jacobs et al. 1991	48	6/23 (26)	3/25 (12)
Ford et al. 1992	39	11/12 (92)	1/3 (33)
Morrissey et al. 1993	64	37/57 (65)	1/32 (3)
Beck et al. 1993	24	16/56 (29)	2/62 (3)[c]
Total		136/318 (43)	10/229 (4)

[a]Clinically or laboratory supported definite MS.
[b]Includes cases of clinically probable MS and chronic progressive myelopathy.
[c]Includes minor abnormalities, all small or non-periventricular.

isolated optic neuritis (Miller et al. 1988a). New symptoms and/or signs allowing a diagnosis of clinically definite or probable MS (Poser et al. 1983) were seen in 12/34 (35%) with abnormal brain MRI at presentation but in none of 19 with a normal scan. The same research team also reported their findings after a mean of 16 months in 56 patients who had presented with an isolated syndrome of the spinal cord or brainstem (Miller et al. 1989). New relapses allowed a diagnosis of clinically probable or definite MS in 17/35 (49%) with an abnormal initial scan and in only 1/21 (5%) with a normal scan. Fredericksen et al. (1991) and Martinelli et al. (1991) reported similar outcomes in their cohorts of patients with optic neuritis: after respective mean follow-ups of 11 and 32 months, clinically definite MS had developed in 7/31 (23%) and 7/21 (33%) with abnormal MRI but in none of 41 patients with a normal initial scan.

More recently, Morrissey performed a 5-year follow-up of the same cohort of patients studied by Miller after 12–16 months (Morrissey et al. 1993). By this time, progression to clinically definite MS had occurred in 37/57 (65%) with an abnormal MRI and in only 1/32 (3%) with a normal scan. The outcome was similar for each subgroup of patients. Thus for optic neuritis patients, MS developed in 23/28 with an abnormal MRI and 1/16 without disseminated lesions; the corresponding outcomes for those with spinal cord syndromes were 10/17 and 1/11, and for brainstem syndromes 8/12 and 0/5.

Ford et al. (1992) examined 15 patients with an isolated partial myelitis. Brain MRI was abnormal in 12 and normal in three; at follow-up after a mean of 38 months 11/12 with MRI abnormalities had developed clinically or laboratory supported definite MS compared with only 1/3 without lesions.

The study of Beck et al. (1993) is important as it was a particularly large study of patients recruited into the North American Optic Neuritis Treatment Trial. The primary aim was to ascertain whether or not a course of steroids improved visual outcome in comparison with placebo. Although the speed of recovery was hastened by a short course of intravenous methylprednisolone (IVMP) followed by oral prednisolone (Beck et al. 1992), the final visual outcome was not affected (Beck and Cleary 1993). An unexpected observation was that the rate of progression to MS after 2 years was halved in the group treated by IVMP (Beck et al. 1993). Most patients had brain MRI scans at entry, but, because of the apparent modifying effect of IVMP on progression to MS, evaluation of the predictive value of MRI is best ascertained in the placebo group. In this group, clinically definite MS had developed after two years of follow-up in only 2/62 (3%) with either a normal brain MRI or only small or non-periventricular abnormalities. In contrast, 16/51 (31%) with more extensive MRI abnormalities had developed MS.

Both Morrissey's and Beck's studies have shown that the number or grade of MRI abnormalities influences the risk for developing MS. Thus, in the London cohort, progression to MS was seen in 13/24 (54%) with one to three lesions and in 28/33 (85%) with four or more lesions. In the placebo arm of the American trial, MS developed after 2 years in 2/12 (17%) with one periventricular or ovoid lesion at least 3 mm in size and in 14/39 (36%) with 2 or more periventricular or ovoid lesions at least 3 mm in size.

Lee et al. (1991b) reported their 2-year follow-up findings on a group of 200 patients in whom MS was suspected at presentation but could not be classified as definite. This cohort was more heterogeneous than the studies already mentioned. It included not only those with an isolated acute syndrome such as optic neuritis but also patients with chronic progressive myelopathy and those with clinically probable MS. Nevertheless, the follow-up findings are remarkably consistent with the series of Morrissey et al. (1993) and Beck et al. (1993). After 2 years, 16 were proved to have an alternative diagnosis. Of the remaining 184, 55 had developed clinically definite MS by having "clinical relapses, appropriate clinical progression or both". Clinically definite disease developed in 46/94 (49%) in whom the initial MRI was classified as "strongly suggestive of MS" (four lesions present, all non-periventricular; or three lesions present with at least one periventricular), 6/24 (25%) with one to three lesions, none of which was periventricular, and in only 3/66 (5%) with normal MRI.

The study of Jacobs et al. (1991) is exceptional in that MRI findings did not alter the risk for developing MS. Patients with isolated optic neuritis were followed up for a mean of 4 years. As reported in all other studies, there was a low frequency of progression to MS in those with normal MRI at presentation (3/25 (12%)). However, only 6/23 (26%) with abnormal MRI had converted to MS in the same period. In seeking an explanation for this discrepancy, it is relevant to note that the range of follow-up in Jacobs' series was extremely variable, ranging between 2 months and 15.5 years from the onset of optic neuritis. The inclusion of patients who were first scanned several years after the onset of optic neuritis introduces the bias that some were excluded in whom clinical conversion to MS had already taken place. On the other hand, patients who have been followed up for only a few months will naturally exhibit a lower rate of clinical conversion.

Implications for Patient Management

Considered as a whole, the evidence is compelling that brain MRI findings at presentation with an acute isolated syndrome are highly predictive of the likelihood of conversion to definite disease in the next 1–5 years. This information is of practical importance in counselling individual patients. For example, in patients with normal MRI, an optimistic prognosis can be given; only about 5% will develop MS in the next 5 years (though much longer follow-up is needed to elucidate the final risk for this cohort). The MRI results will also be useful in selecting appropriate patients for trials of therapy aimed at preventing the conversion from suspected to definite MS. It would make good sense to restrict recruitment to those with four or more lesions because a high event rate in the placebo group (conversion to MS) will mean that fewer patients are needed to demonstrate a designated treatment effect (e.g. 50% reduction in conversion to MS) and those with a lower risk of conversion to MS will not be exposed to possible treatment side effects.

Should patients with clinically isolated syndromes undergo MRI? The answer will be "yes" in most cases of brainstem and spinal cord syndromes (examining both brain and spinal cord in the latter instance), there being a pressing need to identify remediable causes. In optic neuritis, the clinical picture is often so characteristic that imaging is not required for diagnosis. It would be useful if the patient wants a prognostic statement regarding progression to MS in the next 5 years. Also, if a treatment was available that delayed conversion from isolated optic neuritis to MS, brain MRI would be indicated to select appropriate patients for treatment (i.e. those with cerebral abnormalities). One study (Beck et al. 1993) has reported that a short course of IVMP followed by oral prednisolone delays conversion to MS. However, this was an unexpected finding in a study whose primary aim was to assess the effect of treatment on visual recovery, and it needs to be confirmed in further studies designed to look particularly at conversion to MS.

Gadolinium-Enhanced Brain Magnetic Resonance Imaging and Risk for Multiple Sclerosis

Patients with optic neuritis can be divided into three groups of roughly equal size, according to the combined T2-weighted and gadolinium-enhanced brain MRI findings at presentation: one-third have normal imaging, another third have multiple non-enhancing lesions, and one-third have a mixture of enhancing and non-enhancing lesions (Christiansen et al. 1992; Miller et al. 1987b; Youl 1992). A question arising is whether or not enhancement is associated with an altered risk for future progression to MS.

Barkhof et al. (1994) has addressed this issue by the follow-up of a cohort of 67 patients presenting with a clinically isolated syndrome who had undergone T2-weighted and gadolinium-enhanced MRI. After a median follow-up of 14 months, 22 (33%) had developed clinically definite MS, which also became evident in 21/45 (47%) with MRI abnormalities "typical of MS" on T2-weighted images (four lesions, all non-periventricular, or three lesions, one of which is periventricular (Paty et al. 1988)), and in only 1/22 (5%) with lesser degrees of abnormality or a normal scan. One or more gadolinium-enhancing lesions were seen in 18 patients, of whom 14 (78%) had developed MS at follow-up. However, 7/27 (26%) with only non-enhancing T2-weighted lesions had also developed MS. While this suggests that the presence of gadolinium-enhancing lesions increases the likelihood of early conversion, it is also apparent that enhancement is less sensitive than "classical" T2-weighted abnormalities in identifying patients who will develop MS. Longer follow-up data are needed to establish whether or not the prognostic data obtained from gadolinium enhancement is a useful addition to that provided by T2-weighted imaging alone.

Conventional Brain Magnetic Resonance Imaging and Risk for Disability

To date, there have been much less data concerning MRI and the subsequent risk for disability. This is hardly surprising, since very few patients become severely disabled within the first 5 years from disease onset. The experience of the National Hospital cohort in London is the most informative source of data at the present time. After 5 years, only 8% had developed a severe disability (Expanded Disability Status Scale (EDSS) ≥ 6) but 20% had at least moderate disability (EDSS ≥ 3). The likelihood of acquiring a moderate disability did correlate significantly with the initial number of T2-weighted MRI lesions (Morrissey et al. 1993) and with the total T2-weighted lesion load (Filippi et al. 1994), the latter being measured using a semiautomated thresholding technique (Wicks et al. 1992). No patient without lesions or with one lesion at presentation had an EDSS ≥ 3 after 5 years; however, 17% with two to three lesions did, as did 30% with four to ten lesions, and 56% with more than ten lesions (Morrissey et al. 1993). The quantified initial T2-weighted lesion load correlated moderately with the EDSS after 5 years ($r = 0.62$, $P < 0.0001$) (Table 9.2, Figure 9.2) and with the increase of lesion load over the 5 years ($r = 0.61$, $P < 0.0001$) (Filippi et al. 1994).

Table 9.2. Clinically isolated syndromes: 5-year follow-up

	Group A ($n = 21$) (%)	Group B ($n = 31$) (%)	Group C ($n = 32$) (%)
Progression to MS*	19 (90)	17 (55)	2 (6)
Clinically definite	18 (86)	15 (48)	1 (3)
Clinically probable	1 (4)	2 (7)	1 (3)
EDSS ≥ 3**	11 (52)	7 (23)	0 (0)
Increased lesion load ≥ 1 cm^3***	18 (86)	11 (35)	2 (6)

Group A: Initial lesion load >1.23 cm^3; Group B: Initial MR abnormal, lesion load <1.23 cm^3; Group C: Initial MR normal.

*A vs B $P < 0.01$; A vs C $P < 0.001$; B vs C $P < 0.001$.

**A vs B $P < 0.05$; A vs C $P < 0.001$; B vs C $P < 0.005$.

***A vs B $P < 0.001$; A vs C $P < 0.001$; B vs C $P < 0.005$.

(All statistical comparisons performed using chi-squared test.)

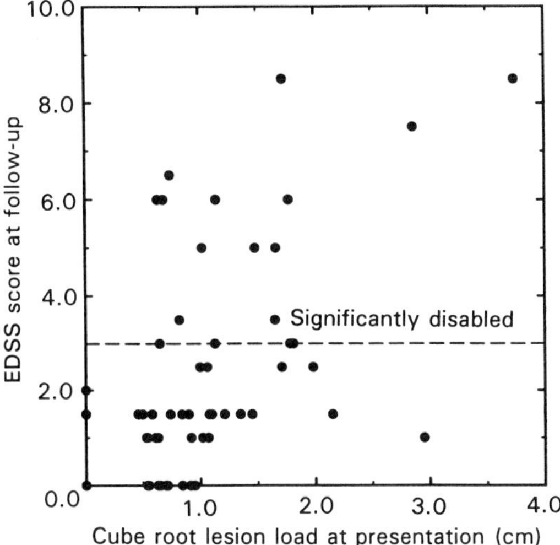

Figure 9.2. Correlation between total brain lesion load at presentation and disability at 5-year follow-up (24 patients had a normal MRI at presentation and EDSS = 0 at follow-up). Statistical analysis: Spearman rank correlation coefficient = 0.619; $P < 0.0001$. (Lesion volumes are presented as cube roots of lesion volumes in order to show the correlation more clearly.)

These data suggest an important predictive value of T2-weighted MRI for subsequent neurologic impairment and disability when obtained at or near the clinical onset of the disease (there are as yet no data available on the predictive value of gadolinium-enhancing lesions for disability). Further studies are now needed with follow-up longer than 5 years. This is especially needed to ascertain the relationship between intial MRI findings and the more severe locomotor disabilities, which for most patients develop only after 10–15 years or longer.

Magnetic Resonance Imaging of the Acute Symptomatic Lesion

Using current MRI technology, it is possible to detect the majority of symptomatic lesions in in the brainstem, spinal cord and optic nerves. Surface coils are required to visualize spinal lesions, and spinal multi-array coils combined with fast spin echo images provide rapid and sensitive screening of the entire spinal cord (Kidd et al. 1993; Thorpe et al. 1993) (Figure 9.3). Detection of lesions within the intraorbital optic nerve requires effective suppression of the orbital fat signal, either using a STIR (short conversion time inversion recovery) sequence (Miller et al. 1988b) or a chemical shift selective fat saturation pulse (Gass et al. 1995; Lee et al. 1991a) (Figure 9.4). Lesions judged clinically to be less than 1 month old usually display gadolinium enhancement (Youl et al. 1991) and sometimes swelling. Detection of the symptomatic lesion consolidates the clinical diagnosis of demyelination. It also provides an opportunity to explore patho

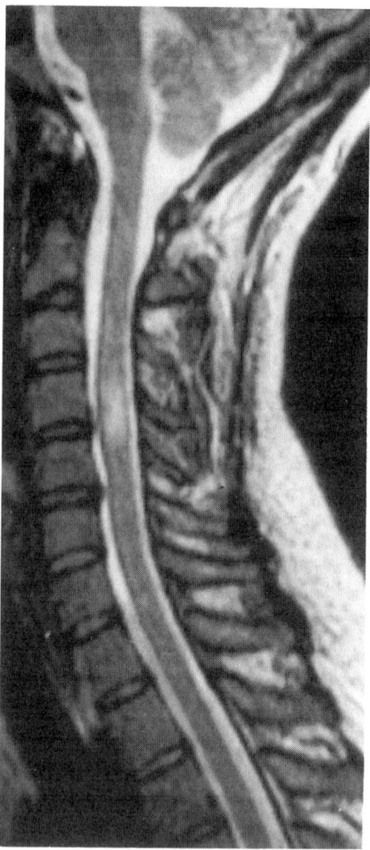

Figure 9.3. Sagittal T2-weighted fast spin echo image of the spinal cord using a multi-array receiver coil in a patient with an isolated partial cord syndrome. There is a single intrinsic lesion at the C4–C5 level.

physiologic mechanisms in demyelinating disease; this is especially so in the optic nerve, where pathology (MRI), nerve conduction (visual evoked potentials) and clinical deficit (neuro-ophthalmologic examination) can be elegantly correlated. It has been observed, for example, that incomplete or slow recovery of vision after an attack of optic neuritis is more likely to occur with long lesions (at least 1.5 cm) that extend into the optic canal (Miller et al. 1988b). Further studies of these clinically eloquent lesions should be performed using the range of nuclear magnetic resonance (NMR) techniques to improve pathologic specificity that are now available.

Chronic Progressive Myelopathy

The differential diagnosis of chronic progressive myelopathy (CPM) is extensive, and it first behoves the physician to exclude a remediable compressive lesion.

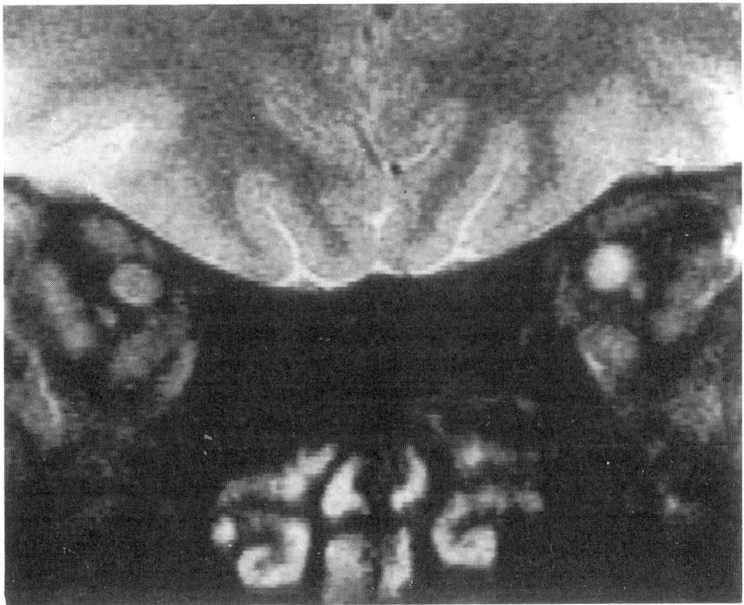

Figure 9.4. Coronal fat suppressed high resolution T2-weighted fast spin echo image of the optic nerves in a patient with acute left optic neuritis. There is high signal in the affected nerve.

High resolution spinal MRI is the best way of doing this. Modern techniques will even detect the majority of spinal arteriovenous malformations (Thorpe et al. 1994), traditionally a difficult diagnosis. In CPM patients without an identifiable structural lesion, MS is a common cause; one postmortem series reported demyelinating lesions in 12/19 (63%) of such patients (Marshall 1955). In one series of patients with non-compressive CPM, who were aged less than 50 years, there were cerebral MRI lesions compatible with demyelination in 21/29 (72%) (Miller et al. 1987a). Another study described brain MRI abnormalities "strongly suggestive of MS" in 31/52 (60%) patients (Paty et al. 1988).

In older adults, cerebral white matter abnormalities need to be interpreted cautiously, because of their increasing frequency due to small vessel disease in the general population. However, in younger adults with non-compressive CPM, the presence of multiple brain lesions characteristic of demyelination and CSF oligoclonal bands provide strong support for the diagnosis of MS. The presence of multiple intrinsic cord lesions adds further confidence to the diagnosis. Multiple cord lesions are a particularly valuable finding in older adults, since they do not develop with aging per se in the same way as cerebral lesions (Thorpe et al. 1993). In summary, a combination of characteristic brain and spinal MRI and CSF abnormalities can establish a confident diagnosis of MS in many patients with CPM.

Conclusion: Current Status and Future Perspectives

It has been consistently demonstrated that the presence and extent of cerebral white matter lesions at presentation with an acute clinically isolated syndrome of the optic nerves, spinal cord or brainstem has a strong predictive value for the development of clinically definite MS in the next 5 years. The extent of abnormalities is also moderately predictive of disability after 5 years. These data suggest a valuable role of MRI in counselling individual patients at presentation, selecting suitable candidates for trials of treatments aimed at delaying conversion to definite MS, and monitoring the effects of treatment. Longer follow-up is needed to ascertain more clearly the prognosis for disability. Studies are also needed to evaluate the prognostic influence of other NMR parameters that are more specific to pathology. For example, proton MR spectroscopy, magnetization transfer imaging and T1-weighted imaging probably all provide a measure of demyelination and/or axonal loss, the pathologic substrates of disability in MS. Preliminary studies using these techniques in established MS suggests a stronger correlation with clinical status than occurs with conventional T2-weighted images (Davie et al. 1994; Gass et al. 1994; van Walderveen et al. 1995).

References

Barkhof F, Filippi M, Tas MW et al. (1994) Towards specific MR imaging criteria for early MS. Proceedings of the European Committee for Treatment and Research in Multiple Sclerosis, 10th Congress. University Studio Press, Athens. p 9

Beck RW, Cleary PA (1993) Optic neuritis treatment trial: one-year follow up results. Arch Ophthalmol 111:773–775

Beck RW, Cleary PA, Anderson MM et al. (1992) A randomised, controlled trial of corticosteroids in the treatment of acute optic neuritis. N Engl J Med 326:581–588

Beck RW, Cleary PA, Trobe JD et al. (1993) The effect of corticosteroids for acute optic neuritis on the subsequent development of multiple sclerosis. N Engl J Med 329:1764–1769

Bradley WG, Whitty CW (1968) Acute optic neuritis: prognosis for the development of multiple sclerosis. J Neurol Neurosurg Psychiatry 31:10–18

Christiansen P, Frederiksen JL, Henriksen O, Larsson HBW (1992) Gd-DTPA enhanced lesions in the brain of patients with acute optic neuritis. Acta Neurol Scand 85:141–146

Cohen MM, Lessell S, Wolf PA (1979) A prospective study of the risk of developing multiple sclerosis in uncomplicated optic neuritis. Neurology 29:208–213

Compston DAS, Batchelor JR, Earl CJ, McDonald WI (1978) Factors influencing the risk of multiple sclerosis developing in patients with optic neuritis. Brain 101:495–511

Davie CA, Barker GJ, Webb S et al. (1994) Proton magnetic resonance spectroscopy (MRS) study of cerebellar dysfunction in multiple sclerosis. J Neurol 341(Suppl 1):S151

Filippi M, Horsfield MA, Morrissey SP et al. (1994) Quantitative brain MRI lesion load predicts the course of clinically isolated syndromes suggestive of multiple sclerosis. Neurology 44:635–641

Ford B, Tampieri D, Francis G (1992) Long term follow-up of acute partial transverse myelopathy. Neurology 42:250–252

Francis DA, Compston DAS, Batchelor JR, McDonald WI (1987) A reassessment of the risk of multiple sclerosis developing in patients with optic neuritis after extended follow-up. J Neurol Neurosurg Psychiatry 50:758–765

Frederiksen JL, Larsson HBW, Olesen J, Stigsby B (1991) MRI, VEP, SEP and biothesiometry suggest monosymptomatic acute optic neuritis to be a first manifestation of multiple sclerosis. Acta Neurol Scand 83:343–350

Gass A, Barker GJ, Kidd D et al. (1994) Correlation of magnetisation transfer ratio with clinical disability in multiple sclerosis. Ann Neurol 36:62–67

Gass A, Barker GJ, Moseley IF et al. (1995) High resolution MRI of the anterior visual pathways in patients with optic neuropathies. J Neurol Neurosurg Psychiatry 58:562–569

Jacobs L, Kinkel PR, Kinkel WR (1986) Silent brain lesions in patients with isolated optic neuritis. A clinical and nuclear magnetic resonance imaging study. Arch Neurol 43:452–455

Jacobs L, Munschauer FE, Kaba SE (1991) Clinical and magnetic resonance imaging in optic neuritis. Neurology 41:15–19

Kesselring J, Miller DH, Robb SA et al. (1990) Acute disseminated encephalomyelitis: MRI findings and the distinction from multiple sclerosis. Brain 113:291–320

Kidd D, Thorpe JW, Thompson AJ et al. (1993) Spinal cord MRI using multi-array coils and fast spin echo: II. Findings in MS. Neurology 43:2632–2637

Kurtzke JF, Beebe GW, Nagler B et al. (1977) Studies on the natural history of multiple sclerosis: 8. Early prognostic features of the later course of the illness. J Chron Dis 30:819–830

Landy PJ (1983) A prospective study of the risk of developing multiple sclerosis in optic neuritis in a tropical and subtropical area. J Neurol Neurosurg Psychiatry 46:659–661

Lee DH, Simon JH, Szumowski J et al. (1991a) Optic neuritis and orbital lesions: lipid-suppressed and chemical shift MR imaging. Radiology 179:543–546

Lee KH, Hashimoto SA, Hooge JP et al. (1991b) Magnetic resonance imaging of the head in the diagnosis of multiple sclerosis: a prospective 2-year follow-up with comparison of clinical evaluation, evoked potentials, oligoclonal banding, and CT. Neurology 41:657–660

Lipton HL, Teasdall RD (1973) Acute transverse myelopathy in adults. Arch Neurol 28:252–257

Marshall J (1955) Spastic paraplegia of middle age. Lancet i:643–646

Martinelli V, Comi G, Filippi M et al. (1991) Paraclinical tests in acute-onset optic neuritis: basal data and results of short term follow up. Acta Neurol Scand 84:231–236

Matthews WB (1991) Clinical aspects. In: Matthews WB (ed) McAlpine's multiple sclerosis, 2nd edn. Churchill Livingstone, London, pp 43–300

McAlpine D (1964) The benign form of multiple sclerosis. Br Med J ii:1029–1032

Miller DH, McDonald WI, Blumhardt LD et al. (1987a) MRI of brain and spinal cord in isolated noncompressive spinal cord syndromes. Ann Neurol 22:714–723

Miller DH, McDonald WI, Johnson G et al. (1987b) Gadolinium-DTPA enhanced MRI of the brain and orbits in patients with clinically isolated optic neuritis. Proceedings of the Society of Magnetic Resonance in Medicine, 6th annual meeting, vol 1. Society of Magnetic Resonance in Medicine, Berkeley, p 143

Miller DH, Ormerod IEC, McDonald WI et al. (1988a) The early risk of multiple sclerosis after optic neuritis. J Neurol Neurosurg Psychiatry 51:1569–1571

Miller DH, Newton MR, van der Poel JC et al. (1988b) Magnetic resonance imaging of the optic nerve in optic neuritis. Neurology 38:175–179

Miller DH, Ormerod IEC, Rudge P et al. (1989) The early risk of multiple sclerosis following isolated acute syndromes of the brainstem and spinal cord. Ann Neurol 26:635–639

Miller DH, Hornabrook RW, Purdie G (1992) The natural history of multiple sclerosis: a regional study with some longitudinal data. J Neurol Neurosurg Psychiatry 55:341–346

Morrissey SP, Miller DH, Kendall BE et al. (1993) The significance of brain magnetic resonance imaging abnormalities at presentation with clinically isolated syndromes suggestive of multiple sclerosis. A 5-year follow-up study. Brain 116:135–146

Morrissey SP, Borruat FX, Miller DH et al. (1995) Bilateral simultaneous optic neuropathy in adults: clinical, imaging serological, and genetic studies. J Neurol Neurosurg Psychiatry 58:70–74

Moulin D, Paty D, Ebers GC (1983) The predictive value of cerebrospinal fluid electrophoresis in "possible" multiple sclerosis. Brain 106:809–816

Nikolskelainen E, Frey H, Salmi A (1981) Prognosis of optic neuritis with special reference to cerebrospinal fluid immunoglobulins and measles virus antibodies. Ann Neurol 9:545–550

Ormerod IEC, McDonald WI, du Boulay GH et al. (1986a) Disseminated lesions at presentation in patients with optic neuritis. J Neurol Neurosurg Psychiatry 49:124–127

Ormerod IEC, Bronstein A, Rudge P et al. (1986b) Magnetic resonance imaging in clinically isolated lesions of the brain stem. J Neurol Neurosurg Psychiatry 49:737–743

Parkin PJ, Heirons R, McDonald WI (1984) Bilateral optic neuritis: a long term follow up. Brain 107:951–964

Paty DW, Oger JJF, Kastrukoff LF et al. (1988) MRI in the diagnosis of MS: a prospective study with comparison of clinical evaluation, evoked potentials, oligoclonal banding, and CT. Neurology 38:180–185

Perkin GD, Rose FC (1979) Optic neuritis and its differential diagnosis. Oxford University Press, Oxford

Phadke JG (1987) Survivial pattern and cause of death in patients with multiple sclerosis: results from an epidemiological study in north east Scotland. J Neurol Neurosurg Psychiatry 50:523–531

Poser CM, Paty DW, Scheinberg L et al. (1983) New diagnostic criteria for multiple sclerosis: guidelines for research protocols. Ann Neurol 13:227–231

Poser S, Raun NE, Poser W (1982) Age at onset, initial symptomatology, and the course of multiple sclerosis. Acta Neurol Scand 66:355–362

Rizzo JF, Lessell S (1988) Risk of developing multiple sclerosis after uncomplicated optic neuritis: a long-term prospective study. Neurology 38:185–190

Sandberg-Wollheim M, Bynke H, Cronqvist S et al. (1990) A long-term prospective study of optic neuritis: evaluation of risk factors. Ann Neurol 27:386–393

Sharief MK, Thompson EJ (1991) The predictive value of intrathecal immunoglobulin synthesis and magnetic resonance imaging in acute isolated syndromes for subsequent development of multiple sclerosis. Ann Neurol 29:147–151

Stadt D, Kappos L, Rohrach E et al. (1990) Occurrence of MRI abnormalities in patients with isolated optic neuritis. Eur Neurol 30:305–309

Thompson AJ, Miller DH (1992) Magnetic resonance imaging in clinical practice. In: Kennard C (ed) Recent advances in clinical neurology, vol 7. Churchill Livingstone, London, pp 199–219

Thompson AJ, Hutchison M, Brazil J et al. (1986) A clinical and laboratory study of benign multiple sclerosis. Q J Med 58:69–80

Thorpe JW, Kidd D, Kendall BE et al. (1993) Spinal cord MRI using mult-array coils and fast spin echo. I. Technical aspects and findings in healthy adults. Neurology 43:2625–2631

Thorpe JW, Kendall BE, MacManus DG, McDonald WI, Miller DH (1994) Dynamic gadolinium-enhanced MRI in detection of spinal arteriovenous malformations. Neuroradiology 36:522–529

van Walderveen MAA, Barkhof F, Hommes OR et al. (1995) Correlating MR imaging and clinical disease activity in multiple sclerosis: relevance of hypointense lesions on short TR/TE ("T1-weighted") spin-echo images. Neurology 45:1684–1690

Visscher BR, Liv K-S, Clarke VA et al. (1984) Onset of symptoms as predictors of mortality and disability in multiple sclerosis. Acta Neurol Scand 70:321–328

Wicks DA, Tofts P, Miller DH et al. (1992) Volume measuresment of multiple sclerosis lesions with magnetisation images: a preliminary study. Neuroradiology 34:475–479

Youl BD (1992) Magnetic resonance imaging studies of optic neuritis [thesis]. University of Melbourne, Melbourne

Youl BD, Turano G, Miller DH et al. (1991) The pathophysiology of optic neuritis: an association of gadolinium leakage with clinical and electrophysiological deficits. Brain 114:2437–2450

10 Strategies to Delay the Onset of Clinically Definite Multiple Sclerosis in Patients with Monosymptomatic Presentations of Optic Neuritis, Brainstem Syndromes or Myelopathy

Roy W. Beck

Introduction

Converging lines of evidence suggest that it is now possible definitively to test strategies to delay the onset of clinically definite multiple sclerosis (CDMS) in patients who experience first attacks of optic neuritis, brainstem syndromes or myelitis. It has been demonstrated that brain magnetic resonance imaging (MRI) can identify patients with monosymptomatic presentations who subsequently are at high risk to develop CDMS. There is also evidence to suggest that the development of CDMS following isolated optic neuritis can be delayed by administering intravenous corticosteroids. A study to investigate this question further in monosymptomatic patients is now particularly relevant for several reasons. It has been shown that treatment can have a beneficial effect on the course of early relapsing-remitting MS and in vitro data from studies of experimental allergic encephalomyelitis (an animal model of multiple sclerosis) provide a potential explanation for why treatment at the time of an initial monosymptomatic event (e.g. optic neuritis) might have greater efficacy than treatment once CDMS is well established. In this chapter we will review evidence supporting the need for such a study as well as aspects of study design that must be properly addressed to assure its successful completion.

Identification of High Risk Patients

Brain MRI has greatly enhanced the ability to predict which patients with optic neuritis are likely to develop MS. The presence of "clinically silent" brain lesions on MRI at the time of onset of optic neuritis has been shown to increase the short-term risk of subsequent conversion to CDMS as well as the development of new brain MRI lesions in all studies in which this has been analyzed (Beck et al. 1993c; Frederiksen et al. 1989; Jacobs et al. 1991; Martinelli et al. 1991; Morrissey et al. 1993).

Table 10.1. Cumulative incidence of CDMS in ONTT patients by baseline MRI status

Time period (years)	Baseline MRI (%)		
	Grade 0–I ($n = 202$)	Grade II–III ($n = 61$)	Grade IV ($n = 89$)
0.5	1.0	6.8	17.2
1	2.6	14.0	25.6
2	4.9	19.7	31.7
3	9.3	27.7	43.1
4[a]	13.3	35.4	49.8

Grade 0 = normal; I = non-specific changes; II = generally 1 lesion; III = generally 2 lesions; IV = 3 or more lesions (lesions defined as >3 mm; for grades III and IV, at least 1 lesion required to be periventricular or ovoid).
[a]4-year follow-up not yet completed for all patients.

Table 10.2. Development of CDMS after optic neuritis relative to MRI abnormality from literature

	Length of follow-up (mean years)	Abnormal MRI[a] (%)	Normal MRI[a] (%)
Jacobs et al. (1991)	4.0	6/23 (26)	3/25 (12)
Jacobs (unpublished)	5.5	17/40 (43)	4/32 (13)
Martinelli et al. (1991)	2.7	7/21 (33)	0/16 (0)
Frederiksen et al. (1989)	0.9	7/30 (23)	0/20 (0)
Miller et al. (1988)	1.0	12/34 (35)	0/19 (0)
Morrisey et al. (1993)	5.5	23/28 (82)	1/16 (6)

[a]No. patients developing CDMS/total no. at risk.

The Optic Neuritis Treatment Trial (ONTT) found the 2-year risk of CDMS to be 25% in 150 patients with one or more brain MRI lesions, compared with 5% in 202 patients without lesions (Beck et al. 1993c). Data from extended follow-up of the ONTT cohort are provided in Table 10.1. A tabulation of other studies is provided in Table 10.2.

Differences in the reported rates between studies can be explained by the variable length of follow-up and differing diagnostic criteria, definitions of brain MRI abnormality and timing of MRI relative to the onset of optic neuritis. Despite the variations in methodology, there is reasonable consistency between studies.

The study of Morrissey et al. (1993) represents a longer follow-up of the series reported by Miller et al. (1988). This study indicates that, with sufficiently long follow-up most, if not all optic neuritis patients who have silent brain MRI signal abnormalities will ultimately develop additional clinical manifestations sufficient for a diagnosis of CDMS. In addition, this study and the others indicate that the risk of MS, at least within the first 5 years after optic neuritis, is low in patients with normal brain MRI; it is too low to be able to evaluate treatment efficacy within the confines of a feasible sample size.

With regard to spinal cord syndromes, Ford et al. (1992) showed that among 15 patients with partial myelopathy followed for a mean of 3.2 years, 11 of 12 (92%) with brain MRI signal abnormalities and one of three with a normal scan converted to CDMS. In the study of Morrissey et al. (1993) 59% of myelopathy patients with positive head MRI converted to MS, whereas only 9% of those with negative MRI converted during follow-up approximating 5 years.

With regard to brainstem syndromes, Morrissey et al. (1993) included 17 patients with isolated brainstem syndromes, and found that with a mean follow-up of 5.8 years, CDMS developed in 67% of the 12 patients who had an initial abnormal brain MRI (in addition to a lesion causing brainstem syndrome) and in none of the five patients with a normal scan.

Two studies have grouped together patients with neurologic events suggestive of MS. Lee et al. (1991a) performed a 2-year follow-up of 200 patients with suspected MS who underwent brain MRI at presentation. Conversion to CDMS occurred in 41% of those with one or more brain lesions compatible with MS and in only 5% with normal brain MRI. The study of Filippi et al. (1994) further demonstrates the value of quantitative MRI by showing that 90% of patients presenting with an acute clinically isolated syndrome of the optic nerves, brainstem or spinal cord, and a with brain lesion load $>1.23\,cm^3$, converted during 5 years' follow-up, whereas conversions to MS occurred in 55% of those with a lesion load of $<1.23\,cm^3$ and only 6% with normal MRI.

From these reports, it is apparent that a study of patients who develop optic neuritis or other acute neurologic events, and who have silent lesions on brain MRI, is in essence a study of patients most of whom are destined to develop additional attacks of demyelination and be diagnosed as CDMS. It is also apparent that for patients with normal brain MRI, their short-term risk of developing CDMS is sufficiently low that it would not be feasible to determine whether they would benefit from prophylactic treatment.

Optic Neuritis Treatment Trial

The Optic Neuritis Treatment Trial (ONTT) found a reduction in the 2-year rate of development of CDMS in patients treated with intravenous followed by oral corticosteroids at the time of optic neuritis. The mechanism by which a single intravenous methylprednisolone (IVMP) course could induce a 2-year clinical benefit is unknown, but may relate to the timing of its administration and its widespread effects on the immune system (Kupersmith et al. 1994; Reder et al. 1994).

The ONTT enrolled 389 patients with acute monosymptomatic optic neuritis who did not meet diagnostic criteria for clinically probable or CDMS at the time of study entry (Poser et al. 1983). Entry criteria included the diagnosis of acute unilateral optic neuritis with visual symptoms of 8 days or less, age between 18 and 46 years, no previous history of optic neuritis or ophthalmoscopic signs of optic atrophy in the affected eye, no evidence of a systemic disease that might be associated with the optic neuritis, and no previous treatment with corticosteroids for optic neuritis in the fellow eye.

Patients were randomly assigned to one of three treatment regimens:

1. IVMP 250 mg every 6 hours for 3 days followed by oral prednisone 1 mg/kg per day for 11 days (the intravenous group);
2. Oral prednisone 1 mg/kg per day for 14 days (the prednisone group);
3. Oral placebo for 14 days (the placebo group).

Regimens 1 and 2 were followed by a short oral prednisone taper consisting of 20 mg on day 15 and 10 mg on days 16 and 18. Whereas patients in the prednisone and placebo groups were masked to their treatment allocation, patients in the intravenous group were not.

Structured, detailed neurologic examinations were performed at baseline and at follow-up after 6 months, 1 year and then yearly. Additional examinations were performed at times when patients developed symptoms of new neurologic disease or recurrences of optic neuritis.

Of the 389 patients included in this study, 134 were randomly assigned to the intravenous group, 129 to the prednisone group, and 126 to the placebo group. The number enrolled at individual clinical centers ranged from 12 to 40 (median 27). The mean age was 31.7 ± 6.7 years; 77% were female and 85.1% Caucasian. Patients entered the trial within a mean of 5.0 ± 1.6 days from the onset of visual symptoms.

The ONTT found that, compared with the placebo regimen, the intravenous regimen showed more rapid recovery of vision but no long-term visual benefit (Beck et al. 1992, 1993b). Most of the difference in rate of visual recovery between groups was seen in the first 2 weeks. Thereafter, differences in visual function between groups were small. After 1 year of follow-up, there were no significant differences between the groups in visual acuity, contrast sensitivity, color vision, or visual field (Beck et al. 1993b). The regimen of oral prednisone alone not only provided no benefit to vision but was also associated with an increased rate of new attacks of optic neuritis in both the initially affected and fellow eyes. Within the first 2 years of follow-up, new attacks of optic neuritis in either eye occurred in 30% of the patients in the oral prednisone group, compared with 16% in the placebo group and 14% in the intravenous group.

Unexpectedly, the study found that the intravenous group had a lower rate of development of MS within the first 2 years than did the placebo or prednisone groups (Beck et al. 1993c). Among the patients in the intravenous group, MS developed within 2 years in only 7.5% compared with 16.7% of the placebo group and 14.7% of the prednisone group. The 2-year adjusted rate ratio for the development of CDMS in the intravenous group was 0.34 (95% confidence interval 0.16–0.74; $P = 0.0063$) compared with the placebo group and 0.38 (95% confidence interval 0.17–0.83; $P = 0.015$) compared with the prednisone group. When the outcome was redefined to be either: development of clinically definite or probable MS, or development of CDMS or a new attack of optic neuritis in the fellow eye, the results were similar as indicated in Table 10.3.

Most of the beneficial treatment effect was manifested in the patients with abnormal brain MRI at study entry. Among those patients with two or more MRI signal abnormalities, CDMS developed within 2 years in 35.9% of the 39 patients in the placebo group, 32.4 per cent of the 37 patients in the prednisone group, and only 16.2% of the 37 patients in the intravenous group. Independent of treatment, the rate of development of CDMS in patients with a normal or non-specifically abnormal scan was so low that therapeutic efficacy for these patients could not be judged.

As expected, the apparent beneficial effect of treatment was not permanent. Table 10.4 provides the group-specific cumulative incidences of development of MS by time period, indicating that after the third year of follow-up there was no longer a beneficial treatment effect.

Table 10.3. Comparison of 2-year rate of CDMS in ONTT by treatment groups

Outcome	Treatment groups compared	
	IV versus placebo	IV versus prednisone
	RR (95% CI)[a] *P*-value	RR (95% CI)[a] *P*-value
Definite MS	0.34 (0.16–0.74) 0.006	0.38 (0.17–0.83) 0.01
Probable or definite MS	0.40 (0.22–0.72) 0.002	0.45 (0.25–0.80) 0.007
Definite MS or new fellow eye optic neuritis	0.37 (0.20–0.70) 0.002	0.32 (0.17–0.58) 0.0002
Definite MS or new either eye optic neuritis	0.50 (0.29–0.84) 0.009	0.37 (0.23–0.61) 0.0001

IV: intravenous; RR: relative risk.
[a]Relative risk and 95% confidence interval from proportional hazards model controlling for MRI grade, previous optic neuritis in the fellow eye, family history of MS, and prior neurologic symptoms.

Table 10.4. Cumulative percentage of ONTT patients with CDMS by treatment group

Time period (years)	Treatment group (%)		
	Intravenous ($n = 134$)	Placebo ($n = 126$)	Prednisone ($n = 129$)
0.5	3.1	7.4	7.3
1	6.4	13.5	10.7
2	8.1	18.0	16.0
3	18.1	21.3	26.9

Interpretation of the Optic Neuritis Treatment Trial Results

Although the study was designed primarily to assess visual recovery, the assessment of MS was a preplanned secondary objective. Recognizing the potential importance of the trial's findings, the ONTT Study Group made exhaustive efforts to evaluate all potential sources of bias, confounding, and errors in data recording or analysis as possible explanations for the surprising treatment effect. These efforts included:

1. Review of all neurologic data by a masked observer to classify each patient regarding whether CDMS had developed;
2. Phone contact of patients who had missed the 2-year follow-up visit to determine whether any symptoms of MS had developed;
3. Survey of examining neurologists to determine whether they had any suspicion of a beneficial treatment effect;
4. Assessment of all potential confounding variables;
5. Complete evaluation of the integrity of the dataset and replication of all data analysis at a second biostatistical center.

The 2-year rate of development of CDMS in the placebo group approximated that of other reported series; therefore the ONTT findings reflect the intravenous group faring better than expected, not the placebo group faring worse. In assessing how this finding should be interpreted, the investigators considered the following possibilities as explanations before concluding that the apparent treatment effect was most likely real.

Could the Patients in the Intravenous Group Have Under-reported New Symptoms of Multiple Sclerosis Relative to the Placebo Group?

This is unlikely. There is no reason to believe that any patient had a preconceived notion that treatment would benefit the neurologic course. Since visual recovery began quickly in all three groups, there should not have been a greater belief on the part of any patient group that treatment was affecting neurologic status.

Because the Neurologists Were not Completely Masked, Could They Have Under-interpreted New Symptoms and Established Signs of Multiple Sclerosis in the Intravenous Group Relative to the Other Groups?

This is also unlikely. First, the neurologists were not generally aware of the patient treatment group at follow-up visits. Secondly, a formal survey of the neurologists provided no indication that they expected treatment to benefit the neurologic course. Thirdly, all of the neurologic examinations were conducted by a detailed, standardized protocol, and completed forms were reviewed in a masked fashion by an authority in MS (Donald W Paty) to ascertain that the appropriate criteria for classification of MS status had been applied.

Could a Placebo Effect Have Produced the Results?

This is unlikely. This question is relevant because it has been shown that immunologic changes can occur in MS patients treated with a placebo (Camenga et al. 1986; Giang in press), but it is improbable that the brief intravenous regimen or patient awareness of treatment assignment could have produced physiologic effects powerful enough to account for such a large difference in the rate of MS between groups. Moreover, virtually all patients in all three groups were starting to show improvement in vision after the first few days. Thus, they should all have been expected to believe that they were receiving an active drug.

Could the Apparent Treatment Effect Have Been Due to an Imbalance in Risk Factors Among the Three Groups?

This is unlikely. This was extensively evaluated in the data analysis. Controlling for potential confounding variables, including age, gender, race, family history of multiple sclerosis, previous history of optic neuritis in the fellow eye, prior nonspecific neurologic symptoms, and number of signal abnormalities on brain MRI, did not alter the results. In fact, the intravenous group had a slightly higher baseline risk for MS than the other groups; controlling for this slightly increased the magnitude of the treatment effect estimate.

Had the treatment effect not abated in time, there would have been concern that the intravenous group was, in some unmeasurable way, inherently at lower risk for MS than were the other two groups, despite randomization and control for potential confounders in the analyses.

Could the Apparent Treatment Effect Have Been Due to Chance?

This is unlikely. The 2-year time period for analysis was preplanned. The *P*-values for the treatment group comparisons were very small. The treatment effect was remarkably consistent across clinical centers and levels of baseline covariates. An effect of similar magnitude to that found at 2 years was found after 6 months and 1 year of follow-up (Table 10.4)).

Why Did Intravenous Corticosteroid Treatment Exert a Beneficial Effect While Oral Prednisone Treatment Exerted No Benefit and Actually Predisposed to More Frequent Optic Neuritis Recurrences?

Although a definitive answer is not available, it is well recognized that high dose corticosteroid treatment produces immunomodulatory effects that are not seen with low dose corticosteroid treatment (Kupersmith et al. 1994). The intravenous regimen may, for example, have achieved higher trough levels, which had a greater effect on reducing helper/inducer CD4+ T-cell subsets known to be active in demyelination associated with optic neuritis and MS. The adverse effect of prednisone may have resulted from a preferential reduction in suppressor/inducer CD4+ T-cell subsets (Corbett and Cruse 1993; Haynes et al. 1978; Mix et al. 1990; Wucherpfennig et al. 1991). In experimental allergic encephalomyelitis, Reder et al. (1994) demonstrated that varying the corticosteroid treatment regimen can produce markedly different effects on relapse rate.

Review Panel's Conclusions

The National Institutes of Health convened a review panel (three biostatisticians: Marian Fisher, Daniel Seigel and Roy Milton; and five MS experts: Stephen Reingold, Henry McFarland, Kenneth Johnson, George Ebers, and John Whitaker) critically to evaluate the study results prior to publication. The panel shared the study investigators' reservations with regard to the fact that the study had not been primarily designed to assess the development of MS and that the finding was unexpected without a firm physiologic basis. They nevertheless concluded that the results were likely to be valid and the treatment effect was likely to be real (Kupersmith et al. 1994).

Rationale for Treatment at the Time of the First Clinical Event

Although the etiology of MS is uncertain, evidence suggests that it is in part an autoimmune disease directed against protein components of myelin.

The autoimmune hypothesis has been the central rationale for immunosuppressive and immunomodulatory treatments used for patients with established MS. A review of MS clinical trials suggests that intervention may be more effective at earlier stages of the disease and relatively less effective as the disease progresses (Kinkel and Goodkin 1994). In this regard, pilot studies of copolymer 1 (COP 1) found greater effectiveness in patients with low disability at the onset of the study (defined as Expanded Disability Status Scale (EDSS) 0–2) (Bornstein et al. 1987). Furthermore, no efficacy for COP 1 was noted in chronic progressive MS patients with a relatively long duration of disease (Bornstein et al. 1991). Studies of type I interferons have demonstrated efficacy in early relapsing-remitting MS, (Durelli et al. 1994; IFNB Multiple Sclerosis Study Group 1993) but preliminary studies have not demonstrated a benefit for longer duration, chronic progressive MS (Kastrukoff et al. 1990). These studies raise the possibility that treatment early in the disease is more effective than treatment in well established cases of long duration.

The autoreactive T-cell repertoire in animal models of autoimmunity is dynamic with amplification (i.e. epitope spreading) of the T-cell repertoire shortly after disease induction (Lehman et al. 1992). If epitope spreading plays a role in the progression of MS, it may provide a strong rationale for initiating immunotherapy as soon as possible after disease induction. Studies attempting to define the autoimmune T-cell repertoire in MS have been guided by parallel investigations of experimental autoimmune encephalomyelitis (EAE), an animal model that shares many clinicopathologic features with MS (Alvord et al. 1984; Raine 1984). Data obtained from acute EAE following immunization with MBP raised the possibility that the autoreactive T-cell response was highly restricted in terms of T-cell receptor usage and determinant specificity (Acha Orbea, et al. 1988; Urban et al. 1988). Initial studies of the autoreactive T-cell repertoire in MS attempted to identify immunodominant determinants of myelin proteins and restricted usage of T-cell receptors that could be potentially targeted with specific forms of immunotherapy. These investigations have produced conflicting results, with some evidence for a restricted T-cell response (Kotzin et al. 1991; Lee et al. 1991b; Ota et al. 1990; Wucherpfennig et al. 1990) but more evidence of significant heterogeneity (Allegrett et al. 1990; Kitze et al. 1988; Martin et al. 1991, 1992; Pette et al. 1990a, 1990b; Richert et al. 1991). These conflicting results can be reconciled by data demonstrating that the T-cell repertoire in experimental autoimmune disease is restricted only during the early, inductive events of the disease (Cross et al. 1993; Kaufmann et al. 1993; Lehmann et al. 1992). Following the initial tissue injury, the T-cell response spreads from an initiating antigenic domain (such as a peptide determinant of myelin basic protein) to other cryptic antigens present on the same protein (i.e. intramolecular epitope spreading) or other proteins present in the injured tissue (i.e. intermolecular spreading). In separate studies these cryptic, second wave determinants were found to be pathogenic when injected into animals, suggesting that epitope spreading represents an amplification event in disease pathogenesis and not merely an epiphenomena of tissue injury (Hood et al. 1989). Preliminary studies have suggested that lymphokine release (i.e. IL-2 and INF-γ) during initial tissue injury upregulates antigen presentation and generates a microenvironment in the target organ, which favors priming (i.e. activation to a pathogenic state) of naive T cells recruited to the site of tissue injury (Heath et al. 1992; Sarvetnick et al. 1990). This may explain the worsening seen in MS patients treated with intravenous INF-γ (Panitch et al. 1987). It also provides a scientific rationale for early treatments designed to arrest the process prior to disease progression.

Design Considerations for Future Studies Examining Treatment Effects in Monosymptomatic Patients

Recruitment of patients into a prevention trial will take considerable effort. Such a study will involve incident, rather than prevalent cases, unlike any other large multicenter clinical trial performed within the MS medical community. A large number of patients will need to be screened to identify a cohort that is eligible for this study. Because of the need to evaluate potential patients quickly after the onset of symptoms, a community-based approach with a large number of centers may be necessary to try to identify a sufficient number of eligible patients.

Eligibility Criteria

As with any clinical trial, criteria must be established for patient eligibility in an attempt to maintain a high level of internal validity, while at the same time attempting to maximize generalizability. The age range of patients should encompass the usual range within which first neurologic events consistent with MS generally occur. A range of 18–45 years would seem to be reasonable. A wider age range would increase the likelihood that patients with disorders other than MS might be included. The inclusion of older patients also would increase the proportion of patients with a chronic progressive course from the onset, which would complicate the analysis and interpretation of the results.

As discussed earlier, brain MRI is a powerful predictor of the risk of MS in patients with optic neuritis. Because the 5-year risk of MS appears to be so low in patients with normal brain MRI, there is not a good justification for prophylactically treating such patients. In addition, from a study design point of view, inclusion of only patients at higher risk for MS substantially reduces the sample size required. Therefore, eligibility for a prevention trial should require the presence of signal abnormalities on brain MRI. Since the MS risk is closely related to the number of brain MRI signal abnormalities present at the time of optic neuritis, the risk of MS will be directly related to the severity of MRI disease, and the sample size will be inversely related. However, the more restrictive the MRI criteria, the greater will be the number of patients that will need to be screened for eligibility. Both Morrissey et al. (1993) and Beck et al. (1993c) found that, with one lesion only, the expected risk of MS within 2 years was relatively low. In addition, Beck et al. (1993a) showed that the inter-rater and intra-rater reliability, when classifying a scan as normal or abnormal, was only fair when a single lesion was present. Based on this experience, it would seem reasonable to require two or more brain MRI signal abnormalities, meeting certain specifications in regard to size, shape, and location. The desire to enter patients as soon after the onset of symptoms as possible would prelude quantifying lesion load at a central MRI reading center as an entry criterion. Based on the ONTT experience, it is expected that approximately one-third of patients with optic neuritis who would otherwise be eligible for the trial would have the requisite MRI abnormalities (e.g. two or more signal abnormalities).

In the ONTT, it was not unusual for patients to report previous transient neurologic symptoms, usually sensory, that were too vague to classify as an MS attack. Among the ONTT patients with two or more brain MRI lesions (i.e. patients who would be eligible for this trial), on baseline questioning, 38% reported some type of neurologic symptom in the past. Exclusion of such a large number of patients because of these vague symptoms would be likely to make recruitment for a trial unfeasible. Since there is no way to know whether previous symptoms of this type were due to demyelination, it is probably most reasonable to include in a trial patients who report ill-defined previous neurologic symptoms that were insufficient to classify them as having probable MS.

Since it is postulated that the timing of treatment relative to disease onset may be critical, it will be important to try to enroll patients as soon after the appearance of symptoms as possible. This desire must be weighed against the practicality that there will be a time delay between the onset of symptoms and the patient seeking medical attention and being evaluated for eligibility. Limiting entry to patients with symptoms of 14 days or less would seem to represent a reasonable compromise. In the ONTT, the time window for entry was a maximum of 8 days from the onset of visual symptoms. This did not prove to be a deterrent to recruitment; the average number of days of symptoms at the time of study entry was five. In the "prevention trial", however, a longer time window may be needed because: patients with non-visual events may not seek medical attention as quickly as those with visual loss, particularly if symptoms take several days to develop fully; and brain MRI must be performed before a patient can be determined to be eligible.

Potential Treatments to Be Evaluated in a Future Study

Results of recent studies suggest that there are three treatments that warrant consideration for evaluation in a "prevention" trial: intravenous corticosteroids, beta interferons, and COP 1. Other treatments that in the future are demonstrated to have benefit in MS, particularly for the relapsing-remitting form of the disease, should also be considered for a prevention trial. The rationale for evaluating beta interferons (IFNB Multiple Sclerosis Study Group 1993; Jacobs et al. 1993, 1994; Paty et al. 1993) and COP 1 (Bornstein and Johnson 1992) relate to their demonstrated efficacy in recent studies of relapsing-remitting MS. These studies are extensively detailed in Chapters 11 and 13.

The rationale for evaluating corticosteroids relates to the results of the ONTT, which were reviewed earlier. The dosage and duration of corticosteroid treatment in inflammatory diseases has been for the most part empirical (Troiano et al. 1987). The corticosteroid dosage administered in the ONTT was selected based on the dosage that was most commonly used in clinical practice at the time the study was initiated: 3 days of IVMP 250 mg every 6 hours, followed by a short course of oral prednisone. It has subsequently been shown that an intravenous dose of 1 g is similarly well tolerated and easily administered in an outpatient setting. Ease of outpatient administration, the limited adverse effects, and the reduced cost make this an attractive treatment approach for a study protocol.

The principal rationale for administering IVMP at intervals relates to the ONTT finding that the treatment effect was time-limited. There does not appear to be a physiologic basis for determining the proper frequency of sequential treatment. Based on the ONTT data which demonstrate that the rate of MS increases after the first 6 months (Table 10.5), treatment at 6-month intervals would seem reasonable.

Initial Treatment of all Patients with Corticosteroids

One design issue to be addressed is whether all patients should receive initial treatment with IVMP. The major detrimental effect of this would be that it would not provide for a replication of the ONTT finding of a beneficial effect of IVMP compared with placebo on delaying the development of CDMS (Beck et al. 1993c). However, there are several drawbacks to the inclusion of a group that has received no active treatment at all.

First, since IVMP treatment has been shown conclusively to be beneficial in providing more rapid recovery of function following an acute demyelinating event and since serious side effects are rare, there are potential ethical concerns about withholding a treatment that, at least in one study, has also been shown to benefit the longer term neurologic course as well, even if this has not been corroborated in other studies.

Secondly, eligible patients and referring physicians might be less likely to support a study that was perceived to constitute a barrier to receiving widely available standard care for an acute demyelinating syndrome.

Thirdly, although many MS trials have included a control group that received no active treatment, patients who are experiencing their first clinical manifestation of MS are quite different. Thus, experience in randomizing patients with established MS to a group receiving no active treatment is not directly applicable. Monosymptomatic patients are generally less functionally impaired, do not recognize that they have a potentially chronic disease, and are likely to be told by their neurologists that they have a more favorable prognosis than patients with

Table 10.5. Conditional probability of CDMS by time interval in ONTT[a]

Time period (years)	Treatment group		
	Intravenous ($n = 134$)	Placebo ($n = 126$)	Prednisone ($n = 129$)
0.5	0.06 ± 0.04	0.14 ± 0.06	0.17 ± 0.07
0.5–1.0	0.10 ± 0.06	0.28 ± 0.08	0.15 ± 0.07
1–2	0.09 ± 0.06	0.18 ± 0.09	0.22 ± 0.10

[a]Including those patients with abnormal brain MRI (≥2 signal abnormalities); definition of CDMS includes fellow eye optic neuritis.

established CDMS. For these reasons, monosymptomatic patients, in contrast to patients with CDMS, may be unwilling to accept a study design in which no active treatment might be received.

Fourthly, inclusion of a group receiving no active treatment could harm the external validity of the results if patients with severe visual or neurologic deficits were more likely to be treated with IVMP and thus not entered into the study. The study population would then be over-represented by patients with mild deficits.

Fifthly, as stated above, the main purpose of a group that did not receive initial intravenous corticosteroids for the acute event would be to replicate the ONTT findings. The clinical importance of doing this will be reduced by the results of this trial. If there is no beneficial effect of intravenous corticosteroids at 6-month intervals compared with intravenous corticosteroid treatment at study entry only, then the clinical importance (although perhaps not the scientific importance), even if it is real, is lessened. If the study finds that the sequential corticosteroid treatments are beneficial compared with the initial treatment alone, then whether the initial treatment alone is beneficial in and of itself is a moot point.

Although from a strictly scientific viewpoint it would be valuable to have a control group that received no active treatment whatsoever, on weighing the pros and cons of inclusion of such a group, this would almost certainly prove to be unfeasible. Recruitment for an MS prevention trial will be difficult as it is. Inclusion of a group that received no active treatment would be likely to so impede recruitment for the study that the study's objectives would not be realized.

Masking the Treatment Assignments

Assuming that all patients receive initial treatment with open-label corticosteroids, a decision needs to be made in designing a trial about whether the subsequent treatments that are to be assessed for efficacy and safety should be compared with placebo-treated controls or untreated controls. Although it is always preferable to include placebo controls in a study, the decision about whether this should be done in a monosymptomatic prevention trial is not straightforward. The pros and cons of masking the active treatment groups by inclusion of placebo-treated controls are discussed below.

Pros

1. Immunologic changes might occur that are differential between treatment groups if one group perceives that it is receiving a more beneficial treatment compared with the other groups (Camenga et al. 1986; Giang et al. in press). The impact of differences in patient behavior related to their knowing their treatment group upon outcome assessment can be minimized by having a clearly defined clinical endpoint, having the examining neurologists masked,

and using MRI as a second outcome measure. Noseworthy et al. (1994) evaluated the effect on the results of patient blinding and physician blinding in the Canadian co-operative MS trial of cyclophosphamide and plasma exchange. They found that patient unblinding did not seem to produce appreciable bias, unlike physician unblinding. Therefore, they concluded that having examiners blinded was far more important than having patients blinded. Thus, even if patients are "unblinded" by side effects, it is not likely that this will impact significantly on the results as long as the examiners remain blinded.

2. Although neurologists performing endpoint examinations could be kept masked regarding treatment group without placebo, patient masking provides additional assurance that neurologists are masked.
3. Results from a double-masked study would be more readily accepted than those from a single-masked study.

Cons

1. The complexity of conducting the study would be increased considerably, particularly with a study design utilizing multiple community-based centers.
2. With untreated rather than placebo-treated controls, the study design would be very similar to clinical practice. Therefore, it would be easier to gain community-based neurologist support for participating in the study, possibly easier to get health maintenance organizations to agree to participate, and lessen potential for problems in trying to get insurance companies to pay for the visits that could be considered part of routine care.
3. With placebos, it would be likely to be more difficult to get patients to agree to be randomized. Patients may be less likely to participate knowing that the frequent injections might be placebo. This is particularly true when the drugs being used in the study are readily available without study participation.
4. Even in a placebo-controlled study, many patients would probably guess their treatment group because of the side effects. In the ONTT, with intravenous steroids, some weight gain was almost universal and minor side effects much more common than encountered in the placebo group (Chrousos et al. 1993). In the Betaseron study (IFNB Multiple Sclerosis Study Group 1993), patients generally could identify that they were receiving active drug, because of local skin reaction and other side effects, although they could not necessarily distinguish between the higher and lower doses (D. Paty, personal communication). Although a placebo for intravenous methylprednisolone containing nicotinic acid (Ellison et al. 1989) could be used to produce facial flushing, other side effects of corticosteroids could still serve to identify the treatment group assignment.
5. The use of placebos would most likely have a detrimental effect on patient compliance during follow-up, since most patients will be relatively asymptomatic after the first month and may not be inclined to continue taking regular injections knowing that they may be receiving placebo. Patients who decide not to comply with their randomized treatments may also be inclined to drop out of the study. As discussed in a prior section, an important point to con-

sider is that patients in this trial are very different to patients in trials of established MS. They almost certainly do not have the mindset of a patient with a chronic disease. At study entry, they will have just learned about the possibility (or probability) of MS and will not have had time to deal emotionally with this at the time they have to decide whether to participate in the trial. Also, within a few weeks of study entry, most of the patients will have little or no visual or neurologic disability and will feel physically normal. Both of these factors may produce difficulty in continued patient acceptance of a blinded treatment and thus impact upon patient adherence to the protocol.

6. One of the outcome assessments of interest would be a measure of quality of life, specifically related to medication administration and side effects, on feeling of well-being and costs of missed work time for treatment (see Chapter 6). Having all patients receive the same treatment schedules would limit the utility of this assessment. If the control group received no treatment (active or placebo) beyond the initial corticosteroid regimen, the impact of the frequent beta interferon injections on quality of life could be more readily assessed.

In summary, the cons for having a placebo-treated control group rather than an untreated control group seemingly outweigh the pros. It is likely that internal validity could be maintained without their use of placebos and that their use could reduce patient compliance to an extent such that the benefits to enhanced validity would be overshadowed by the detractions. From a practical standpoint, the feasibility of successfully completing such a study may be determined ultimately by the referring neurologists. Their willingness to accept results from a study of untreated rather than placebo-treated controls will probably be a significant factor in recruiting the necessary patients to meet the required sample size.

Outcome Determinations

The outcome of treatments can be evaluated in several ways including:

1. Slowing of the rate of development of new neurologic events;
2. Reduction in the development of neurologic disability;
3. Reduction in the development of signal abnormalities on brain MRI;
4. Improved quality of life.

The consensus reached at a workshop on MS clinical trial design (Whitaker et al. in press) was that clinical measures should serve as the primary outcomes in full scale randomized trials and serial cranial MRI should serve as a secondary outcome measure.

If development of a new neurologic event is considered as the primary outcome, then assuming that all patients are treated initially with corticosteroids, a fixed period of time should be established before a second event is counted. This will allow for the possibility that some patients might initially worsen after completion of the corticosteroids. In the ONTT, it was found that four of the 151 patients who received the intravenous followed by the oral regimen had two or more lines of decrease in visual acuity between the day 15 and day 30 visits. It would therefore seem reasonable to exclude a second event for 30 days after the onset of optic neuritis.

A decision needs to be made about whether a new attack of optic neuritis in the fellow eye, which occurs at least 30 days after the onset of the initial treatment should be considered sufficient for diagnosis of CDMS. Although diagnostic criteria are vague about this (Poser et al. 1983), they do suggest that consecutive optic neuritis in each eye, separated by at least 15 days, constitutes evidence of two events sufficient for diagnosis of CDMS. However, recurrent optic neuritis in the same eye does not appear to be sufficient for diagnosis. The inclusion of fellow eye optic neuritis in the definition of outcome would have the favorable effect of reducing the sample size requirement by increasing the expected event rate in the control group. If a new attack of optic neuritis in the fellow eye is considered part of the study's primary outcome definition, then patients who experienced previous optic neuritis that recurs at the time of study entry should be excluded.

The time period for assessing the study outcome must be established as a compromise between the need to have a sufficiently long time period to obtain a sufficient number of outcomes and not too long a period, such that losses to follow-up and patient non-compliance become a validity-threatening problem. If the development of a new neurologic event is chosen to be the primary study outcome, then either a 2- or 3-year follow-up period would seem most reasonable. Review of the older literature (1950–1976) as summarized by Perkin and Rose (1979) showed that the majority of patients who converted to clinical MS after optic neuritis did so within the first 2 years. This is corroborated in Paty's data, which indicated that, among patients with monosymptomatic onsets who develop CDMS within 15 years, 50%–60% do so within 2 years (D. Paty, personal communication) A 2-year follow-up period would have the advantage of enhanced patient compliance and a shorter term of study. A 3-year follow-up period would have the advantage of a reduced sample size because of the higher event rate in 3 versus 2 years and might be more clinically meaningful. A follow-up period longer than 3 years would be likely to prove to be unfeasible because of the large proportion of patients who would be relatively asymptomatic and almost certainly unwilling to comply with such a long-term, unproven treatment regimen.

A major problem in assessing any outcome other than the development of a new neurologic event is that maintaining the integrity of the treatment groups would be likely to prove to be unfeasible. Once a new neurologic event occurs that is sufficient for classifying the patient as having CDMS, it may be necessary on either ethical or practical grounds to treat the acute event with corticosteroids and to consider long-term treatment with an FDA-approved drug such as Betaseron. In such cases, it may not be possible to maintain the patient in a masked treatment group. Since it is probable that this will be the case for a substantial number of patients who develop a new neurologic event, the validity of any treatment group outcome comparisons that rely on data collected beyond the initial neurologic event will be impaired.

Neurologic Disability

Although neurologic disability, in theory, would be a preferable outcome measure to the development of a new clinical event, it is not practical to select this as a primary outcome measure. First, as discussed above, once a patient develops a new neurologic event and almost certainly once neurologic disability is sustained, open-label therapy will probably be substituted for the masked protocol treatment in a substantial number of patients. Secondly, assuming that patients with CDMS are excluded from the study, the frequency of development of the measurable neurologic disability that would be expected to occur within the first 2–3 years of follow-up would be low. In the ONTT, among patients with two or more signal abnormalities on the baseline brain MRI, an EDSS score ≥2 was present in only 14% of 74 patients at 3 years and in only 10% of 46 patients who completed 5 years of follow-up. Thus, based on the ONTT experience, even extending the follow-up period to 5 years would not provide a sufficient amount of disability in the control group to assess treatment benefit with a feasible sample size.

Magnetic Resonance Imaging

A number of recent studies have shown that serial MRI studies both complement the clinical impression of a treatment effect (if one is seen) and improve the likelihood that a subclinical treatment effect will not go undetected.

Serial cranial MRI studies at 6-month intervals may represent a practical compromise between the ideal, yet prohibitively expensive, position that scans must be done every 4–6 weeks on all patients to detect subtle and transient changes in lesion size and to identify areas of intermittent gadolinium enhancement (indicative of blood–brain barrier disruption) (Harris et al. 1991; McFarland et al. 1992; Smith et al. 1993), and the less costly, but less sensitive, annual MRI design. MRI studies every 6 months provide an acceptably sensitive, fiscally responsible and lasting quantifiable index of MS disease activity, as complete disappearance of MRI-detected T2-weighted signal abnormalities occur very rarely, if at all, provided that studies are done at high field (e.g. 1.5 T), using contiguous, interleaved 5 mm sections (Noseworthy et al. 1993; Wiebe et al. 1992). Serial studies suggest that most patients with early relapsing–remitting MS will show evidence of new gadolinium-enhancing lesions within a 6-month period (5/7 in Isaac's series (Isaac et al. 1988), 6/9 in Willoughby's series (Willoughby et al. 1989) and 15/17 in Thompson's series (Miller et al. 1991)).

The interpretation of MRI results will have the same problem as discussed for disability data, namely that, once a new clinical event is reached, the integrity of the treatment groups likely will be likey to be corrupted. Methods of addressing this in the analysis of the MRI data need investigation.

Quality of Life

The majority of patients in a monosymptomatic MS trial will have experienced limited physical disability at study entry, quick resolution of those symptoms, and may remain relatively asymptomatic from a visual and neurologic point of view for the duration of the trial. Thus, assessment of the impact of the treatments on quality of life will be valuable and any benefit found with treatment must be weighed against the potential adverse effect of the treatments on quality of life. Quality of life may be unrelated or inversely related to positive long-term treatment impact, and negatively related to participation in specific arms of the clinical trial, depending on the treatment regimens that are being evaluated. The definition and measurement of quality of life outcomes in the context of clinical trials are discussed in Chapter 6.

Sample Size and Power Considerations

The sample size estimate is highly dependent on the expected outcome rate in the control group. As discussed in earlier sections, it is proposed that the primary outcome be the development of a new neurologic event sufficient for diagnosis of CDMS. It is also proposed that all patients receive initial treatment with intravenous corticosteroids.

Assuming that all patients would receive initial corticosteroid treatment, for a 2-year follow-up study, the ONTT provides the only systematically collected data on patients who would be eligible for the proposed trial. For the ONTT patients in the intravenous group who would be eligible for the proposed trial (e.g. those without clinical MS at baseline and without two or more brain MRI lesions), the 2-year rate of CDMS (including fellow eye optic neuritis in the definition of CDMS) was 25% (95% confidence interval 18–32). If the ONTT finding of a beneficial effect from intravenous corticosteroids was spurious and not a true treatment effect, then the control group rate, based on the ONTT placebo and prednisone groups, would be expected to be about 45%.

If the follow-up period were to be 3 years, then data from other studies as well as the ONTT are applicable since by 3 years there was no longer a benefit to intravenous treatment in the ONTT. For optic neuritis patients, the ONTT data suggest that the 3-year control-group outcome rate would be 45%. From the data reviewed earlier, it is likely that the outcome rate following a brainstem syndrome or myelitis would be likely to be higher, perhaps as high as 75% (Ford et al. 1992; Lee et al. 1991a; Morrissey et al. 1993).

For a study that would compare one treatment against a control, with an alpha level of 0.05, 90% power, adjustment for 10% losses to follow-up over a 2-year period, a 2-year control group outcome rate of 25% and the ability to detect a 50% treatment effect, the necessary sample size would be about 240 in each of the two groups. If a 3-year follow-up study was conducted such that the control group outcome rate was projected to be 50%, then the sample size requirement would be 100 in each of two groups to detect a 50% treatment effect (alpha = 0.05, 90% power, and adjustment for 20% losses to follow-up), and 225 in each of two groups to detect a 33% treatment effect.

Serial MRI can be expected to detect changes that suggest ongoing disease activity earlier and in a greater proportion of enrolled patients than will be identified by neurologic evaluations alone. Thus, MRI should provide increased statistical power compared with a clinical outcome. This may be valuable in identifying subgroups in which there is a differential treatment effect.

Acknowledgements

Much of this chapter is derived from a manual for procedures written for the Monosymptomatic MS Treatment Trial (MMSTT) by a planning committee consisting of Roy Beck, Carol Brownscheidle, Lawrence Jacobs, Rip Kinkel, John Noseworthy, Donald Goodkin, Robert Herndon and Donald Paty. The section "Rationale for treatment at the time of the first clinical event" is attributable to Rip Kinkel, and the section "Outcome determinations: magnetic resonance imaging" to John Noseworthy. The section "Interpretation of the Optic Neuritis Treatment Trial Results" was written in collaboration with Jonathan Trobe and is included as part of a manuscript published in the *Journal of Clinical Neuro-ophthalmology*.

References

Acha Orbea H, Mitchell DJ, Timmermann L et al. (1988) Limited heterogeneity of T cell receptors from lymphocytes mediating autoimmune encephalomyelitis allows specific immune intervention. Cell 54:263

Allegrett M, Nicklas JA, Sriram S et al. (1990) T cells responsive to myelin basic protein in patients with multiple sclerosis. Science 247:718

Alvord EC, Kies MW, Suckling AJ (ed) (1984) Experimental allergic encephalomyelitis: a useful model for multiple sclerosis. New York: Liss (Progress in clinical and biological reseach)

Beck RW, Trobe JD (1995) The Optic Neuritis Treatment Trial: putting the results in perspective. J Clin Neuro-ophthalmol 15:131–135

Beck RW, Cleary PA, Anderson MMJ et al (1992) A randomized, controlled trial of corticosteroids in the treatment of acute optic neuritis. N Engl J Med 326:581–588

Beck RW, Arrington J, Murtagh FR, Cleary PA, Kaufman DI (1993a) Optic neuritis study: brain MRI in acute optic neuritis. Experience of the Optic Neuritis Study Group. Arch Neurol 8:841–846

Beck RW, Cleary PA, Optic Neuritis Study Group (1993b) Optic neuritis treatment trial: one-year follow-up results. Arch Ophthalmol 111:773–775

Beck RW, Cleary PA, Trobe JD et al. (1993c) The effect of corticosteroids for acute optic neuritis on the subsequent development of multiple sclerosis. New Engl J Med 329:1764–1769

Bornstein MB, Johnson KP (1992) Treatment of multiple sclerosis with copolymer 1. In: Rudick RA, Goodkin DE (eds) Treatment of multiple sclerosis. Springer-Verlag, New York, pp 173–198

Bornstein MB, Miller A, Slagle S et al. (1987) A pilot trial of COP 1 in exacerbating-remitting multiple sclerosis. N Engl J Med 317:408–414

Bornstein MB, Miller A, Slagle S et al. (1991) A placebo controlled, double-blind, randomized, two-center pilot trial of COP I in chronic progressive multiple sclerosis. Neurology 41:533–539

Camenga DL, Johnson KP, Alter M (1986) Systemic recombinant alpha-2 interferon therapy in relapsing multiple sclerosis. Arch Neurol 43:1239–1246

Chrousos GA, Kattah JC, Beck RW, Cleary PA, Optic Neuritis Study Group (1993) Side effects of glucocorticoid treatment: experience of the Optic Neuritis Treatment Trial. JAMA 269:2110–2112

Corbett JJ, Cruse JM (1993) Corticosteroids and optic neuritis. Neurology 43:634

Cross AH, Tuohy VK, Raine CS (1993) Development of reactivity to new myelin antigens during chronic relapsing autoimmune demyelination. Cell Immunol 146:261

Durelli L, Bongioanni MR, Cavalo R et al. (1994) Chronic systemic high-dose recombinant interferon alfa-2a reduces exacerbation rate, MRI signs of disease activity and lymphocyte interferon gamma production in relapsing-remitting multiple sclerosis. Neurology 44:406–413

Ellison GW, Meyers LW, McKey MR et al. (1989) A placebo-controlled, randomized, double-masked, variable dosage, clinical trial of azathioprine with and without methylprednisolone in multiple sclerosis. Neurology 39:1087–1126

Filippi M, Horsfield MA, Morrissey SP et al. (1994) Quantitative brain MRI lesion load predicts the course of clinically isolated syndromes suggestive of multiple sclerosis. Neurology 44:635–641

Ford B, Tampieri D, Francis G (1992) Long-term follow-up of acute partial transverse myelopathy. Neurology 42:250–252

Frederiksen JL, Larsson HBW, Henriksen O, Olesen J (1989) Magnetic resonance imaging of the brain in patients with acute monosymptomatic optic neuritis. Acta Neurol Scand 80:512–517

Giang D, Goodman A, Mattson D, Schiffer R, Cohen N, Ader R (1996) Can immunomodulatory effects of cyclophosphamide be conditioned in humans? J Neuropsychiatr Clin Neurosci (in press)

Harris JO, Frank JA, Patronas N, McFarlin DE, McFarland HF (1991) Serial gadolinium-enhanced magnetic resonance imaging scans in patients with early, relapsing-remitting multiple sclerosis: implications for clinical trials and natural history. Ann Neurol 29:548–555

Haynes BF, Fauci AS (1978) The differential effect of in vivo hydrocortisone on the kinetics of subpopulations of human peripheral blood thymus-derived lymphocytes. J Clin Invest 61:703–707

Heath WR, Allison J, Hoffmann MW et al. (1992) Autoimmune diabetes as a consequence of locally produced interleukin-2. Nature 359:547

Hood L, Kumar V, Osaman G et al. (1989) Autoimmune disease and T-cell immunologic recognition. Cold Spring Harb Symp Quant Biol 54:859

IFN-B Multiple Sclerosis Study Group (1993) Interferon beta-1b is effective in relapsing-remitting multiple sclerosis: I. Clinical results of a multicenter, randomized, double-blind, placebo-controlled trial. Neurology 48:655–661

Isaac C, Li DK, Genton M et al. (1988) Multiple sclerosis: a serial study using MRI in relapsing patients. Neurology 38:1511–1515

Jacobs L, Munschauer FE, Kaba SE (1991) Clinical and magnetic resonance imaging in optic neuritis. Neurology 41:15–19

Jacobs L, Cookfair D, Rudick R, Herndon R et al. (1993) A phase III trial of recombinant beta interferon as treatment for multiple sclerosis. Ann Neurol 34:310

Jacobs L, Brownscheidle C, Cookfair D, Rudick RA, The Multiple Sclerosis Collaborative Research Group (1994) Recombinant interferon-beta as treatment for multiple sclerosis. Arthritis Foundation, Atlanta, GA, pp 103–112 (Proceedings: Early decisions in DMARD development: III. Biologic agents in autoimmune disease vol. 3)

Kastrukoff LF, Oger JJ, Hashimoto SA et al. (1990) Systemic lymphoblastoid interferon therapy in chronic progressive multiple sclerois. I. Clinical and MRI evaluation. Neurology 40:479–486

Kaufmann DL, Clare-Salzler M, Tian J et al. (1993) Spontaneous loss of T-cell tolerance to glutamic acid decarboxylase in insulin-dependent diabetes. Nature 366:69

Kinkel RP, Goodkin DE (1994) Immunotherapy for multiple sclerosis: a review of the clinical experience. Clin Immunother 1:117–134

Kitze B, Pette M, Rohrbach E et al. (1988) Myelin-specific T lymphocytes in multiple sclerosis patients and healthy individuals. J Neuroimmunol 20:237

Kotzin BL, Karuturi S, Chou YK et al. (1991) Preferential T-cell receptor beta-chain variable gene use in myelin basic protein-reactive T-cell clones from patients with multiple sclerosis. Proc Natl Acad Sci USA 88:9161

Kupersmith MJ, Kaufman D, Paty DW et al. (1994) Megadose corticosteroids in multiple sclerosis. Neurology 44:1–4

Lee KH, Hashimoto SA, Hooge JP et al. (1991a) Magnetic resonance imaging of the head in the diagnosis of multiple sclerosis. Neurology 41:657–660

Lee SJ, Wucherpfennig KW, Brod SA et al. (1991b) Common T cell receptor V beta usage in oligoclonal T lymphocytes derived from cerebrospinal fluid and blood of patients with multiple sclerosis. Ann Neurol 29:23

Lehmann PV, Forsthuber T, Miller A et al. (1992) Spreading of T-cell autoimmunity to cryptic determinants of an autoantigen. Nature 358:155

Martin R, Howell MD, Jaraquemada D et al. (1991) A myelin basic protein peptide is recognized by cytotoxic T-cells in the context of four HLA-DR types associated with multiple sclerosis. J Exp Med 173:19

Martin R, Utz U, Coligan JE et al. (1992) Diversity in fine specificity and T cell receptor usage of the human CD4+ cytotoxic T cell response specific for the immunodominant myelin basic protein peptide 87–106. J Immunol 148:1359

Martinelli V, Comi G, Filippi M, et al. (1991) Paraclinical tests in acute-onset optic neuritis, basal data and results of a short follow up. Acta Neurol Scand 84:231–236

McFarland HF, Frank JA, Alber PS et al. (1992) Using gadolinium-enhanced magnetic resonance imaging lesions to monitor disease activity in multiple sclerosis. Ann Neurol 32:758–766

Miller DH, Ormerod IEC, McDonald WI et al. (1988) The early risk of multiple sclerosis after optic neuritis. J Neurol Neurosurg Psychiatry 51:1569–1571

Miller DH, Barkhof F, Kappos L, Scotti G, Thompson AJ (1991) Magnetic resonance imaging in monitoring the treatment of multiple sclerosis: concerted action guidelines. J Neurol Neurosurg Psychiatry 54:683–688

Mix E, Olsson T, Correale J et al. (1990) CD4+, CD8+, and CD4–, CD8– T-cells in CSF and blood of patients with multiple sclerosis and tension headache. Scand J Immunol 31:493–501

Morrissey SP, Miller DH, Kendall BE et al. (1993) The significance of brain magnetic resonance imaging abnormalities at presentation with clinically isolated syndromes suggestive of multiple sclerosis. Brain 116:135–146

Noseworthy JH, Hopkins MB, Vandervoort MK et al. (1993) An open-trial evaluation of mitoxantrone in the treatment of progressive MS. Neurology 43:1401–1406

Noseworthy JH, Ebers GC, Vandervoort MK, Farquhar RE, Yetisir E, Roberts R (1994) The impact of blinding on the results of a randomized, placebo-controlled multiple sclerosis clinical trial. Neurology 44:16–20

Ota K, Matsui M, Milford EL et al. (1990) T-cell recognition of an immunodominant myelin basic protein epitope in multiple sclerosis. Nature 346:183

Panitch HS, Hirsh RL, Haley AS et al. (1987) Exacerbations of multiple sclerosis in patients treated with gamma interferon. Lancet i:893–895

Paty DW, Li DKB, UBC MS/MRI Study Group, IFNB Multiple Sclerosis Study Group (1993) Interferon beta-1b is effective in relapsing-remitting multiple sclerosis: II. MRI analysis results of a multicenter, randomized, double-blind, placebo-controlled trial. Neurology 43:662–667

Perkin GD, Rose FC (1979) Optic neuritis and its differential diagnosis. New York: Oxford University Press

Pette M, Fujita K, Kitze B et al. (1990a) Myelin basic protein-specific T lymphocyte lines from MS patients and healthy individuals. Neurology 40:1770

Pette M, Fujita K, Wilkinson D et al. (1990b) Myelin autoreactivity in multiple sclerosis: recognition of myelin basic protein in the context of HLA-DR2 products by T lymphocytes of multiple-sclerosis patient and healthy donors. Proc Natl Acad Sci USA 87:7968

Poser CM, Paty DW, Scheinberg L, McDonald WI et al. (1983) New diagnostic criteria for multiple sclerosis: guidelines for research protocols. Ann Neurol 13:227–231

Raine CS (1984) Biology of disease. Analysis of autoimmune demyelination: its impact upon multiple sclerosis. Lab Invest 50:608–635

Reder AT, Thapar M, Jensen MA (1994) A reduction in serum glucocorticoids provokes experimental allergic encephalomyelitis: implications for treatment of inflammatory brain disease. Neurology 44:2289–2294

Richert JR, Robinson ED, Johnson AH et al. (1991) Heterogeneity of the T-cell receptor beta gene rearrangements generated in myelin basic protein-specific T-cell clones isolated from a patient with multiple sclerosis. Ann Neurol 29:299

Sarvetnick N, Shizuru J, Liggit D et al. (1990) Loss of pancreatic islet tolerance induced by beta-cell expression of interferon-gamma. Nature 346:844

Smith ME, Stone LA, Albert PS et al. (1993). Clinical worsening in multiple sclerosis is associated with increased frequency and area of gadopentetate dimeglumine-enhancing magnetic resonance imaging lesions. Ann Neurol 33:480–489

Troiano JR, Cook SD, Dowling PC (1987) Steroid therapy in multiple sclerosis [Point of view]. Arch Neurol 44:803–807

Urban JL, Kumar V, Kono DH et al. (1988) Restricted use of T cell receptor V genes in immune autoimmune encephalomyelitis raises possibilities for antibody therapy. Cell 54:577

Whitaker JN, McFarland HF, Rudge P, Reingold SC (1996) Outcomes assessment in multiple sclerosis clinical trials: a critical analysis. Multiple Sclerosis (in press)

Wiebe S, Lee DH, Karlik SJ et al. (1992) Serial cranial and spinal cord magnetic resonance imaging in multiple sclerosis. Ann Neurol 32:643–650

Willoughby EW, Grochowski E, Li DK, Oger J, Kastrukoff LF, Paty DW (1989) Serial magnetic resonance scanning in multiple sclerosis: a second prospective study in relapsing patients. Ann Neurol 25:43–49

Wucherpfennig KW, Ota K, Endo N et al. (1990) Shared human T cell receptor V beta usage to immunodominant regions of myelin basic protein. Science 248:1016

Wucherpfennig KW, Newcombe J, Cuzner L et al. (1991) Analysis of T-cell receptors in MS plaques. Neurology 41(Suppl):380

11 Treatment of Multiple Sclerosis with Type I Interferons

Richard A. Rudick, William Sibley and Luca Durelli

Background

Overview of Interferons

Interferons (IFNs) were first detected based on their antiviral properties (Isaacs and Lindenmann 1957), and classified as leukocyte, fibroblast or immune IFN, according to their cellular source. IFNs are now known to comprise a family of more than 20 different proteins, categorized as type I IFN (leukocyte and fibroblast IFN) and type II IFN (immune IFN). Current nomenclature (Table 11.1) is based on sequence analysis of the IFN genes. There are four distinct varieties of type I IFN (IFN-α, IFN-β, IFN-τ and IFN-ω) and a single type II IFN (IFN-γ). In humans, there are at least 18 non-allelic IFN-α genes, four of which are pseudogenes, at least six non-allelic IFN-ω genes, five of which are pseudogenes, but only a single IFN-β gene. Type I IFN genes lack introns and are located on the short arm of chromosome 9. IFN-γ is encoded by a single gene with three introns on chromosome 12. Trophoblast IFN (IFN-τ), a recently described IFN, functions to maintain the gravid state in pregnant female ruminants. IFN-τ has not yet been described in humans. It interacts with the IFN-α/β receptor, although its expression is regulated quite differently (Li and Roberts 1994).

History of Interferon Treatment in MS

During the 20 years that followed the discovery of IFN, there was intense speculation that multiple sclerosis (MS) might be due to a persistent "slow" virus infection, and hope that IFN's antiviral effects might prove therapeutic in MS. Unsuccessful attempts to identify antiviral activity in MS brain (Sibley and Tourtellotte 1968), or to transmit MS to adult (Gibbs et al. 1969) or newborn (Sibley et al. 1980) non-human primates made the possibility of direct viral infection as the etiology of MS seem less likely, but did not eliminate it; consequently, the principal rationale for early IFN trials was the possibility that MS might be due to a virus.

Table 11.1. Classification of the interferons (modified from Baron et al. 1992)

	Type I	Type II
Main types	α and β	γ
Other types	τ and ω	None
Structure	Monomer	Dimer
Cellular source	α: any virus-infected cell	Activated T cells
	β: fibroblasts	NK cells

The earliest MS clinical trials employed natural IFN-α and IFN-β in relatively small numbers of patients because of difficulties in producing large quantities of the agents. Fog (1980) carried out the first trial, treating five progressive MS patients with intramuscular (IM) natural IFN-α, 5 million international units (MIU) daily for 2 weeks, followed by 2.5 MIU daily for 5–15 months. He noted continued clinical deterioration in all patients. Results of larger subsequent studies using IFN-α were also negative or equivocal. Knobler et al. (1984) treated 24 patients with frequent exacerbations with 5 MIU of natural IFN-α or placebo daily by IM injections for 6-month periods in a cross-over design. There were fewer exacerbations during IFN-α treatment in patients with relapsing–remitting MS, but the results did not reach statistical significance, and disability was not demonstrably affected. Camenga et al. (1986) first used recombinant IFN-α in a double-blind, randomized, placebo-controlled trial in 98 MS patients lasting 1 year, using a dosing regimen of 2 MIU, three times weekly by subcutaneous (SC) injection. No clear benefit was demonstrated. A subsequent Australian study (AUSTIMS Research Group 1989) compared natural IFN-α, transfer factor and placebo in a three-arm study. The maximum dosage of IFN-α in this study was 3 MIU twice weekly for 2 months, then weekly for 10 months, and then biweekly for 24 months. There was no significant difference in exacerbation rate or progression of disability in the three groups at the end of the study.

The earliest trial of natural IFN-β was conducted by Jacobs et al. (1981) who gave 1 MIU natural IFN-β intrathecally (IT) twice weekly for 4 weeks, and then monthly for 5 months in a pilot study with ten MS patients. Ten unblinded MS patients who did not have serial lumbar punctures were used as controls. There were significantly fewer exacerbations in IT IFN-β recipients compared with both pre-treatment exacerbation rates (ERs) and to the rates in the untreated controls. Later, Jacobs et al. (1986) reported a larger multicenter trial using similar methods and doses (IFN-β was given IT only once weekly during the first month). Sixty-nine patients were entered into a double-blind, placebo-controlled, randomized study. Control patients had true lumbar punctures at the beginning, at 6 months, and at the end of the study. They had "sham" lumbar punctures corresponding to the other treatment times in the actively treated group. Again the results indicated a significantly greater reduction in ERs in IT IFN-β recipients compared with controls.

Positive results from the latter two studies, initially equivocal results with IFN-α, and the emergence of recombinant IFN-β preparations resulted in two major efforts to test systemic recombinant IFN-β in MS. Johnson et al. (1990) reported the results of a pilot study treating a small group of MS patients with varying doses of SC IFN-β-1b (Betaseron®), a serine-substituted, nonglycosylated recombinant IFN-β preparation produced by *Escherichia coli*. Patients tolerated IFN-β at a dosage of 45 MIU every other day (equivalent to 8 MIU by the new World Health Organization reference standard for recombinant IFN – references to this dose throughout this chapter will use 8 MIU). A final report of the pilot study was reported in 1993 (Knobler et al. 1993). The multicenter Betaseron® study began in 1988 and was completed and first reported in 1993 (IFN-β MS Study Group 1993; Paty et al. 1993). Around the same time as the Betaseron® pilot study, Jacobs and colleagues designed a study of another recombinant IFN-β, IFN-β-1a, a glycosylated recombinant product with an amino acid sequence identical to native IFN-β made by Chinese hamster ovary cells. A pilot study of IFN-β-1a established that an IM injection of 6 MIU, together with oral acetominophen, had few side effects but elicited increased levels of β_2-microglobulin evident for almost 1 week (Jacobs and Munschauer 1992). The multicenter IFN-β-1a (Avonex™) study, conducted by the Multiple Sclerosis Collaborative Research Group (MSCRG), began in 1990 and was completed in 1994 (Jacobs et al. 1994). At the same time, interest in IFN-α was rekindled by a smaller study of recombinant IFN-α that showed beneficial clinical, imaging and immunologic effects (Durelli et al. 1996). These studies have firmly established a therapeutic role for type I IFN in exacerbating-remitting MS patients, and have driven interest in the mechanisms whereby type I IFN exerts a therapeutic response.

Recombinant Interferon-β-1b (Betaseron®) American/Canadian Multicenter Trial

Design and Methodology

This trial was conducted in seven American and four Canadian centers. Three hundred and seventy-two patients were accrued between 1988 and July 1989 and randomized to placebo, 1.6 MIU Betaseron®, and 8 MIU Betaseron® self-administered by SC injections every other day. Patients had relapsing-remitting MS, were ambulatory with mild to moderate disability (mean Kurtzke Expanded Disability Status Scale (EDSS) 2.9) and had MS for a mean period of 4.4 years. The trial was designed to last for 2 years, but patients were given the option to continue for an additional year at the end of years 2, 3 and 4. Because patient accrual was gradual and some subjects elected to leave the trial after 2 or 3 years, the on-study time was variable, ranging from 3.5–5.0 years (Table 11.2). In late 1992, results from the first 3 years were analyzed and an unblinded external advisory committee suggested in January 1993 that the trial be discontinued and all patients offered treatment at a dose 8 MIU.

In addition to determining ERs, the neurologic rating scale (NRS) (Sipe et al 1984) was used to grade exacerbation severity as mild, moderate or severe. Subjects were considered to have disability progression when there was an increase from baseline of ≥1.0 EDSS point (Kurtzke 1983) confirmed on two successive examinations separated by 3 months. Disability measured during an

Table 11.2. Betaseron® in relapsing-remitting MS: number of patients completing each year of study (based on data from IFNB Multiple Sclerosis Study Group 1993)

	Placebo	1.6 MIU	8 MIU
No. enrolled (%)	123 (100)	125 (100)	124 (100)
No. completing (%)			
Year 1	110 (89)	114 (91)	107 (86)
Year 2	96 (78)	95 (76)	95 (77)
Year 3	82 (67)	76 (61)	89 (72)
Year 4	56 (46)	52 (42)	58 (47)
Year 5	2 (2)	2 (2)	1 (1)
Time on study (months)			
Mean	40.3	39.4	40.6
Median	46	45	48
SEM	1.48	1.47	1.61

exacerbation was excluded, unless the symptoms and signs of the exacerbation persisted for longer than 6 months. Computer assisted evaluation of the total T2 lesion area in annual magnetic resonance imaging (MRI) scans was performed by the University of British Columbia analysis group in a blinded fashion. In 1994, all scans on a given patient were reanalyzed simultaneously to confirm reports in the original publication. In the 217 patients having a fourth or fifth year annual scan, the statistical significance of change from baseline in total lesion burden was calculated within treatment groups, as was the difference in change between placebo and 8 MIU Betaseron® recipients. Patients were followed to the point of dropout and all data derived to that point were included in the analysis. Data were also analyzed separately for the 159 dropouts, to evaluate any systematic bias that they may have introduced into the study.

Exacerbations Rates

Exacerbation rates in 8 MIU Betaseron® recipients were approximately 30% lower than placebo recipients during the entire blinded study (Table 11.3). When the data were analyzed by study year, the differences were highly significant only during the first 2 years of the study, although the 8 MIU group continued to have approximately 30% fewer exacerbations than the placebo group in years 3–5. Loss of statistical significance occurred for several reasons. There appeared to be a drop in ER in all arms of the study during years 3–5, which may be in part due to the natural decline in ER commonly observed in untreated MS patients. An additional reason, however, was that dropouts with the highest ERs were in the placebo group. Annual ERs in dropouts were 1.6 for placebo recipients, 1.35 for 1.6 MIU Betaseron® recipients and 1.02 for 8 MIU Betaseron® recipients during the study. These factors and the smaller sample sizes diminished the power to show statistically significant treatment effects on ERs in the later years, even though annually there were always about one-third fewer exacerbations in the 8 MIU group.

Table 11.3. Pooled data: annual exacerbation rates during entire blinded Betaseron® trial (based on data from IFNB Multiple Sclerosis Study Group 1993)

Group	Rate	95% CI
Placebo	1.12	1.02–1.23
1.6 MIU	0.96	0.87–1.06
8.0 MIU	0.78	0.70–0.88

Placebo vs 8 MIU $p = 0.0006$
Placebo vs 1.6 MIU $p = 0.0057$
1.6 MIU vs 8 MIU $p = 0.3323$

Table 11.4. Exacerbation severity: Betaseron® study (based on data from IFNB Multiple Sclerosis Study Group 1993)

Severity	Annual exacerbation rate		
	Placebo	1.6 MIU	8 MIU
Mild	0.49	0.50	0.41
Moderate	0.23	0.16	0.16
Severe	0.14	0.11	0.08
Unknown	0.27	0.19	0.14

Significance of rate of moderate and severe exacerbations:
Placebo vs 8 MIU $p = 0.012$
Placebo vs 1.6 MIU $p = 0.023$
1.6 MIU vs 8 MIU $p = 0.875$

Exacerbation Severity

Subjects treated with Betaseron® during the entire blinded trial also had fewer moderate/severe attacks than patients in the placebo group (Table 11.4, above), consistent with the original 1993 report. The "unknowns" listed in this table represent patients in whom examinations were not performed until at least several days after new symptoms reached their peak, when objective assessment of peak severity was no longer possible. The combined effect of fewer exacerbations and fewer severe exacerbations resulted in significantly fewer hospitalizations for Betaseron® recipients, as previously reported.

Effect on Disability

At the end of 3 years, 28% (34/123) of placebo recipients had confirmed disability progression, compared with 20% (25/124) of the 8 MIU Betaseron® recipients. During the entire blinded trial (median follow-up approximately 4 years) confirmed progression occurred in fewer 8 MIU Betaseron® recipients than placebo recipients, but the differences did not reach statistical significance. Fifty-six (46%) of 123 placebo recipients progressed, compared with 43 (35%) of 124 8 MIU Betaseron® recipients, and the median time to progression in those placebo patients who progressed was 4.18 years, compared with 4.79 years in the 8 MIU treatment arm ($p = 0.096$). Progression rates did not vary according to entry EDSS. For patients with entry EDSS <3.0, 45% of placebo recipients progressed compared with only 36% of 8 MIU Betaseron® recipients. For patients with entry EDSS ≥3.0, 47% of placebo recipients progressed compared with only 34% of the 8 MIU Betaseron® recipients.

Effect on Magnetic Resonance Imaging Activity and Total T2 Lesion Area

The most dramatic effects seen in the Betaseron® trial were in a 52-patient cohort having unenhanced brian MRI scans every 6 weeks for 2 years. The median percentage active scans (new or enlarging T2-weighted lesions) was 29.4% in placebo recipients and 5.9% in the 8 MIU Betaseron® recipients, which was a sixfold reduction. Likewise, the median number of new T2-weighted lesions per year in this cohort was 2.0 in placebo recipients and 0.5 in 8 MIU Betaseron® recipients, which was a fourfold reduction. At the end of the first year, the MRI total T2-weighted lesion burden, as measured from annual scans performed on all patients, increased from baseline by 12.2% in the placebo group and *decreased* by 1.1% in the 8 MIU Betaseron® recipients. At the end of the second year, there was a 20% increase in placebo recipients, and a 0.1% decrease in the 8 MIU Betaseron® recipients.

The analysis of the final results of the blinded trial (IFNB Multiple Sclerosis Study Group 1995) included a detailed study of 217 patients having either a fourth or fifth year evaluable scan after baseline. A modified version of this analysis is included in Table 11.5. The *p*-values in parentheses refer to the significance of year to year changes in MRI lesion burden within treatment arms. Note that the yearly increase in MRI lesion burden remained significant in the placebo group and in the 1.6 MIU Betaseron® group (with one exception), but there was no significant yearly increase in MRI lesion burden in the 8 MIU Betaseron® group. The differences between the placebo and 8 MIU Betaseron® groups remained highly significant each year.

The Effect of Dropouts on the Interpretation of Results

A number of patients chose to discontinue the protocol at the end of the second or third years; in some cases, patients saw no change in existing symptoms and the results of the study were at that time unknown to them; some patients dropped out because of continuing activity of MS or because of side effects (IFNB Multiple Sclerosis Study Group and UBC/MRI Analysis Group 1995). Data on dropouts were analyzed and compared with results in study completers to evaluate any possible bias that might have been introduced by the dropouts. Patients with more severe MS tended to drop out of all of the treatment arms, but this was especially true in the placebo group, as evidenced by higher exacerbation rates, greater annual increases in EDSS, and higher new annual MRI lesion burden in dropouts compared with completers in the placebo arm (Table 11.6). This pattern would have the effect of decreasing the power of the study for showing treatment effects in the later years. The median annual EDSS change was: 0.24 in placebo group dropouts compared with no change in placebo group completers; 0.20 in the 1.6 MIU

Table 11.5. Median percentage change from baseline in MRI T2 lesion area in 217 patients having a year 4 or year 5 scan after baseline (based on data from IFNB Multiple Sclerosis Study Group 1993)

Timing of MRI	Placebo	1.6 MIU	8 MIU	Placebo vs 8 MIU
Baseline				
n	73	66	78	
Median % change (mm^2)	1503	1086	1525	
p				0.1996
1 year				
n	72	62	77	
Median % change (mm^2)	6.7	5.7	–4.9	
p	0.001	0.001	0.072	0.0012
2 years				
n	72	61	73	
Median % change (mm^2)	11.9	12.4	–5.6	
p	0.0001	0.001	0.259	0.0015
3 years				
n	70	59	73	
Median % change (mm^2)	21.0	6.1	–3.8	
p	0.0001	0.012	0.993	0.0002
4 years				
n	72	61	75	
Median % change (mm^2)	18.7	11.7	–0.8	
p	0.0001	0.001	0.917	0.0055
5 years				
n	14	16	19	
Median % change (mm^2)	30.2	10.6	3.6	
p	0.003	0.0833	0.374	0.0363

Notes:

1. The variability in "n" is due to differences in the number of patients with evaluable scans at a given time: e.g. a patient could have a year 5 scan but not a year 4 scan.
2. The *p*-values in columns 2–4 are for change from baseline MRI, within a treatment group.
3. Numbers are not identical to those in Table 11.2: All patients having a scan within 6 months of the anniversary of their study entry date were included for that year; therefore, the *n* is greater for each year than in Table 11.2, which refers to the number of patients completing each year.

Table 11.6. Dropouts and completers from the Betaseron® study (based on data from IFNB Multiple Sclerosis Study Group 1993)

	Dropouts	Completers
Annual exacerbation rates		
Placebo	1.6	0.98
1.6 MIU	1.35	0.80
8.0 MIU	1.02	0.72
EDSS: median annual change		
Placebo	0.24	0.0
1.6 MIU	0.20	0.13
8.0 MIU	0.07	0.0
MRI: median annual % change		
Placebo	13.7	4.6
1.6 MIU	5.0	3.0
8.0 MIU	–2.2	–0.1

Betaseron® group dropouts compared with 0.13 in completers; and 0.07 in the 8 MIU Betaseron® group dropouts compared with no change in the completers. The median annual percentage change in MRI lesion area was: 13.7 in placebo group dropouts compared with 4.6 for completers; 5.0 for the 1.6 MIU Betaseron® group dropouts compared with 3.0 for completers; and –2.2 in the 8 MIU Betaseron® group dropouts compared with –0.1 in completers. Thus, patients remaining in the placebo group throughout the study were those with less severe disability and MRI progression in the early years of the trial. It is likely that this helped to obscure any demonstrable treatment effect on disability, and lessened the magnitude of the observed MRI treatment effects.

Side Effects

In general, Betaseron® was well tolerated. Flu-like symptoms after injections with body aching and slight fever were the principal side effects. Flu-like symptoms were seen to some extent in the majority of patients in the first few weeks of the trial. These symptoms gradually subsided and were seldom troublesome after the second month of treatment. The frequency of flu-like symptoms was less in older patients (Table 11.7) and in patients with large body size (Table 11.8). Postmarketing experience with Betaseron® has indicated that flu-like symptoms are transient and continue indefinitely in only 4% of patients, and that they can be markedly reduced in severity by treatment with ibuprofen before and during the first 8–24 hours after injection. The slight fever experienced by some patients, especially after the first injection, is almost certainly a major cause of anecdotal reports of transient worsening of old MS symptoms during this period.

The other main side effect was injection site swelling and redness, which was variable in severity, being slight or modest in most patients. Injection site reactions tended to become somewhat less with time but generally continued to occur after each injection in affected patients. Injection site necrosis occurred at some time in 5% of patients, but only rarely after each injection. In some patients, poor injection technique may be a contributing factor. Laboratory abnormalities such as mild leukopenia and lymphopenia, and elevation of liver enzymes, normally subsided after the first several weeks and approached the rate seen in placebo recipients after 3 months. There have been no cases of clinical liver

Table 11.7. Effect of age on incidence of flu-like symptoms in MS patients treated with Betaseron® (based on data from IFNB Multiple Sclerosis Study Group 1993)

Age[a] (years)	% of subjects		
	Placebo	1.6 MIU	8 MIU
18–28	22	22	60
29–33	19	30	68
34–36	25	33	60
37–41	24	17	47
42–50	28	23	37

[a]Each age category represents 20% of overall patient population in the trial.

Table 11.8. Effect of body size on incidence of flu-like symptoms in MS patients treated with Betaseron® (based on data from IFNB Multiple Sclerosis Study Group 1993)

Surface area (m^2)[a]	% of subjects		
	Placebo	1.6 MIU	8 MIU
1.290–1.582	19	24	70
1.583–1.694	25	33	52
1.695–1.813	14	26	61
1.814–1.980	35	12	56
1.981–2.540	28	22	38

[a]Each category represents 20% of overall patient population in the trial.

disease induced by Betaseron®, and no opportunistic infections. Feelings of depression were reported with about the same frequency in all treatment arms in the first 2 years of the trial, although all of the three suicide attempts occurred during this period in Betaseron® recipients. In contrast to the first 2 years of the trial, feelings of depression were about twice as common in Betaseron® recipients during the last 3 years (5.26% placebo, 9.4% 1.6 MIU, and 11.7% 8 MIU Betaseron® recipients). The meaning of this is unclear, since many of the patients with more severe MS dropped out of the placebo group before the last 3 years of the study.

During the study, neutralizing antibodies (NABs) were measured quarterly. In some patients, a positive titer was seen sporadically but a sustained increase did not develop. Patients were classified as NAB-positive when there were two successive positive serum specimens. By this criterion, 38% of the patients remaining in the 8 MIU treatment arm were NAB-positive by the end of the third year. Development of NAB positivity usually occurred in the first year; after its development, the annual exacerbation rates of patients were the same as in the placebo arm. Thus, the group data reflecting reduction of exacerbation rates in the Betaseron® trial was almost entirely attributable to the NAB-negative patients (62% of treated patients). This group of patients experienced about a 50% reduction in exacerbation rate. The full clinical significance of NAB positivity, including the subsequent use of Betaseron® or other interferon preparations in these patients, is not known.

Recombinant Interferon-β-1a (Avonex™): the Multiple Sclerosis Collaborative Research Group Study

Design and Methodology

Recombinant IFN-β-1a (Avonex™) is a recombinant beta interferon product expressed by a mammalian cell line: the Chinese hampster ovary cell. IFN-β-1a is amino acid sequence-identical to human IFN-β and is glycosylated. The MSCRG conducted a multicenter, double-blind, randomized, placebo-controlled trial of IFN-β-1a at four clinical sites (Jacobs et al. 1996). Patients were randomized to two treatment arms: IFN-β–1a and placebo. Study subjects had definite MS of ≥1 year duration, were 18–55 years of age, had entry EDSS scores between 1.0 and

3.5, inclusive, had relapsing–remitting MS with ≥2 exacerbations in the prior 3 years, and were free of exacerbations or corticosteroid use for ≥2 months. The patients were well matched by treatment arm at baseline (Table 11.9).

The primary outcome was time to worsening from baseline EDSS of ≥1.0 point, persisting for two successive scheduled visits ≥6 months apart. The time to worsening was calculated as the number of days from randomization to the first EDSS score that was ≥1.0 points worse than baseline. The statistical analysis for this outcome variable used the Mantel–Cox statistic of Kaplan–Meier survival plots. Secondary outcomes included protocol-defined exacerbations, quantitative measures of upper and lower extremity function, neuropsychologic test perform ance, measurements of MS-related quality of life, the number and volume of gadolinium-enhanced MRI lesions on yearly MRI scans, and the volume of T2-weighted lesions on yearly MRI scans (Jacobs et al. 1996).

Treatment consisted of IFN-β-1a, 6 MIU IM, once weekly for up to 2 years. Weekly study injections were administered by a study nurse at each site, or by a designate (usually a local doctor or office nurse) under the study nurse's direction. Patients were not permitted to self-inject during the study. Acetominophen 650 mg orally was administered 6 hours prior to and for 24 hours after each IM injection to minimize flu-like side effects. The IFN-β-1a used in the study was supplied by Biogen, Inc. as a lyophilized product in vials containing 6×10^6 IU IFN-β-1a/30 μg protein. Subjects were evaluated by the examining neurologist every 6 months, or at the time of suspected exacerbation, throughout the study. A separate blinded treating neurologist provided standard MS treatment such as physiotherapy and symptomatic medications. At the time of suspected exacerbations, subjects were treated with IM corticotrophin gel, or with intravenous methylprednisolone at the discretion of the treating neurologist.

Table 11.9. Baseline characteristics for MSCRG IFN-β-1a study

	Placebo	IFN-β-1a
Total accrual no. (%)	143 (48)	158 (52)
Buffalo	38 (27)	48 (30)
Cleveland	39 (27)	41 (26)
Portland	37 (26)	42 (27)
Washington, DC	29 (20)	27 (17)
Male no. (%)	40 (28)	40 (25)
Female no. (%)	103 (72)	118 (75)
Caucasian no. (%)	131 (92)	147 (93)
Black no. (%)	9 (6)	11 (7)
Other no. (%)	3 (2)	0 (0)
Age		
Mean (SEM)	36.9 (0.64)	36.7 (0.57)
Range	16–54	18–55
Disease duration		
Years (SEM)	6.4 (0.49)	6.6 (0.46)
Range	1.0–31.0	1.0–30.7
Prestudy ER		
Mean (SEM)	1.2 (0.048)	1.2 (0.046)
Range	0.67–3.2	0.67–3.7
Entry EDSS		
Mean (SEM)	2.3 (0.069)	2.4 (0.064)
Range	1.0–3.5	1.0–3.5

Table 11.10. Duration of follow-up and dropouts: MSCRG IFN-β-1a study

	Placebo	IFN-β-1a	Total
No. patients enrolled[a]	143	158	301
No. patients who dropped out before end of study (%)[b]	3 (2.1)	10 (6.3)	13 (4.3)
No. patients who stopped injections early (%)[c]	9 (6.3)	14 (8.9)	23 (7.6)
Time on study[d] (weeks)			
≥26	142	157	299
≥52	132	150	282
≥78	110	119	229
≥104[e]	87	85	172
≥130	53	54	107
≥156	14	14	28

[a]All subjects enrolled in the study were included in the primary outcome and time-to-first-exacerbation analyses.
[b]A total of 140 placebo and 148 IFN-β-1a subjects completed the study. Of those subjects who discontinued follow-up before the study ended, one placebo and four IFN-β-1a subjects failed to complete at least 52 weeks on study.
[c]Of the nine placebo recipients who stopped injections early, eight continued to be followed until the end of the study. Of the 14 IFN-β-1a recipients who stopped injections early, four continued to be followed until the end of the study.
[d]Per study protocol, subjects had variable lengths of follow-up.
[e]82 placebo and 83 IFN-β-1a subjects underwent year 2 MRIs.

Accrual began in November 1990 and ended with 301 patients in April 1993. The study ended on 15 February 1994. According to the study design, patients were followed for variable lengths of time, depending on when they entered the study. Table 11.10 (above) shows the duration of follow-up by study arm, and the number and distribution of patients who discontinued injections or dropped out of the study. Only 13 (4%) of 301 patients withdrew and were therefore lost to follow-up before the end of the study; most of these were followed for ≥1 year. All patients randomized to one of the treatment arms were included in the Kaplan–Meier survival curves. The 13 patients who withdrew from the study were included in the survival curves, but were censored at the time of their last study visit.

Principal Results from the Multiple Sclerosis Collaborative Research Group Interferon-β-1a Study

Figure 11.1 shows the Kaplan–Meier survival curve illustrating the cumulative percentage of subjects who experienced sustained worsening on EDSS of ≥1.0 points during the study. The probability of progressing was significantly ($p = 0.024$) higher in placebo recipients than in IFN-β-1a recipients. Sustained progression rates were estimated from the survival curve using an exponential model. Estimated 1-year sustained progression rates were 20.1% for placebo and 12.0% for IFN-β–1a recipients; estimated 2-year sustained progression rates using the exponential model were 36.2% for placebo recipients and 22.6% in IFN-β-1a recipients. Estimates of the median time to sustained progression using

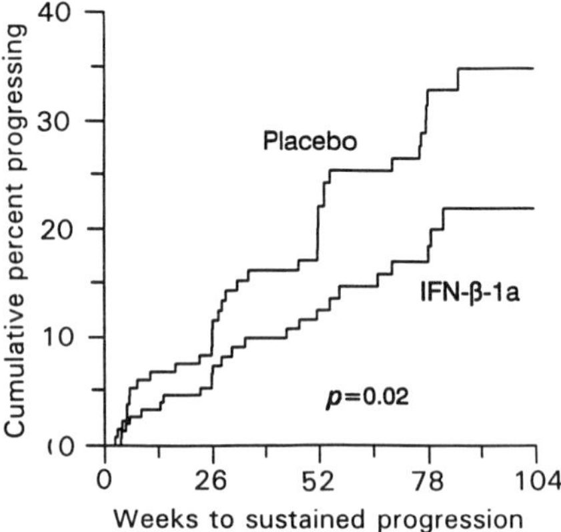

Figure 11.1. Kaplan–Meier failure-time curve showing the cumulative percentage progressing according to number of weeks to beginning of sustained progression.

the exponential model were 3.1 years for placebo recipients compared with 5.4 years for the IFN-β-1a recipients ($p = 0.024$). Thus, IFN-β-1a significantly decreased the rate of sustained progression of neurologic impairment (EDSS) as defined in advance of the study.

Table 11.11. MSCRG IFN-β-1a study: EDSS and exacerbations In subjects completing ≥104 weeks

	Placebo	IFN-β-1a	p-value
No. patients completing week 104	87	85	
Within-subject change in EDSS, baseline to week 104[a]			
Median	0.5	0.0	
Mean (SEM)	0.736 (0.155)	0.247 (0.138)	0.020[b]
No.subjects completing week 130	56	55	
Within-subject sustained change in EDSS, baseline to week 104[c]			
Median	0.25	0.0	
Mean (sem)	0.607 (0.181)	0.018 (0.143)	0.018
No. exacerbations per patient[a] (%)			
0	23 (26)	31 (36)	
1	26 (30)	26 (31)	
2	10 (11)	15 (18)	
3	12 (14)	6 (7)	0.027
On-study exacerbation rate/year	0.90	0.61	0.002

[a]Mean change in actual EDSS score, baseline to 2 years for those persons completing at least 104 weeks on the study.
[b]Mann–Whitney rank sum test.
[c]Sustained change was calculated using the lower of the last two visits (weeks 104 or 130) as the final score, to ensure that the EDSS represented a progression sustained for at least 6 months after the week 104 visit. Therefore, only subjects with both week 104 and week 130 data were included in this analysis (56 placebo subjects and 55 IFN-β-1a subjects).

Several analyses were conducted on 172 patients who completed ≥2 years on study, including: within-person change in EDSS; proportion of patients remaining exacerbation free; distribution of exacerbation numbers per patient; annual ERs; the number and volume of gadolinium-enhancing MRI lesions; the proportion of MRI scans with gadolinium enhancement; within-person absolute and percentage change in total T2 lesion volume; and percentage of subjects with changes in total T2 lesion volumes ≥10%. There were significant benefits in favor of IFN-β–1a in the mean within-person EDSS change from baseline to week 104, the mean *sustained* change from baseline to week 104, ERs, and the distribution of exacerbation numbers by treatment arm (Table 11.11, opposite). For the analysis of EDSS change from baseline, the week 104 EDSS was subtracted from the baseline EDSS to obtain the within-person EDSS change score. The placebo

Table 11.12. MSCRG IFN-β-1a study: gadolinium-enhanced MRI lesions[a]

Lesions	Placebo	IFNβ-1a	*p*-value
Baseline			
No. patients	132	141	
Mean no. lesions (SEM)	2.32 (0.37)	3.17 (0.62)	
Median	1.0	1.0	
Range	0–23	0–56	
Year 1			
No. patients	123	134	
Mean no. lesions (SEM)	1.59 (0.31)	1.04 (0.28)	
Median	0	0	
Range	0–22	0–28	0.024
Year 2			
No. patients	82	83	
Mean no. lesions (SEM)	1.65 (0.48)	0.80 (0.22)	
Median	0	0	
Range	0–34	0–13	
			0.051
Lesion volume			
Baseline			
No. patients	132	140	
Mean vol. (mm^2) (SEM)	219 (36.2)	255 (45.1)	
Median (mm^2)	13	27	
Range (mm^2)	0–2752	0–2858	
Year 1			
No. patients	123	134	
Mean vol. (mm^2) (SEM)	96.5 (21.1)	70.0 (24.9)	
Median (mm^2)	0	0	
Range	0–1977	0–2797	0.020
Year 2			
No. patients	82	82	
Mean vol. (mm^2) (SEM)	122.4 (48.5)	74.1 (38.3)	
Median (mm^2)	0	0	
Range (mm^2)	0–3791	0–2847	0.032

[a]All available MRI scans were analyzed at each time point.

group worsened an average of 0.736 ± 0.155 versus 0.247 ± 0.138 in the IFN-β-1a group ($p = 0.02$). In order to eliminate transient fluctuations the sustained EDSS change was calculated for each patient by subtracting the baseline EDSS score from the lower of the week 104 and week 130 EDSS score. Using this method, the mean sustained worsening in the placebo arm was 0.607 ± 0.181 compared with 0.018 ± 0.143 ($p = 0.018$). The benefit on EDSS change was equally distributed across all entry EDSS scores.

There was a significant decline in the proportion of scans showing gadolinium enhancement in the IFN-β-1a recipients. There was also a decrease in the number and volume of gadolinium-enhancing MRI lesions in both placebo and IFN-β-1a recipients (Table 11.12, p. 235), but this was significantly greater in the IFN-β-1a recipients. Reasons for the decline in the placebo recipients are not entirely clear, but they probably include regression to the mean, steroid treatment used in this closely followed group of MS patients, and possibly declining gadolinium enhancement as a function of the natural history of the disease. In contrast to the Betaseron® study, the IFN-β-1a study found no significant change in T2 lesion volumes between baseline and year 2, either within the placebo arm or between treatment arms. The explanation for the differences in T2 lesion volumes in the placebo arms of the Betaseron® and the MSCRG IFN-β-1a studies is unclear at the present time, but may in part reflect differences in measurement technique.

A significant aspect related to the internal validity of the MSCRG IFN-β-1a study result was compliance with the protocol and the limited numbers of subjects who were lost to follow-up (Table 11.10). One hundred and thirty-four placebo subjects (94%) and 144 IFN-β-1a subjects (91%) completed the intramuscular injection schedule as planned, and 140 placebo subjects (98%) and 148 IFN-β-1a subjects (94%) completed the entire study as scheduled. Only 13 patients withdrew before their final study visit; most of these patients were followed for at least 1 year. As a result of the unusually low dropout rate, the study results are not likely to be contaminated by differential dropout from the study arms, which may have influenced the results of the Betaseron® study, as discussed above.

Toxicity

Compliance with the study protocol also suggested that IFN-β-1a was well tolerated. Flu-like symptoms occurred in 31% of placebo and 56% of recombinant IFN-β-1a recipients; in the recombinant IFN-β-1a recipients who experienced flu-like symptoms, the median number of on-study days was only 8.0. Mild anemia was more commonly observed in IFN-β-1a recipients, but did not require dosage adjustment or transfusion in any patient. Injection site reactions, depressive symptoms, transaminase elevations and menstrual disorders were seen in <10% of subjects and were equally distributed between the two treatment arms. Anti-interferon activity was detected by a biologic assay in 14% of recombinant IFN-β-1a recipients at year 1 and 23% at year 2. Thus, IFN-β-1a recipients experienced flu-like symptoms similar to other IFN study recipients, but, unlike the experience with the Betaseron® study, there was no evidence for injection site reactions, transaminase elevation or clinical depression.

Recombinant Alpha Interferon

Recombinant IFN-α became available during the early 1980s and clinical trials have established its efficacy in many diseases (Johnson et al. 1994; Tyring 1992). Durelli and colleagues (Durelli et al. 1994) tested the effects of high dose chronic systemic recombinant IFN-α in relapsing-remitting MS. A dose of 9 MIU was chosen because studies using lower doses of IFN-α had failed to demonstrate clinical efficacy (AUSTIMS Research Group 1989; Camenga et al. 1986; Kastrukoff et al. 1990; Knobler et al. 1984), because 9 MIU had been associated with acceptable side effects in patients with viral or neoplastic diseases (Quesada 1992), and because of previously established immunologic effects at that dose (Krown 1987).

Design and Methodology

Twenty MS subjects with ≥2 exacerbations in the preceding 2 years were stratified by EDSS and by gender, and randomized to 9 MIU recombinant IFN-α (Roferon-A, Roche S.p.A., Milano, Italy) (12 patients) or placebo (eight patients). The drug was given by IM injection between 8 p.m. and 9 p.m. every other day for 6 months. Acetaminophen 1000 mg p.o. was taken 2 hours before, 2 hours after and 8 hours after each injection. Patients were examined by blinded physicians without knowledge of the treatment or side effects. Six months of injections were followed by 6 months of observation without injections. Neurologic examinations were repeated monthly or whenever a patient felt that an exacerbation might be occurring. Disease activity was also monitored with serial unenhanced cranial MRI scans (Koopmans et al. 1989; McFarland et al. 1992; Miller et al. 1991; Nauta et al. 1994) carried out before treatment, at treatment end, and 6 months after treatment end. Scans demonstrating new or enlarging lesions on T2-weighted spin-echo sequences (Paty et al. 1993) were categorized as showing disease activity. The effect of treatment on serum β_2 microglobulin, a class I major histocompatibility complex (MHC)-associated protein known to be induced by IFNs (Borden et al. 1986), was monitored using a commercially available enzyme-linked immunosorbent assay (ELISA) kit.

Clinical Results from the Alpha Interferon Study

During IFN-α treatment, two exacerbations occurred in the IFN-α group and eight in the placebo group (Table 11.13). The calculated ER was significantly higher in placebo recipients (1.0 exacerbation/patient/6 months) than in IFN-α recipients (0.17 exacerbations/patient/six months). Compared with the rate prior to entering the study, the ER was significantly decreased in the IFN-α group but unchanged in the placebo group. The median time to first exacerbation was higher in the IFN-α group than the placebo group (111 versus 58 days), although this did not reach statistical significance due to the small number of subjects. Exacerbation severity, rated according to NRS score (Sipe et al. 1984), was lower in IFN-α group. IFN-α recipients had significantly fewer moderately severe or

Table 11.13. Clinical and MRI results from IFN-α study (based on data from Durelli et al. 1994)

Measure	IFN-α			Placebo		
	Baseline	6 mo[a]	12 mo[a]	Baseline	6 mo	12 mo
Exacerbations	9	2[b]	3	7	8	4
Exacerbation rate	0.75	0.17[b]	0.25	0.88	1.0	0.5
Active MRI lesions	-	1[b]	14[c]	-	27	17
Active MRI lesions per patient	-	0.08[b]	1.17[c]	-	3.38	2.13
% subjects with active MRI lesions	-	8.3[b]	50[c]	-	75	75
% subjects with disease activity	-	16.7[b]	66.7[c]	-	87.5	75

[a]6 mo = end of the 6-month treatment period; 12 mo = end of the 6-month follow-up after treatment period.
[b]Significantly different from placebo.
[c]Significantly different from treatment period.

severe exacerbations (Fisher's exact test $p < 0.03$). No exacerbation in IFN-α recipients required treatment; three severe exacerbations in placebo recipients required hospitalization and high dose IV methylprednisolone treatment.

Magnetic Resonance Imaging Results from the Alpha Interferon Study

The proportion of active MRI scans was 1/12 in IFN-α recipients and 6/8 in placebo recipients ($p < 0.005$). There was only one active lesion in the 12 IFN-α recipients, but 27 active lesions in eight placebo recipients. The mean number of active lesions per patient (±SEM) was 0.08 ± 0.08 in the IFN-α group and 3.37 ± 1.03 in the placebo group ($p < 0.01$). Based on either clinical or MRI evidence, active disease was observed in 2/12 subjects in the IFN-α group and in 7/8 subjects in the placebo group ($p < 0.005$).

Multiple Sclerosis Activity After Stopping Alpha Interferon Injections

During the 6 months after stopping treatment, three exacerbations were observed in the previously IFN-α-treated group and four in the previously placebo-treated group; exacerbation severity and median time to first exacerbation after discontinuing injections were similar in both groups (Table 11.13). At the final MRI scan, 14 active lesions could be detected in the IFN-α-treated group versus 17 in the placebo-treated group. The proportion of patients with active MRI lesions was 6/12 in the IFN-α-treated group and 6/8 in the placebo-treated group. By combining the clinical and MRI data, the proportion of patients with either clinical or MRI signs of disease activity was 7/12 in the IFN-α-treated group versus 6/8 in the placebo-treated group. Serum levels of β_2-microglobulin returned to baseline values, and, as indicated in Table 11.14, there were no significant differences between the two groups. These data suggest that the therapeutic effects

Table 11.14. Immunologic results from IFN-α study (based on data from Durelli et al. 1994)

Measure	IFN-α			Placebo		
	Baseline	6 mo[a]	12 mo[a]	Baseline	6 mo	12 mo
Serum β_2-microglobulin (ng/ml)	1091	1791[b,c]	1098[d]	1200	1086	1053
Lymphocyte IFN-γ (u/ml)	19.1	3.0[b,c]	12.4[d]	21.7	15.4	12.2
Lymphocyte TNF-α (pg/ml)	18.1	5.8[b,c]	18.9	21.0	20.6	28.2
Macrophage HLA-DR antigen expression[e]						
IFN-γ 500 u/ml	959	807	944	1169	1134	977
Without IFN-γ	440	418	450	488	549	589
PB mononuclear cells (cells/mm^3)	2165	1646[b]	1892	1958	1840	1977
CSF CD4+ cells (cells/mm^3)	0.97	0.75[b]	-	1.91	2.04	-
% CSF CD8+ CD11b+	2.39	6.91[b]	-	3.97	4.35	-
% CSF CD3- CD56+	6.02	16.67[b]	-	21.13	18.25	-

[a]6 mo = end of the 6-month treatment period; 12 mo = end of the 6-month follow-up after treatment period.
[b]Significantly different from baseline.
[c]Significantly different from placebo.
[d]Significantly different from treatment period.
[e]Mean fluorescence intensity.

of IFN-α persisted only during treatment, and that MS activity rebounded to baseline levels after treatment was discontinued.

Immunologic Results from the Alpha Interferon Study

Serum levels of β_2-microglobulin were significantly increased in IFN-α-treated subjects but unchanged in placebo-treated subjects, indicating a biologic response to IFN-α treatment. The immunologic effects of IFN-α in vivo were assessed by measuring cytokine secretion by peripheral blood (PB) lymphocyte cultures, MHC II molecule expression by PB monocytes, and by determining surface antigen expression by PB lymphocytes and cerebrospinal fluid (CSF) lymphocytes (Durelli et al. 1994). Immunologic studies were performed before treatment, at treatment end, and 6 months after treatment end. Spontaneous cytokine production was determined by radioimmunoassay (IFN-γ) or by commercially available ELISA kits (tumor necrosis factor (TNF)-α, transforming growth factor (TGF-β), interleukin (IL)-4 and IL-10). Monocytes were cultured for 24 hours in the presence or absence of IFN-γ, 500 iu/ml, and then labeled for CD14 and human leukocyte antigen (HLA)-DR antigen expression. Lymphocyte differentiation antigens were analyzed with a direct immunofluorescence technique using fluoroescein isothiocyanate or phycoerythrin-conjugated monoclonal antibodies. Particular attention was given to the CD8+ CD11b+ population that identifies a CD8+ subset with suppressor–effector function, particularly when the cytofluorometer window is set to study cells with CD8 high and CD11b low fluorescent staining intensity ($CD8+^{high}$ $CD11b+^{low}$) (Durelli et al. 1991).

Baseline cytokine production by lymphocyte cultures was similar in both study groups (Table 11.14). After 6 months of treatment, IFN-γ and TNF-α secretion by PB lymphocytes from IFN-α recipients was significantly decreased from baseline ($p < 0.04$), while it was unchanged in controls. In addition, IFN-γ and TNF-α production of the treated group was significantly lower than that of the placebo group at the end of treatment ($p < 0.04$). In contrast, TGF-β levels were slightly, but not significantly, elevated, IL-10 was unchanged and IL-4 was undetectable in culture supernatants both before and after therapy. PB monocyte HLA-DR antigen expression of both unstimulated and IFN-γ-stimulated cultures was unchanged from baseline in both study groups and not different between the study arms. After treatment with IFN-α, PB lymphocyte and CSF CD4+ T-cell counts were significantly decreased and the percentages of CSF CD8+, CD8+^{high} CD11b+^{low} T cells (suppressor–effector subset), and CD3– CD56+ cells (natural killer lymphocytes) were significantly increased from baseline, but were unchanged in the placebo recipients. Six months after stopping treatment, PB lymphocyte counts and cytokine levels of the previously IFN-α-treated patients returned to baseline values. Lumbar punctures were not repeated.

Toxicity

Side effects were the major limitation for use of chronic high dose IFN-α therapy in these patients. All the common side effects of IFN-α therapy (Quesada 1992) were observed. A flu-like syndrome (fever, headache, arthralgias and myalgias) occurred in more than 60% of subjects and progressively disappeared 1–3 months after starting treatment. Laboratory abnormalities included mild neutropenia (cells 1000–2000/mm^3) (50%), and mild (twice normal) or moderate (three times normal) hepatic enzyme elevation (50%). Hair loss (25%) and skin rashes (9%) were less common. Fatigue (50%) and depression (9%) were major problems that usually started after 1–3 months of treatment, and did not disappear during treatment. Since fatigue and depression are common symptoms in MS patients, these side effects from IFN-α injections are likely to limit the use of the drug; in two of 12 patients, fatigue with injections was sufficiently debilitating to affect employment during treatment and to discourage using injections for a longer period. Fatigue was particularly severe in subjects already suffering from this symptom before starting recombinant IFN-α. The selection of patients without pre-existing fatigue and the use of symptomatic drugs or the reduction of recombinant IFN-α dose at the onset of fatigue may be appropriate strategies in future recombinant IFN-α MS trials. A more prolonged interval between injections, such as the weekly dose interval used in the MSCRG IFN-β-1a study may not be feasible with IFN-α because tachyphylaxis to fever only develops if repeated drug injections are given at frequent intervals (<72 hours) (Gauci 1987). A multicenter trial comparing high dose (9 MIU) and intermediate dose (4.5 MIU) recombinant IFN-α-2a in relapsing–remitting MS is under way in Europe (R. Nilsen, personal communication). Longer follow-up of MS patients treated long term with IFN-α is also needed. From the long-term trials with IFN-α in chronic hepatitis patients (Quesada 1992) and from increasing experience with MS patients treated with recombinant IFN-α for more than 6 months, it appears that adaptation to chronic side effects occurs to some extent in many patients.

Significance of the Studies Summarized in this Chapter

Type I Interferon Decreases the Exacerbation Rate

The Betaseron® (IFN-β-1b) and Avonex™ (IFN-β-1a) studies both demonstrated approximately a one-third reduction in exacerbations; the Betaseron® study group demonstrated less severe exacerbations with 8 MIU Betaseron® compared with placebo. The Roferon-A (IFN-α) study showed a significantly decreased ER in treated patients, despite a small sample size. Thus, three separate studies with systemically administered type I IFN all showed significantly reduced ERs compared with placebo. These studies were consistent with each other and also confirmed prior studies with different designs and routes of administration. While questions remain about the clinical relevance of a 30% reduction in ER, there seems to be little doubt that type I IFN reduces the rate of exacerbation.

Type I Interferon Decreases Multiple Sclerosis Activity Demonstrated by Magnetic Resonance Imaging

The Betaseron® study group was the first to demonstrate convincing effects on unenhanced MS lesions visualized by MRI. In fact, the MRI findings were significant in obtaining US FDA approval for Betaseron® in relapsing–remitting MS patients. This has significance beyond the study itself; it ushered in a new era in MS clinical trials, in which MRI has assumed a key role in assessing therapeutic responses to intervention. In the Betaseron® study, the MRI findings were critical, in view of the uncertain significance of a partial effect on the ER. While the findings were generally accepted as valid, in part because prior large trials of cyclosporine and lymphoblastoid IFN had failed to find any differences between quantitative serial MRI scans in actively treated compared with placebo-treated patients' scans (Kastrukoff et al. 1990; Multiple Sclerosis Study Group 1990), the relationship between MRI changes and subsequent clinical change is unknown.

The MSCRG Avonex™ study was the first to demonstrate reduced gadolinium-enhancing lesion number and volume. The findings were consistent with the 52-patient cohort scanned frequently without gadolinium during the Betaseron® study. Within that cohort, new and enlarging T2 lesions were observed less frequently in 8 MIU Betaseron® recipients. Since new or enlarging MRI lesions are thought to start with a phase of gadolinium enhancement, the findings from the Avonex™ study suggest that type I IFN acts at an early stage of lesion formation.

The Betaseron® study group found that T2 lesion areas progressively increased year to year in placebo recipients, while the MSCRG was unable to demonstrate a change from baseline to year 2 in T2 volumes within placebo recipients. In the MSCRG study, there was a slight *decrease* in median T2 volume (median change $-325\,mm^3$; –6.5%) between baseline and year 2 in placebo recipients. The discrepancy in study results cannot be explained by dropouts; there were almost none in the MSCRG study, and the dropouts from the placebo group of the Betaseron® study had a *larger* degree of worsening on their MRI scans. It also seems unlikely that the patients were significantly different, since the entry criteria were strongly overlapping and the clinical behavior of the groups during the study was very similar. The difference seems more likely to be due to technical differences in the MRI scans and the image analysis.

The discrepant MRI T2 lesion results in the MSCRG Avonex™ and Betaseron® studies raise important questions about the significance of MRI changes and the role of MRI scanning in testing new treatments. The Betaseron® study showed a significant effect on T2 lesion progression, but not on disability progression, while the MSCRG showed the opposite. Which is the more meaningful outcome? Is it conceivable that a study could result in a positive effect on clinical measures but a worsening of the MRI findings? How would we interpret that finding? What is the relative importance of an effect on new gadolinium enhancement compared with new and enlarging T2 lesions? As the ability improves to measure T2 lesion volume more precisely, what will the behavior of these lesions be over time? What is the relationship between T2 lesion changes and clinical changes? These and other issues related to the use of MRI in clinical trials are the subject of a National Multiple Sclerosis Society task force charged with making recommendations about the optimal use of MRI in MS trials.

Interferon β-1a Decreased Progression of Disability

Using survival analysis and carefully optimizing the use of the EDSS, the MSCRG was able to demonstrate a statistically significant effect on sustained worsening by ≥1.0 point on the EDSS. Survival analysis has not been commonly used in MS clinical trials; the MSCRG study may be the first Phase III MS trial to use this method for the primary outcome variable. Survival analysis is a powerful technique since it allows the use of all patient time on study, regardless of whether an individual patient has completed a particular amount of time. Further, survival analysis allows different follow-up times for patients and can significantly shorten trials. The treatment effect on the EDSS in the MSCRG trial was not dependent on the survival analysis, however. The within-subject mean EDSS change from baseline to year 2 was significantly less for the IFN-β-1a than for the placebo recipients. The finding that IFN-β-1a decreased progression along the EDSS is considered highly significant, since it seems likely (although does not prove) that this effect predicts less severe disability for the IFN-β-1a recipients in subsequent years.

It does not follow, however, that the IFN-β-1a study established this agent as a more effective drug, however. The Betaseron® study was designed to detect an effect on ER, while the MSCRG study was designed to detect an effect on EDSS. Additionally, the severity of disease progression in placebo dropouts in the Betaseron® study may have obscured an effect on the EDSS.

These Studies Suggest a Dose-Response to Type I Interferon and Some Variability in the Individual Response to Interferon Injections

The results of the Betaseron® study directly demonstrated a dose–response treatment effect for ER and progression of MRI T2 lesion burden. Recombinant IFN-α, 9 MIU q.o.d., was effective by clinical and imaging measures, while lower doses were ineffective (AUSTIMS Research Group 1989; Camenga et al. 1986; Kastrukoff et al. 1990; Knobler et al. 1984). These results suggest that higher doses of type I IFN may achieve more significant clinical results. The limiting factor may be adverse reactions at higher doses, as was evident in the IFN-α trial, and possibly in the high dose arm of the Betaseron® study. IFN-β-1a, however, was tested at low dose (6 MIU weekly) compared with either IFN-α (31.5 MIU weekly) or Betaseron® (28 MIU weekly). It would seem that a dose comparison study with IFN-β-1a would be warranted. The Betaseron® study provided some insight into the variability of individual response to a fixed dose. The incidence of side effects was inversely related to body size. Perhaps the dose of type I IFN will need to be individualized, at least to body size and, perhaps, to targeted IFN biologic effects that can be measured following injections.

Type I Interferon is Associated with Measurable Immunologic Effects

IFN-α treatment was associated with decreased production of the proinflammatory cytokines IFN-γ and TNF-α, and Betaseron® has been associated with increased non-specific suppressor activity (Noronha et al. 1991). These results suggest the possibility that type I IFN therapy may shift the immune response from a proinflammatory to an immunoregulatory pattern. The molecular mechanisms underlying the therapeutic effects of IFN in MS patients remain to be elucidated, however (see Chapter 2).

The Alpha Interferon Study Suggests that Treatment May Have to be Continued to Sustain Clinical Effects

Six months after stopping IFN-α treatment, clinical and imaging evidence for disease activity recurred. Reappearance of clinical or laboratory signs of disease activity after stopping IFN-α treatment has been well documented in chronic hepatitits and lymphoproliferative disease, in which the efficacy of IFN-α treatment is well established (Borden et al. 1986; Platanias and Golomb 1992; Quesada 1992; Saracco et al. 1993). In the latter studies, recurrence of disease activity after stopping treatment was associated with the disappearance of all the biologic signs of IFN-α treatment (such as increased β_2-microglobulin serum levels or lymphopenia). Similarly, in the IFN-α MS study, after stopping treatment, disease activity recurred and lymphokine changes and β_2-microglobulin serum levels reverted toward pretreatment levels. Long-term type I IFN therapy may be needed in MS patients to maintain immunologic and therapeutic effects.

Biologic Effects of Interferons and Possible Mechanisms of Action in Multiple Sclerosis

Mechanisms of the Effects of Interferon

At the same time that large scale studies of type I IFN were ongoing in MS patients, interferon biologists were defining the molecular mechanisms used by IFNs to exert biologic effects. IFNs act by binding specific high affinity surface receptors (Shearer and Taylor-Papadimitriou 1987). IFN-α and IFN-β utilize the same receptor complex; two separate receptor proteins can bind IFN-α/β (Novick et al. 1994). IFN ligand-binding receptor subunits lack enzymatic activity and require the function of two cytoplasmic protein tyrosine kinases (tyk 2 and JAK 1) for signaling (Muller et al. 1993). IFN-γ binds to a distinct receptor, coded by a gene located on chromosome 6 (Aguet et al. 1988). An additional transmembrane subunit located on chromosome 21, and, functioning in a species-specific fashion, is required for IFN-γ signaling (Hemmi et al. 1994; Soh et al. 1994). Two cytoplasmic protein tyrosine kinases, JAK 1 and JAK 2, are necessary for IFN-γ signaling through this receptor (Muller et al. 1993; Watling et al. 1993). Thus the IFN-α/β and IFN-γ multisubunit receptor complexes have structural homology and are considered to represent a distinct cytokine receptor family.

Type I IFN-receptor binding leads directly to transcription of a set of immediate response genes, termed the interferon stimulated genes (ISGs) (Darnell et al. 1994). This pathway involves protein–protein interactions to form a transcriptional activator, ISGF3 (IFN stimulated gene factor-3). ISGF3 activates transcription via an inducible enhancer, the ISRE (IFN stimulated response element). Upon receptor binding by IFN-α or IFN-β, latent cytoplasmic transcription factors, collectively termed ISGF3-α, are phosphorylated on tyrosine residues and accumulate in the nucleus, where they form a complex with a 48 kDa DNA-binding protein, designated ISGF3-γ. These components comprise ISGF3, which is necessary and sufficient to induce transcription from ISG promoter/enhancer elements containing ISREs.

The family of cytoplasmic proteins that are activated by tyrosine phosphorylation and serve as transcription activators have been termed STATs (signal transducers and activators of transcription) (Shuai et al. 1993). The STAT complex that interacts with the IFN-α/β receptor consists of STAT 1α/β (p91/p84) and STAT 2 (p113). Either STAT 1α or STAT 1β can associate with STAT 2 to form ISGF3-α; this complex joins with a DNA-binding protein termed p48 in the cell nucleus to form an active transcription factor. This complex, once activated, binds to the ISRE, inducing transcription of ISGs. The IFN-α/β STAT pathway at least partially overlaps with one STAT pathway used for IFN-γ signaling. IFN-γ stimulates phosphorylation, dimerization and nuclear translocation of p91 (Shuai et al. 1994). IFN-γ signaling does not require p113, p84, p48 or Tyk 2. It does, however, require JAK 1 and another tyrosine kinase, JAK 2, both of which are phosphorylated in response to IFN-γ.

The effects of IFNs are mediated by induction of ISGs. Types I and II IFNs induce the transcription of overlapping sets of genes. Differential hybridization to cDNA libraries has resulted in the identification of 20–30 IFN-regulated genes. The number of such genes can be expected to increase with the development of newer techniques. Assigning functions to individual IFN-inducible gene products continues to be the great challenge in IFN research.

Antiviral Properties

Antiviral properties are the best recognized and intensively studied effects of IFNs and have been recently elucidated at the molecular level (reviewed in Vilcek and Sen 1995). The fundamental principle is that specific antiviral proteins are induced by IFNs and these proteins exert inhibitory effects on selected steps in the replicative cycle of individual viruses, including viral replication, penetration, uncoating, transcription, translation, assembly of progeny viruses and release of virions from infected cells (Lengyel 1982; Pestka et al. 1987; Sen and Lengyel 1992). Induction of 2′5′-oligoadenylate synthetase (2′5′-AS), Mx proteins and the double-stranded RNA-dependent protein kinase (PKR) are required for establishing the antiviral state towards certain RNA viruses (Baron et al. 1991).

Type I IFNs may exert a therapeutic effect in MS via antiviral properties in two ways. First, IFN may exert an inhibitory effect on an as-yet unidentified pathogen in MS tissue. This possibility is entirely speculative at present, since there is no current evidence directly implicating a viral etiology for MS. Secondly, type I IFN may reduce the frequency or severity of common viral infections in MS patients (Panitch 1994). Banal viral infections have been reliably associated with MS exacerbations (Sibley et al. 1985), probably as a result of non-specific immune activation. While there is little current evidence to support the notion that type I IFN acts by reducing the frequency of clinically trivial viral infections in MS patients, it remains an attractive possibility.

Antiproliferative Effects

Type I IFNs inhibit proliferation of tumor cells as well as normal cells by prolonging the cell cycle (Borden 1992). In neoplastic Daudi cells, type I IFN may suppress the transcription of c-*myc* by disrupting the association of a positive transcription factor, E2F, with regulatory DNA elements need for c-*myc* expression (Melamed et al. 1993). IFNs may further exert antiproliferative effects by inhibiting the induction of ornithine decarboxylase, decreasing the biosynthesis of putrescine and other essential polyamines (Sekar et al. 1983). Additional antiproliferative activity may be mediated by the induction of 2′5′-AS and the inhibition of various growth factors (Olsson et al, 1992; Tominaga and Lengyel 1985). Since several growth factors and cytokines induce IFNs, it is possible that activation of IFN genes may be part of a negative feedback regulation of cell replication (Borden 1992).

Antiproliferative effects may be relevant to therapeutic effects in MS. Activated antimyelin basis protein lymphocytes are present in MS blood and CSF (Allegretta et al. 1990; Olsson et al. 1992; Soderstrom et al. 1993). Type I IFN may inhibit proliferation of activated myelin-reactive T cells, thereby decreasing their number and their propensity to enter brain parenchyma. Rudick et al. (1993) showed that recombinant IFN-β inhibited mitogen or CD3 monoclonal antibody-driven T-cell proliferation and also surface expression of a number of activation markers (Rudick et al. 1993). Inhibition was observed in CD4 and CD8+ T-cell subsets. The effect was evident *in vitro*, and also in cells isolated from patients who received IFN-β-1a injections.

Immunomodulatory Effects

Immunomodulatory effects of IFN-γ have been relatively well studied compared with type I IFNs, although the clinical efficacy of type I IFNs in MS is accelerating studies of their immune effects. The most prominent immunologic effect of IFN is modulation of MHC antigen expression. All IFNs (IFNα, IFN-β, and IFN-γ) induce increased surface expression of class I MHC antigens and the associated glycoprotein, $\beta_2$microglobulin. Class II antigen and Fc receptor expression are stimulated predominantly by IFN-γ (Friedman et al. 1980). Both Types I and II IFNs activate macrophages, natural killer cells and cytotoxic T cells.

The MS lesion has many of the features of a delayed type hypersensitivity (DTH) reaction (Traugott et al. 1983). Mononuclear cells, predominantly CD4+ lymphocytes, monocyte/macrophages and activated microglia, are readily observed at sites of active demyelination. β_2 and β_1 integrins and proinflammatory cytokines including IFN-γ, TNF-α, and IL-1β are evident with histochemical stains at sites of active inflammation. Oligoclonal T cells with γ/δ receptors (Selmaj et al. 1991) and HLA-DR on activated microglia (Bö et al. 1994) are present. These elements of the DTH-like reaction can be considered potential targets for type I IFN action in MS.

Effects of type I IFNs on these and other components of the cell-mediated immune response are likely to be complex and it will be challenging to relate the effects clearly to therapeutic mechanisms. Since type I and type II IFNs have different clinical effects, it may be informative to focus on biologic effects that differ between these two classes of IFNs. Type II IFN consistently stimulates class II MHC expression by all responsive cell lines tested. Type I IFN, on the other hand, inhibits class II MHC expression by human astrocytes (Barna et al. 1989; Ransohoff et al. 1991, 1992) and murine macrophages (Ling et al. 1985). The inhibitory effects on astrocyte class II MHC expression are relatively specific for class II MHC genes, regulated transcriptionally, and mediated by an uncharacterized IFN-inducible gene product (Ransohoff et al. 1991). It is an attractive possibility that type I IFN is therapeutic in MS by inhibiting class II expression on CNS microglia and macrophages, thereby inhibiting their activation, although this has not been directly addressed.

Suppressor cell function measured by the concanavalin A (ConA) suppressor assay and by pokeweed mitogen-induced immunoglobulin secretion is decreased in patients before and during relapses and in progressive disease (Antel et al.

1979), but is relatively normal in stable patients. Betaseron® and IFN-α, but not IFN-γ, added to lymphocyte cultures improved ConA-driven non-specific suppressor activity in MS patients and in normal subjects (Noronha et al. 1990, 1992). The mechanisms of enhanced non-specific immune suppressor activity in response to type I IFNs and its relationship to disease pathogenesis or IFN efficacy have yet to be elucidated. Durelli's (Durelli et al. 1994) finding of increased suppressor-inducer cells after treatment with IFN-α may relate to these findings.

For peripheral blood mononuclear cells, type I IFN appears to cause early induction of IFN-γ (R. A. Rudick, R. M. Ransohoff, unpublished observations) and IL-2 gene expression (Noronha et al. 1993), although there are reports of IFN-γ inhibition at a later time point (Durelli 1994; Noronha et al. 1993). The effects of type I IFN on suppressor cytokines (e.g. IL-4, IL-10, and TGF-β) remain to be elucidated, although there is some early evidence that type I IFN can induce the IL-10 gene, at least in certain cell populations.

The roles of type I IFN in the cytokine network that governs lymphocyte, monocyte, endothelial cell, and parenchymal cell interactions are likely to be complex, but will be critical in understanding the results of the MS clinical trials reported in this chapter, and in further developing type I IFN as an MS treatment.

References

Aguet M, Dembic Z, Merlin G (1988) Molecular cloning and expression of the human IFN-gamma receptor. Cell 55:273–280

Allegretta M, Nicklas JA, Sriram S, Albertini RJ (1990) T cells responsive to myelin basic protein in patients with multiple sclerosis. Science. 247:718–721

Antel JP, Arnason BGW, Medof ME (1979) Suppressor cell function in multiple sclerosis: correlation with clinical disease activity. Ann Neurol 5:338–342

AUSTIMS Research Group (1989) Interferon-alpha and transfer factor in the treatment of multiple sclerosis: a double-blind, placebo-controlled trial. J Neurol Neurosurg Psychiatry 52:566–574

Barna BP, Chou SM, Jacobs B, Yen-Lieberman B, Ransohoff RM (1989) Interferon-beta impairs induction of HLA-DR antigen expression in cultured adult human astrocytes. J Neuroimmunol 23:45–53

Baron S, Tyiring SK, Fleischmann WR et al. (1991) The interferons, mechanisms of action and clinical applications. JAMA 266:1375–1383

Baron S, Coppenhaver DH, Dianzani F et al. (1992) Introduction to the interferon system. In: Baron S, Coppenhaver DH, Dianzani F et al. (eds) Interferon: principles and medical applications. The University of Texas Medical Branch Department of Microbiology, Galveston, TX, pp 1–15

Bö L, Mork S, Kong PA, Nyland H, Pardo CA, Trapp BD (1994) Detection of MHC class II antigens on macrophages and microglia, but not on astrocytes and endothelia in active multiple sclerosis lesions. J Neuroimmunol 51:135–146

Borden EC (1992) Interferons: pleiotropic cellular modulators. Clin Immunol Immunopathol 62:518–524

Borden E, Paulnock D, Spear G, Byrne G, Merrit J, Brown R (1986) Biological response modification in man: measurement of interferon induced proteins. In: Baron S, Dianzani F, Stanton JC, Fleischmann WR (eds) The interferon system: a current review. University of Texas Press, Austin, TX, pp 1–7

Camenga DL, Johnson KP, Alter M et al. (1986) Systemic recombinant alpha-2 interferon therapy in relapsing multiple sclerosis. Arch Neurol 43:1239–1246

Darnell JE, Kerr IM, Stark GR (1994) Jak–STAT pathways and transcriptional activation in response to IFNs and other extracellular signaling proteins. Science 264:1415–1421

Durelli L, Poccardi G, Cavallo R (1991) CD8+ high CD11b+ low T cells (T suppressor-effectors) in multiple sclerosis cerebrospinal fluid are increased during high dose corticosteroid treatment. J Neuroimmunol 31:221–228

Durelli L, Bongioanni MR, Cavallo R et al. (1994) Chronic systemic high-dose recombinant interferon alfa-2a reduces exacerbation rate, MRI signs of disease activity, and lymphocyte interferon gamma production in relapsing-remitting multiple sclerosis. Neurology 44:406–413

Fog T (1980) Interferon treatment of multiple sclerosis patients. A pilot study. In: Boese A (ed) Search for the cuase of MS and other chronic diseases of the CNS. Weinheim, Verlag Chemie, pp 490–493

Friedman WH, Gresser I, Bandeu MT, Aguet M, Neauport-Sautes C (1980) Interferon enhances the expression of Fc gamma receptors. J Immunol 124:2436–2441

Gauci L (1987) Management of cancer patients receiving interferon alfa-2a. Int J Cancer 1 Suppl:21–30

Gibbs CJ, Gajdusek DC, Alpers MP (1969) Attempts to transmit subacute and chronic neurological diseases to animals. In: Burdzy K, Kallos P (eds) Pathogenesis and etiology of demyelinating diseases. Karger, Basel, pp 519–552

Hemmi S, Bohni R, Stark G, DiMarco F, Aguet M (1994) A novel member of the interferon receptor family complements functionality of the murine interferon gamma receptor. Cell 76:803–810

IFNB Multiple Sclerosis Study Group (1993) Interferon beta-1b is effective in relapsing-remitting multiple sclerosis: I. Clinical results of a multicenter, randomized, double-blind, placebo-controlled trial. Neurology 43:655–661

IFNB Multiple Sclerosis Study Group and the University of British Columbia MS/MRI Analysis Group (1995). Interferon beta-1b in the treatment of multiple sclerosis: final outcome of the randomized controlled trial. Neurology 45:1277–1285

Isaac A, Lindenmann J (1957) Virus interference: I. The interferon. Proc R Soc Lond B Biol Sci 147:258–267

Jacobs L, O'Malley J, Freeman A, Ekes R (1981) Intrathecal interferon reduces exacerbations of multiple sclerosis. Science 214:1026–1028

Jacobs L, Salazar AM, Herndon R, Reese PA, Freeman A et al. (1986) Multicentre double-blind study of effect of intrathecally administered natural human fibroblast interferon on exacerbations of multiple sclerosis. Lancet ii:1411–1413

Jacobs L, Munschauer F (1992) Treatment of multiple sclerosis with interferons. In: Rudick R, Goodkin D (eds) Treatment of multiple sclerosis. Springer-Verlag, London, pp 233–250

Jacobs L, Cookfair D, Rudick R et al. (1996) Intramuscular interferon beta-1-a for disease progression in relapsing multiple sclerosis. Ann Neurol 39:285–294

Johnson HM, Bazer FW, Szente BE, Jarpe RA (1994) How interferons fight disease. Sci Am 5:40–47

Johnson KP, Knobler RL, Greenstein JI et al. (1990) Recombinant human interferon beta treatment of relapsing-remitting multiple sclerosis: pilot study results [abstract]. Neurology 40(Suppl. 1):261

Kastrukoff LF, Oger JJ, Hashimoto SA et al. (1990) Systemic lymphoblastoid interferon therapy in chronic progressive multiple sclerosis: I. Clinical and MRI evaluation. Neurology 40:479–486

Knobler KP, Greenstein JI, Johnson KP et al. (1993) Systemic recombinant human interferon-beta treatment of relapsing-remitting multiple sclerosis: pilot study analysis and six-year follow-up. J Interferon Res 13:333–340

Knobler RL, Panitch HS, Braheny SL et al. (1984) Systemic alpha-interferon therapy of multiple sclerosis. Neurology 34:1273–1279

Koopmans RA, Li DKB, Oger JJF, Mayo J, Paty DW (1989) The lesion of multiple sclerosis: imaging of acute and chronic stages. Neurology 39:959–963

Krown SE (1987) Clinical trials of interferons in human malignancy. In: Pfeffer LM (ed) Mechanisms of interferon actions, vol. II. CRC Press, Boca Raton, FL, pp 144–178

Kurtzke JF (1983) Rating neurologic impairment in multiple sclerosis: an expanded disability status scale (EDSS). Neurology 33:1444–1452

Lengyel P (1982) Biochemistry of interferons and their actions. Ann Rev Biochem 51:251–282

Li J, Roberts RM (1994) Interferon-tau and interferon-alpha interact with the same receptors in bovine endometrium. Use of a readily iodinatable form of recombinant interferon-tau for binding studies. J Biol Chem 269:13544–13550

Ling PD, Warren MK, Vogel SN (1985) Antagonistic effect of interferon-beta on the interferon-gamma-induced expression of Ia antigen in murine macrophages. J Immunol 135:1857–1863

McFarland HF, Frank JA, Albert PS et al. (1992) Using gadolinium-enhanced magnetic resonance imaging lesions to monitor disease activity in multiple sclerosis. Ann Neurol 32:758–766

Melamed D, Tietenbrun N, Yarden A, Kimchi A (1993) Interferons and interleukin-6 suppress the

DNA-binding activity of E2F in growth-sensitive hematopoietic cells. Mol Cell Biol 13:5255–5265

Miller DH, Barkhof F, Berry I, Kappos L, Scotti G, Thompson AJ (1991) Magnetic resonance imaging in monitoring the treatment of multiple sclerosis: concerted action guidelines. J Neurol Neurosurg Psychiatry 54:683–688

Muller M, Briscoe J, Laxton C et al. (1993) The protein tyrosine kinase JAK 1 complements defects in interferon alpha/beta and gamma signal transduction. Nature 366:129–135

Multiple Sclerosis Study Group (1990) Efficacy and toxicity of cyclosporin in chronic progressive multiple sclerosis: a randomized, double-blinded, placebo-controlled clinical trial. Ann Neurol 27:591–605

Nauta JJP, Barkhof F, Thompson AJ, Miller DH (1994) Magnetic resonance imaging in monitoring the treatment of multiple sclerosis patients: statistical power of parallel-groups and crossover designs. J Neurol Sci 122:6–14

Noronha A, Toscas A, Jensen MA (1990) Interferon beta augments suppressor cell function in multiple sclerosis. Ann Neurol 27:207–210

Noronha A, Toscas A, Jensen MA (1991) IFN-beta down-regulates IFN-gamma production by activated T cells in MS [abstract]. Neurology 41(Suppl 1):219

Noronha A, Toscas A, Jensen MA (1992) Contrasting effects of alpha, beta and gamma interferons on nonspecific suppression function in multiple sclerosis. Ann Neurol 31:103–106

Noronha A, Toscas A, Jensen MA (1993) Interferon β decreases T cell activation and interferon γ production in multiple sclerosis. J Neuroimmunol 46:145–154

Novick D, Cohen B, Rubinstein M (1994) The human interferon alpha/beta receptor: characterization and molecular cloning. Cell 77:391–400

Olsson T, Sun J, Hillert J et al. (1992) Increased numbers of T cells recognizing multiple myelin basic protein epitopes in multiple sclerosis. Eur J Immunol 22:1083–1087

Panitch HS (1994) Influence of infection on exacerbations of multiple sclerosis. Ann Neurol 36(Suppl 1):S25–S28

Paty DW, Li DKB, the UBC MS/MRI Study Group, and the IFNB Multiple Sclerosis Study Group (1993) Interferon beta-1b is effective in relapsing–remitting multiple sclerosis: II. MRI analysis results of a multicenter, randomized, double-blind, placebo-controlled trial. Neurology 43:662–667

Pestka S, Langer JA, Zoon KC, Samuel CE. (1987) Interferons and their actions. Annu Rev Biochem 56:727–777

Platanias LC, Golomb HM (1992) Clinical use of interferons: hairy cell, chronic myelogenous and other leukemias. In: Baron S, Coppenhaver DH, Dianzani F et al. (eds) Interferon: principles and medical applications. University of Texas Medical Branch Department of Microbiology, Galveston, TX, pp 487–499

Quesada JR (1992) Toxicity and side effects of interferons. In: Baron S, Coppenhaver DH, Dianzani F et al. (eds) Interferon: principles and medical applications. University of Texas Medical Branch Department of Microbiology, Galveston, TX, pp 427–432

Ransohoff RM, Devajyothi C, Estes ML et al. (1991) Interferon-β specifically inhibits interferon-γ induced class II major histocompatibility complex gene transcription in a human astrocytoma cell line. J Neuroimmunol 33:103–112

Ransohoff RM, Tuohy VK, Barna BP, Rudick RA (1992) Monocytes in active multiple sclerosis: intact regulation of HLA-DR density in vivo. J Neuroimmunol 37:169–176

Rudick RA, Carpenter CS, Cookfair DL, Tuohy VK, Ransohoff RM (1993) In vitro and in vivo inhibition of mitogen-driven T-cell activation by recombinant interferon beta. Neurology 43:2080–2087

Saracco G, Rosina F, Abate ML et al. (1993) Long-term follow-up of patients with chronic hepatitis C treated with different doses of interferon alpha-2b. Hepatology 18:1300–1305

Sekar V, Atmar VJ, Joshi AR, Krim M, Kuehn G (1983) Inhibition of ornithine decarboylase in human fibroblast cells by type I and type II interferons. Biochem Biophys Res Commun 114:950–954

Selmaj K, Brosnan CF, Raine CS (1991) Colocalization of lymphocytes bearing gamma delta T-cell receptor and heat shock protein hsp65+ oligodendrocytes in multiple sclerosis. Proc Natl Acad Sci USA 88:6452–6456

Sen GC, Lengyel P (1992) The interferon system: a bird's eye view of its biochemistry. J Biol Chem 267:5017–5020

Shearer M, Taylor-Papadimitriou J (1987) Regulation of cell growth by interferon. Cancer Metast Rev 6:199–221

Shuai K, Ziemiecki A, Wilks AF et al. (1993) Polypeptide signalling to the nucleus through tyrosine phosphorylation of Jak and Stat protein. Nature 366:580–583

Shuai K, Horvath CM, Huang T, Gureshi SA, Cowburn D, Darnell JE (1994) Interferon activation of the transcription factor Stat91 involves dimerization through SH2-phosphotyrosyl peptide interactions. Cell 76:821–828

Sibley WA, Tourtellotte WW (1968) Interferon assay of multiple sclerosis tissue. Trans Am Neurol Assoc 93:124–126

Sibley WA, Laguna JF, Kalter SS (1980) Attempts to transmit multiple sclerosis to newborn and germ-free non-human primates: a ten-year interim report. In: Bauer HJ, Poser S, Ritter G (eds) Progress in multiple sclerosis research. Springer-Verlag, Berlin, pp 80–85

Sibley WA, Bamford CR, Clark K (1985) Clinical viral infections and multiple sclerosis. Lancet i:1313–1315

Sipe JC, Knobler RL, Braheny SL, Rice GPA, Panitch HS, Oldstone MBA (1984) A neurologic rating scale (NRS) for use in multiple sclerosis. Neurology 34:1368–1372

Soderstrom M, Link H, Sun JB et al. (1993) T cells recognizing multiple peptides of myelin basic protein are found in blood and enriched in cerebrospinal fluid in optic neuritis and multiple sclerosis. Scand J Immunol 37:355–368

Soh J, Donnelly RJ, Kotenko S et al. (1994) Identification and sequence of an accessory factor required for activation of the human interferon gamma receptor. Cell 76:793–802

Tominaga SI, Lengyel P (1985) Beta-interferon alters the pattern of proteins secreted from quiescent and platelet-derived growth factor-treated BALB/C-3T3 cells. J Biol Chem 260:1975–1978

Traugott U, Reinherz EL, Raine CS (1983) Multiple sclerosis: distribution of T cells. T-cell subsets and Ia-positive macrophages in lesions of different ages. J Immunol 4:201–221

Tyring SK (1992) Introduction to clinical uses of interferons. In: Baron S, Coppenhaver DH, Dianzani F et al. (eds) Interferon: principles and medical applications. University of Texas Medical Branch Department of Microbiology, Galveston, TX, pp 399–408

Vilcek J, Sen GC (1995) Interferons and other cytokines. In: Fields BN, Knipe DM, Howley PM (eds) Fields' virology. Raven Press, New York

Watling D, Guschin D, Muller M et al. (1993) Complementation by the protein tyrosine kinase Jak 2 of a mutant cell line defective in the interferon-gamma signal transduction pathway. Nature 366:166–170

12 Treatment of Multiple Sclerosis with Methotrexate

Donald E. Goodkin, Jill S. Fischer, Kenneth P. Johnson and M.B. Bornstein

Background

Considerable evidence supports the hypothesis that multiple sclerosis (MS) is an autoimmune disease associated with heightened immune activity directed against central nervous system antigens (Hafler and Weiner 1989; Olsson 1992) (see Chapter 2). There are a number of reports of the therapeutic benefit of immune suppression in patients with MS, as determined by widely accepted measures of disease progression (Rudick and Goodkin 1992). However, with the exception of copolymer 1 (COP 1) (see Chapter 13) and interferons beta-1b and beta-1a (IFN-β) (see Chapter 11) in ambulatory relapsing-remitting MS patients, and 2-chlorodeoxyadenosine (2-CdA) (see Chapter 14) in patients with chronic progressive MS, limited duration of efficacy and significant toxicity have been problematic (Rudick and Goodkin 1992). COP 1, IFN-β and 2-CdA are each administered parenterally, which is a route of administration less readily accepted by patients than oral ingestion. An effective relatively non-toxic oral therapy for patients with chronic progressive MS is desirable.

Low dose (7.5 mg), weekly oral methotrexate (MTX) has been shown to be a relatively non-toxic, effective treatment for rheumatoid arthritis (RA) (Weinblatt et al. 1992). Clinical investigators originally considered low dose oral MTX to be a potential treatment for MS because of some similarities in the immune alterations and relapsing clinical courses seen in RA and MS patients. The immunologic similarities that were originally appreciated included a reduced number of suppressor-inducer cells and an increased ratio of helper-inducer to suppressor-inducer cells in blood (Goto et al. 1987; Reynolds et al. 1985). Additionally, MTX was shown to inhibit the development of experimental allergic encephalomyelitis (Lisak et al. 1970).

In this chapter, we review the methodology and results of a randomized, placebo-controlled, double-blind clinical trial of oral MTX in chronic progressive MS. The study was designed and initiated in 1989 on the basis of limited earlier experience with MTX in MS patients, the similarity of immune alterations seen in RA and MS, and the successful therapeutic application of low-dose MTX to RA patients without severe toxicity.

Mechanisms of Action

Methotrexate, *N*-10-methylaminopterin, is a potent folate analog. It binds to and inhibits dihydrofolate reductase, an enzyme that is essential for the production of reduced cofactors necessary for the synthesis of both DNA and RNA (Figure 12.1).

Methotrexate enters and exits cells by a carrier-mediated active transport system that is shared by the physiologic reduced folates. Intracellular polyglutamate conjugates of methotrexate inhibit dihydrofolate reductase because they dissociate from dihydrofolate reductase at a much slower rate than native intracellular methotrexate and cannot be removed from the intracellular space by the active transport system (Grosflam et al. 1991). It appears that dihydrofolate reductase inhibition results in toxicity rather than noticeable clinical benefit, since

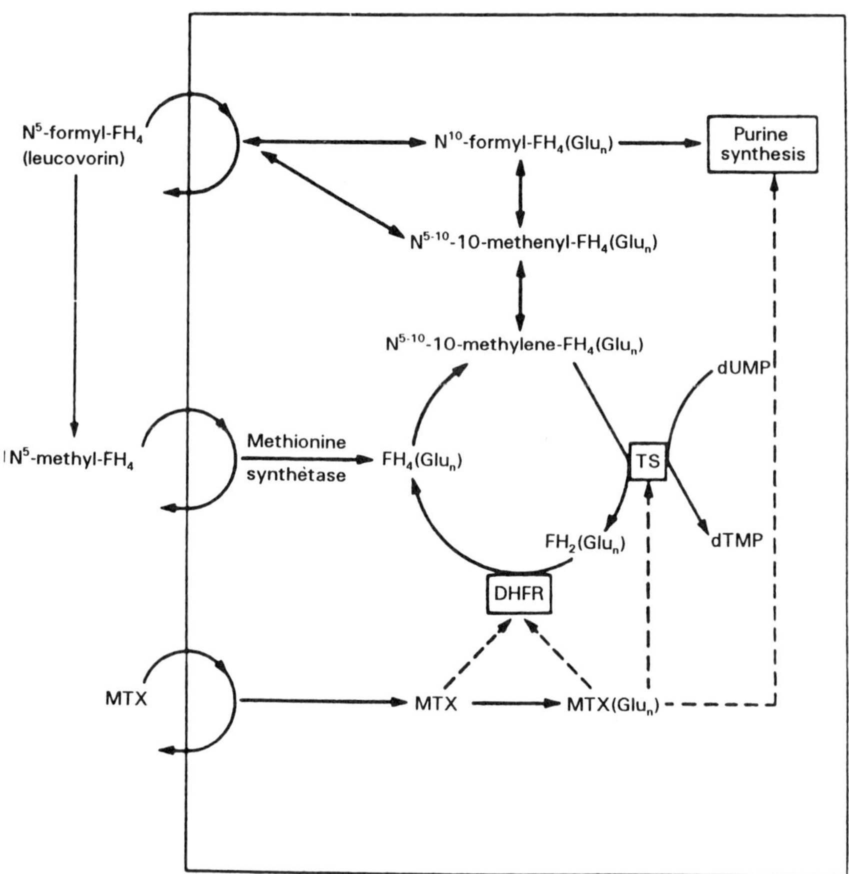

Figure 12.1. Folate-dependent metabolic pathways. (Reprinted with permission from Jolivet et al. *New England Journal of Medicine* 1983;309:1095. Copyright 1983, Massachusetts Medical Society. All rights reserved.)

daily supplementation of methotrexate therapy with oral folic acid 1 mg reduces adverse effects without reducing clinical benefits in patients with RA (Morgan et al. 1990). This suggests that alternative mechanisms of action may account for observed treatment effects. Although the exact mechanism of action of methotrexate in patients with MS is unknown, evidence suggests that methotrexate has potentially relevant immunosuppressive, anti-inflammatory and immunodulatory activities.

Immunosuppressive Activity

An immunosuppressive effect of MTX is supported by the following observations. Significant decreases in immunoglobulin (Ig) M-rheumatoid factor levels have been observed in RA patients who improved clinically during MTX therapy (Alarcon et al. 1990). Serial assessments of T-cell subsets in RA patients treated with weekly, low dose, oral MTX have demonstrated a significant increase in suppressor-effector (CD8+ CD11+) cell numbers and a trend for increases in suppressor-inducer (CD4+ 2H4+) cells that paralleled clinical improvement (Calabrese et al. 1985). Peripheral blood lymphocytes from RA patients receiving MTX grown in low folate culture conditions show in vitro proliferation indices that are lower than those from normal individuals and from RA patients not being treated with MTX (Hine et al. 1990).

Anti-inflammatory Activity

An anti-inflammatory effect of MTX has long been inferred by the observation that clinical manifestations of RA improve within a few weeks after initiating therapy and worsen just as quickly after the drug is discontinued (Weinblatt et al. 1985). The following in vitro observations also support an anti-inflammatory activity for MTX: synthesis of the proinflammatory leukotriene B_4 by peripheral blood neutrophils from MTX-treated RA patients is suppressed (Sperling et al. 1992); and the functional activity of interleukin-1 (IL-1) is decreased by MTX in vitro. This may be on the basis of the binding of IL-1 to MTX by virtue of a 60% sequence homology between IL-1β and dihydrofolate reductase (Segal et al. 1990).

Immunoregulation

MTX may also have significant immunoregulatory activities mediated by its antagonistic effect on histamine receptors located on cytotoxic T cells. It has been demonstrated that histamine binds to histamine-2 (H-2) receptors on cytotoxic T cells, thereby stimulating production of gamma interferon, which upregulates major histocompatibility complex (MHC) class II expression on immunoactive cells (Nielsen and Hammer 1992). H-2 receptor antagonists (H-2RA) have been used with some success in the treatment of psoriasis (Nielson et al. 1991) and pilot studies with H-2RA are already under way in MS. Additionally, MTX therapy is associated with a reduction in levels of IL-6 and soluble IL-2 receptor (sIL-2R) in patients with RA who respond to therapy (Crilly et al. 1995; Rose et al. 1994).

Clinical Pharmacokinetics

Methotexate can be administered orally, subcutaneously, intramuscularly, intravenously or intrathecally. The drug is readily absorbed when administered orally at doses less than 25 mg/m^2 of body surface area. Absorption by a saturable active transport system is erratic at higher doses. The presence of food does not appear to alter the bioavailability of the drug. Peak plasma concentrations are achieved in 1–4 hours after oral administration and significant concentrations of methotrexate can be measured in the serum for periods of 6–12 hours. Elimination pharmacokinetics appear to be linear, such that, given stable renal function, more methotrexate is excreted as the dose is increased. Methotrexate is 50%–60% albumin-bound and approximately 60%–90% of the drug is excreted unchanged in the urine. A small percentage undergoes hepatic metabolism to 7-hydroxymethotrexate, a weak and probably clinically insignificant inhibitor of dihydrofolate reductase (Bannwarth et al. 1994).

Efficacy

Preliminary Studies

There have been two published studies of MTX as a treatment for MS. In the first, oral MTX (2.5 mg/day) and oral 6-mercaptopurine (75 mg/day) were administered to MS patients in alternating 3-month cycles (Neumann and Zeigler 1972). Although the study was randomized and blinded, the patient groups and outcome measures were poorly defined. Additionally, disease duration in the treatment groups was dissimilar. Thus, even though no therapeutic efficacy was evident, design limitations made the results of this study difficult to interpret. The second study suggested a reduction in exacerbation rates for relapsing-remitting MS patients treated with MTX (Currier et al. 1993). No clinical benefit was seen for patients with chronic progressive disease in this pilot study.

Phase II Study of Weekly Low Dose Oral Methotrexate in Chronic Progressive Multiple Sclerosis

Study Methodology

Design and Outcome Measures

The methods and results from the first double-blind, placebo-controlled Phase II clinical trial of low dose (7.5 mg), weekly, oral methotrexate in chronic progressive MS were reported in 1995 (Goodkin et al. 1995). This study was approved by the Institutional Review Board of the Cleveland Clinic Foundation as a placebo-controlled, randomly assigned, double-blinded clinical trial. The MTX group received weekly 7.5 mg oral methotrexate tablets and the placebo group received visually indistinguishable placebo tablets. The primary outcome measure for the study was the proportion of patients experiencing "treatment failure" on the MTX versus the placebo arm of the study, as measured using a composite outcome measure. As defined prior to study onset, patients could meet treatment failure requirements for the composite outcome variable in any of the following ways:

1. Worsening of the entry Expanded Disability Status Scale score (EDSS) (Kurtzke 1983) by ≥1.0 point for patients with an entry score of 3.0–5.0 or by ≥0.5 point for those patients with an entry EDSS score of 5.5–6.5;
2. Worsening of the entry ambulation index (AI) (Hauser et al. 1983) score of 2–6 by ≥1.0 point;
3. Worsening of ≥20% from baseline value on best performance of two successive Box and Block (BBT) or 9-Hole Peg Test (9HPT) scores (Goodkin et al. 1988) obtained with either hand;
4. The appearance of new or enlarging lesions on annual serial magnetic resonance imaging (MRI) scans.

Thus, the composite outcome measure was "disjunctive" (Goodkin et al. 1992a) in that worsening of the designated amount on any of its components was taken to indicate treatment failure. Changes on any of the first four components (EDSS, AI, BBT, 9HPT) of this composite outcome measure had to be sustained for ≥2 months to be designated as treatment failure.

Using data obtained from an earlier study of the natural history of a rigorously characterized MS patient population (Goodkin et al. 1989), it was estimated that 74% (69% on EDSS or AI, 5% on BBT or 9HPT) of the placebo-treated patients would meet clinical criteria for treatment failure within a period of 2 years. It was estimated that an additional 5% of patients would experience treatment failure as measured by new lesions on yearly gadolinium-enhanced brain MRI scans. Thus, the combined clinical and imaging estimated treatment failure rate for the placebo-treated patients was 79%. Based upon the belief that a 50% reduction in the treatment failure rate (for example, 39.5% versus 79%) in the MTX group over 2 years would constitute clinically significant therapeutic efficacy, it was determined that a sample size of 60 patients (30 MTX and 30 placebo) would be sufficient to confirm significance at an alpha level of 0.05 (one-sided) and statistical power of 0.90, allowing for a 20% patient dropout rate. Early in the study it was decided not to include MRI changes as an indication of treatment failure. This was based on concerns regarding the potential contribution of measurement and repositioning error to what is assumed to represent disease activity (Goodkin et al. 1992a). Additionally, the investigators were reluctant to alter therapy based solely upon MRI change. Removing the MRI from the composite outcome measure reduced the projected placebo group treatment failure rate from 79% to 74% and the power from 0.90 to 0.84 with the same sample size, alpha level and expected efficacy.

Participation in this study was offered to clinically definite MS (Poser et al. 1983) patients seen at the Mellen Center for Multiple Sclerosis Treatment and Research at the Cleveland Clinic Foundation between 1988 and 1991. Patients indicating an interest in this trial were evaluated by the study examining physician, who documented evidence of progressive neurologic impairment during a period of 6 months or more prior to study entry. In most instances, patients had been followed at the Mellen Center and increasing neurologic deficit was documented on serial examinations. No patient experienced an exacerbation within 8 months of study entry or had more than one such episode in the 2 years prior to study entry. Exacerbation was defined as a period of acute worsening lasting at least 5 days accompanied by objective changes on standardized neurologic examination (SNE). Deterioration in functional status within 1 month of steroid withdrawal, persisting fever or definable infection were not considered exacerbations prior to study entry or during study participation. At the time of the study entry examination all patients were between the ages of 21 and 60 years, had a disease duration of greater than 1 year, an entry EDSS score of 3.0–6.5, inclusive, and an entry AI score of 2.0–6.0, inclusive. No patient received corticosteroids during the 1 month prior to study entry, immunosuppressant medication for 1 year prior to study entry, or had any prior exposure to lymphoid irradiation. All patients expressed willingness to practice an acceptable method of contraception during the trial. Additionally, patients agreed to keep all necessary protocol appointments, avoid alcohol consumption, and not use probenecid, aspirin, trimethoprim-sulfamethoxazole, phenylbutazone or anticoagulant therapy during the trial. The following patients were excluded from study participation: those who were pregnant, were unwilling to practice acceptable birth control during the study period, had a systemic illness or medical condition that precluded safe administration of MTX, or had clinically evident cognitive impairment for whom a "significant other" could not be present for the duration of the study to help to assure compliance with appointment and medication schedules.

Patients satisfying the entry criteria had an initial SNE, chest radiograph, complete blood cell count (CBC), platelet count, electrolytes, blood urea nitrogen (BUN), serum creatinine, serum aspartate aminotransferase (SGOT), serum alanine aminotransferase (SGPT), serum glucose, urinalysis and an intermediate strength purified protein derivative (PPD) skin test for tuberculosis. Female patients had a pregnancy test, if appropriate. Participants with normal laboratory test results had an educational session regarding the rationale and conduct of the study as well as the potential toxicity of MTX. An informed consent document was read to participents in the presence of an auditor witness and their families when available. Participants who signed the informed consent document were stratified by their ability to walk without assistance (EDSS < 6.0) or with assistance (EDSS ≥ 6.0) and then randomized to MTX or placebo treatment groups. The randomization scheme was developed for each stratum prior to the initiation of the study and was blocked in groups of ten in order to avoid extreme imbalance during the course of the study. Treatment assignments were made by the unblinded study co-ordinator (MMD) once the eligibility of the patient was confirmed. Treatment with weekly oral MTX (7.5 mg) or placebo was initiated within 72 hours after the informed consent document was signed. A repeat baseline examination was performed if the informed consent was signed longer than 1 week after the study screening examination. Sufficient medication was given to the patient for 13 weekly doses.

Throughout this study each participant had the same blinded examining neurologist and treating neurologist. The treating neurologist was permitted access to the treatment code if clinical status suggested toxicity that would potentially require cessation of MTX therapy. Standardized neurologic examinations were recorded at study entry and within 2 weeks of subsequent 6-month intervals. All patients reporting clinical deterioration between 6-month evaluations were seen as soon as possible by the treating neurologist. These patients were then routinely evaluated by the study examining neurologist. The examining neurologist performed all neurologic examinations without reference to earlier examinations and was not permitted to talk to the patient or treating physician about the general progress of the study, clinical events, or therapy provided to any study participant. Following the SNE, the examining neurologist recorded on standard forms Kurtzke functional system scores (FSSs), the EDSS score and the AI score. EDSS determinations were based on FSSs that were clarified and adapted for use in this study (Appendix) to maximize scoring reproducibility (Goodkin et al. 1992c) by the blinded examining physician. The examining neurologist then compared these scores and the 9HPT and BBT scores obtained during the same visit by the study nurse, with the baseline scores for that participant and rendered an opinion whether the participant's clinical status was better, worse or unchanged. Video tapes of the SNE were made by the treating neurologist whenever the examining neurologist could not be present. These were subsequently viewed and scored by the examining neurologist. While in the study, patients were permitted treatment with a standardized steroid protocol under the following circumstances: when experiencing subjective acute worsening for ≥5 days, accompanied by objective deterioration on SNE, or when experiencing subjective worsening sustained for ≥2 weeks without objective change on neurologic examination if treatment was deemed clinically appropriate by the treating neurologist. The standardized treatment regimen consisted of oral prednisone 60 mg administered for 10 days and subsequently tapered by 10 mg/day until discontinued on day 16. When clinically indicated, retreatment was permitted 2 months later with the same regimen or intravenous methylpredisonlone 500 mg for 3 days, followed by oral prednisone 60 mg for 10 days, followed by a 10 mg/day taper until discontinued on day 19. Several widely accepted symptomatic therapies were also permitted when clinically indicated, including vitamins, antispasticity medication, antidepressants, antibiotics, bladder medications, physical and occupational therapy, psychologic counseling, or participation in support groups. The use of amantadine hydrochloride was prohibited when this study was designed because of concerns that it might alter the results of the neurologic examination. The examining physician was blinded to all treatments. Patients were occasionally examined in their homes if they refused or were unable to come to the Mellen Center for the necessary examination.

A comprehensive neuropsychologic testing battery was administered to all patients at study entry and at yearly intervals during the 2-year treatment phase. This battery was an expanded version of that proposed by Peyser et al. (1990) and consisted of measures of verbal abilities and language (Wechler Adult Intelligence Scale - Revised (WAIS-R) Information, Comprehension and Similarities subtests; Multilingual Aphasia Examination Aural Comprehension, Reading Comprehension, and Token Test (abbreviated versions); Boston Diagnostic Aphasia Examination (BDAE), Train Story, and Cookie Theft Picture; Western Aphasia Battery Commands with Auditory Sequencing; Boston Naming Test (15-item version)); verbal fluency (Controlled Oral Word Association Test, Word List Generation (WLG), BDAE Animal Naming); visual perception and construction (Hooper Visual Orientation Test (15-item version), WAIS-R Block Design, Wechsler Memory Scale - Revised (WMS-R) Visual Reproduction Copy); attention and information processing (WMS-R Digit Span and Visual Memory Span subtests; Auditory Trails A; Paced Auditory Serial Addition Test (PASAT-3" and -2"); Symbol–Digit Modalities Test (SDMT); Stroop Test); verbal leaning and memory (WMS-R Logical Memory, California Verbal Leaning Test, Buschke Selective Reminding Test (BSRT); visual learning and memory (WMS-R Visual Reproduction, 7/24 Spatial Recall Test, 10/36 SRT)); and executive functions (Wisconsin Card Sorting Test, Tinkertoy Test). Most of these are standard clinical neuropsychologic measures described in Lezak (1995). The comprehensive battery also included three global screening measures of cognitive function (Mini-Mental State Examination (MMSE; Folstein et al. 1975), Screening Examination for Cognitive Impairment in MS (SECIMS; Beatty et al. 1995), and Quantitative Mental Status Examination (QMSE; Mahler et al. 1989)).

Selected measures of verbal fluency (WLG), attention and information processing (PASAT, SDMT), and leaning and memory (BSRT, 10/36 SRT), were also administered at 6-week intervals for the first 6 months of the treatment phase to 35 patients who were sequentially entered into this study. These measures were part of a separately funded "add-on" study sponsored by the National Multiple Sclerosis Society to assess the relative ability of neuropsychologic testing, gadolinium-enhanced (Gd+) MRI, and various serum and urine tests to detect clinical change in patients enrolled in clinical trials. These 35 patients are hereafter referred to as add-on study patients.

All patients were scheduled for Gd+ MRI brain scans at baseline and at 1 and 2 years. The same 35 add-on study patients who were monitored with a standardized neuropsychologic testing battery were also monitored every 6 weeks with a serial SNE and Gd+ MRI scan for a total of 24 weeks (baseline, 6, 12, 18 and 24 weeks). Patients were imaged on a 1.5 T Signa system (General Electric Medical

Systems, Milwaukee, Wisconsin) using 4X or 5X software. Axial imaging sets were prescribed from a midline sagittal T1-weighted (T1W) image using a line from the bottom of the genu to the bottom of the splenium of the corpus callosum to enable duplication of scan planes in individual patients during the course of the study. For occasional patients who were unable to achieve this degree of flexion, hard copy images demonstrating previous scan locations were used as a reference for subsequent examinations. The following imaging sets were obtained on all patients: axial T1W (TR 500, TE 12, 2 NEX), double echo axial T2-weighted (T2W) (TR 2500, TE 30, 80, 1 NEX), and gadolinium-DPTA enhanced (Magnevist®, Berlex Laboratories, Wayne, NJ, 0.1 mmol/kg) T1W (TR500, TE 12, 1 NEX). All studies were obtained with a circularly polarized head coil, 256×192 matrix, 24 cm or 25 cm field of view, and 5 mm slice thickness with an interslice gap of 2 mm.

MS plaques were identified and marked on the films by the study neuroradiologist (Dr Carolyn Van Dyke) and individual plaque areas were calculated by a single technologist using a hand-drawn cursor-generated region of interest. Each plaque on the initial study was assigned a reference number and tracked over subsequent studies to determine changes in volume. To enable this, slices were matched anatomically and compared visually to determine whether a given plaque was new or corresponded to a previously numbered plaque. Initial and new T2W and Gd+ T1W plaques with a volume $\leq$0.08 cm^2 were excluded from analysis because of unacceptable measurement error, but plaques meeting this initial size criterion were followed to any size. If a plaque could no longer be identified, any subsequent abnormality in a similar location was considered to be a recurring lesion. Plaque enhancement was determined by visual inspection of both Gd+ and unenhanced T1W images. The areas of T2W and Gd+ T1W plaques were summed slice by slice for a total T2W and Gd+ T1W lesion area (cm^2). Both the study neuroradiologist and the technologist were masked to patient treatment assignment and clinical outcome. The intra-rater measurement error for lesion area determination by the study technologist has previously been reported (Goodkin et al. 1992b).

Toxicity Monitoring

Toxicity monitoring with CBC, platelets, SGOT, SGPT, BUN and creatinine was performed monthly in all MTX patients during the 2-year treatment phase. Placebo patients had a phlebotomy to preserve the blinding but no blood analyses were routinely performed after baseline values were obtained. Laboratory values were monitored by the study co-ordinator. Platelet counts of less than 150×10^9/l, a hematocrit of less than 33%, or a white blood cell (WBC) count of less than 3.5×10^9/l were confirmed by immediate repeat testing. Any abnormal laboratory value persisting for three successive determinations was called to the attention of the treating physician and a decision was made regarding the necessity of discontinuing treatment. This decision was made in collaboration with the study advisory committee, which consisted of two rheumatologists experienced in the use of low dose oral MTX in RA and the study biostatistician. Prior to initiating this study it was agreed that medications would be discontinued permanently if the SGOT level was greater than twice the upper limit of normal on a single determination, or temporarily discontinued if the SGOT level was between one and two times the upper limit of normal for three successive months. Patients whose SGOT value returned to normal within 3 weeks of discontinuing medication were permitted to restart MTX therapy at 5.0 mg (or the equivalent number of placebo tablets) weekly. Serum creatinine levels >125 μmol/l (>1.4 mg/100 ml) were also confirmed by repeat testing. The study protocol required that patients with abnormal values should have a creatinine clearance determined and medication permanently discontinued if the clearance was <60 ml/min. In order to preserve the integrity of the blind, whenever a repeat phlebotomy was performed for a laboratory test, or a change in MTX was required, the same procedure was simultaneously followed in a matched patient enrolled in the comparison treatment group.

All patients maintained a daily diary of undesirable events (e.g. viral illnesses), perceived side effects from MTX or other drugs, and procedures experienced during the study. The adverse event diary was checked every 3 months by the study nurse during a clinic visit. The study nurse also counted the remaining MTX tablets at that time to check for compliance with the dosing schedule. Additional medication was then given to the patient for the subsequent 13-week period.

Data Management

Data were entered and maintained in a Paradox database at the Mellen Center and analyzed using SAS. A single, unblinded study co-ordinator was responsible for randomizing patients, monitoring form completeness and flow, entering and maintaining the study database, and scheduling all patient visits, laboratory testing and imaging procedures.

Blinding

In order to evaluate the success of the blinding at the end of the 2-year treatment period, or on discontinuing therapy, the study nurse, patient and examining physician independently made a best guess regarding treatment assignment. The patient and study nurse also rendered a subjective overall assessment of the patient's on-study change in clinical status as being better, the same or worse. The examining physician was permitted to review the entry examination prior to making this global assessment of the patient's clinical course during the study.

Statistical Methods

Baseline characteristics of the two treatment groups were compared using *t*-tests and Wilcoxon rank sum tests (Wilcoxon 1945) for continuous factors, and using chi-square and Fisher's exact tests (Fisher 1992) for categorical factors. Disease progression was defined as the previously specified change from baseline on any one of four parameters: EDSS, AI, 9HPT or BBT. Once this change occurred it had to be sustained for a minimum of 2 months to be labeled a treatment failure. Thus, a progression that was detected only on the last visit did not constitute a treatment failure. Two patients were unable to perform the left hand 9HPT at baseline, therefore these data were not used. The analysis was carried out using only the 2-year treatment phase data in an intent to treat framework, regardless of patient compliance. Based on design considerations, the primary analysis of the efficacy of MTX was carried out using the binomial comparison of proportions.

Secondary analyses examined time to treatment failure, where study time was calculated from the time of initial drug treatment. Time to treatment failure for the composite outcome was taken as the earliest failure time of the four individual parameters. Kaplan–Meier (Kaplan and Meier 1937) methods were used to estimate failure and exacerbation rates throughout the study period and the log-rank test (Peto and Peto 1972) was used to test for differences in distributions between the two treatment groups. Cox proportional hazards regression models (Cox 1922) were used in a stepwise fashion to examine the predictive nature of multiple factors for sustained treatment failure on the composite outcome.

The principal analysis for the neuropsychologic outcome variables consisted of a multivariate analysis of covariance (MANCOVA) of change scores from baseline to year 2 for five dependent variables. Age and education served as covariates, since these are known to influence test performance on many neuropsychologic measures. In order to select variables for the primary neuropsychologic outcome analysis, test–retest correlations for each of the neuropsychologic measures in the comprehensive battery were computed over 1-year and 2-year intervals for placebo subjects only. From these, measures that met predetermined criteria for both reliability ($0.60 > r < 0.90$) over the 2-year treatment phase and independence ($r < 0.50$ with each other) were identified. Given the sample size, the number of dependent variables entered in the MANCOVA was limited to five. These included the Boston Naming Test (BNT, 15-item version), a measure of confrontation naming; WAIS-R Block Design, a measure of visual construction; PASAT-2" (2-second administration), a measure of information processing; Long Delay Free Recall from the California Verbal Leaning Test (CVLT, a measure of verbal list-leaning and memory); and Perseverative Responses from the Wisconsin Card Sorting Test (WCST), a measure of problem-solving flexibility.

Percentage changes and differences in T2W total lesion areas (T2W-TLA) on the annual MRI scans were calculated from the baseline scan and were summarized using median and interquartile range values. Treatment group comparisons for these measures were carried out using the Wilcoxon rank sum test. Gadolinium-enhancement of T1W lesions was defined as present or absent in each scan. The proportion of patients with enhancement at each time period was compared for the two treatment groups using Fisher's exact test.

For the serial 6-weekly MRI scans done in the add-on study, the number and percentage of new and enlarging lesions was calculated for each scan in addition to the T2W-TLA. New lesions were those that had never been seen before. Enlarging lesions were those showing a significant increase in size from a previously stable-appearing lesion. A significant change in size was >45% for lesions of 0.08–0.67 cm^2 and >25% for lesions >0.67 cm^2 (Goodkin et al. 1992b). For tracking these lesions, only those that began larger than 0.08 cm^2 were followed. Additionally, for tracking lesion activity, each scan was compared with the previous scan as its reference point. For consistency of tracking, only patients who had all five 6-weekly scans were used in this portion of the analysis. The effect of MTX on the number of new lesions and number of enlarging lesions was examined using repeated measures regression, utilizing the Generalized Estimated Equations (GEE) approach (Liang 1986). This method accounts for correlations between successive measurements on the same patient, and does not require a normally distributed outcome. The correlation structure chosen for the new and enlarging lesion data was a first-order autoregressive structure, where the correlation between observations on the same patient decreases as the amount of time between observations increases. Because changes in T2W-TLA were calculated from baseline, the correlation structure chosen for these analyses was exchangeable, the correlations between any two measurements on the same person being assumed to be the same.

Results

Accounting of Patients

An account of the study patients is presented in Table 12.1. All 60 patients randomized to treatment began therapy. Seven patients stopped taking the drug for the following reasons: three MTX and one placebo patient felt the drug was not working, one MTX patient felt the study was "too much hassle", one placebo patient required an antibiotic potentially incompatible with study medication, and one MTX patient was found to have an incidental renal cell carcinoma 5 months after initiating therapy. Of the five MTX patients who stopped treatment, two failed treatment before stopping medication and the other three were clinically stable when last seen at 5, 16 and 17 months. Both placebo patients who discontinued treatment did so after meeting treatment failure criteria. Two additional MTX patients met treatment failure criteria while taking therapy before being lost to follow-up. The difference in the proportion of patients in each treatment group who stopped therapy or were lost to follow-up was not statistically significant ($P = 0.15$). Thus, 51 of the 60 patients completed the study strictly according to the protocol. No patient discontinued therapy as a result of drug-related toxicity. All study patients completed an assessment of the blind.

Baseline Patient Characteristics

The clinical and demographic characteristics of the groups at baseline were similar (Table 12.2). There was a slightly larger number of males and primary

Table 12.1. Accounting of patients (reprinted with permission from Goodkin et al. *Annals of Neurology* 1995;37:30–41)

Patient status	Methotrexate (*n*)	Placebo (*n*)	Total (*n*)
Randomized to treatment	31	29	60
Stopped drug[a]	5	2	7
Lost to follow-up	2	0	2
Completed protocol ($P = 0.15$)	24	27	51

[a]See text for specifics

Table 12.2. Baseline characteristics by treatment group (reprinted with permission from Goodkin et al. *Annals of Neurology* 1995;37:30–41)

Characteristic	Methotrexate ($n = 31$)	Placebo ($n = 29$)
Demographics		
Gender ($P^{a} = 0.32$) (%)		
Male	11 (35.5)	14 (48.3)
Female	20 (64.4)	15 (51.7)
Mean (SD) age (years) ($P^{b} = 0.14$)	43 (9.3)	46 (8.8)
Disease duration (years) ($P^{c} = 0.36$)		
Median	11.5	8.3
Interquartile range	6.5–16.6	5.0–15.0
Disease course (*n*) (%) ($P^{a} = 0.91$)		
Primary progressive	7 (22.6)	11 (37.9)
Secondary progressive	24 (77.4)	18 (62.1)
Outcome components		
Expanded Disability Status Scale (*n*) (%)		
2.5	0	1 (3.5)
3.0	1 (3.2)	1 (3.5)
3.5	6 (19.4)	7 (24.1)
4.0	0	1 (3.5)
4.5	2 (6.5)	0
5.0	0	0
5.5	0	0
6.0	10 (32.2)	7 (24.1)
6.5	12 (38.7)	12 (41.3)
Ambulation Index (*n*) (%)		
2	8 (25.8)	8 (27.5)
3	1 (3.2)	3 (10.3)
4	9 (29.0)	5 (17.2)
5	6 (19.4)	1 (3.5)
6	7 (22.6)	12 (41.3)
9-Hole Peg Test mean (SD)		
Right arm ($P^{a} = 0.19$)	30.4 (11.8)	34.3 (10.7)
Left arm ($P^{a} = 0.49$)	33.7 (18.3)	36.7 (13.5)
Box and Block Test mean (SD)		
Right arm ($P^{a} = 0.28$)	51.0 (10.2)	48.4 (8.8)
Left arm ($P^{a} = 0.29$)	48.3 (11.7)	45.2 (10.3)

[a]χ^2 test.
[b]*t*-test.
[c]Wilcoxon rank sum test.

progressive patients assigned to the placebo group, but these differences were not significant. One patient in the placebo group had an EDSS of 3.0 on screening examination for study admission but had a baseline EDSS of 2.5 on a subsequent baseline examination. The second examination for baseline score was required because 8 days had passed between the screening examination and signing the informed consent form. This change in baseline in EDSS was attributed to intraexaminer variability, rather than any change in the MS, as the patient's symptoms had not changed. This patient's most recent EDSS score (2.5) was used as the baseline score before initiating therapy. There were no significant group differences in pretreatment weight, height, WBC, hematocrit, platelet count, SGOT or creatinine (data not shown).

Primary Outcome

There was one primary outcome measure. Sustained (≥2 months) treatment failure rates using the composite outcome measure for each treatment group are shown in Table 12.3. Of the total group of 60 patients, 40 (66.7%) experienced sustained progression on the composite measure at some time during the study. There was a significant relationship between sustained progression and treatment group favoring MTX treatment (MTX = 51.6% versus placebo = 82.8%, $P = 0.011$).

Secondary Outcomes

There were several secondary outcome measures.

Clinical Measures. Sustained treatment failure rates for each component of the composite outcome measure are presented in Table 12.3. Individually, EDSS, 9HPT and BBT components of the composite outcome measure favored MTX therapy. This effect was strongest for the 9HPT ($P = 0.007$), and was seen to a lesser extent for the BBT ($P = 0.068$) and the EDSS ($P = 0.205$). To provide some insight into the clinical significance of the worsening observed on the 9HPT, the magnitude of change was determined for the 19 patients who met criteria for treatment failure as defined by performance on this test. The median change in time from baseline 9HPT performance was 17.7 s and the median percentage change from baseline performance was 45.7%. Sustained treatment failure, as defined by a change in AI, did not differ between the groups.

Table 12.3 also lists the parameters of the composite where sustained failure was first noted. Twenty-five patients first failed on one parameter, 12 failed on two, two failed on three, and one failed on all four parameters simultaneously. Outcomes weighted to ambulatory status (i.e. EDSS, AI) accounted for 47.5% (19/40) of the sustained treatment failures and upper extremity measures accounted for 37.5% (15/40) of the sustained treatment failures.

Sustained treatment failure rates by time on study are shown for the composite outcome measure in Figure 12.2 and for individual components of the composite outcome measure in Figure 12.3. The time elapsed for 50% of patients in each treatment group to achieve sustained treatment failure using the composite outcome measure was 74.4 weeks for MTX and 23.4 weeks for placebo. The difference between overall sustained treatment failure distributions for these

Table 12.3. Sustained treatment failure by treatment group[a] (reprinted with permission from Goodkin et al. *Annals of Neurology* 1995;37:30–41)

Failure parameter	Methotrexate ($n = 31$) no. failing (%)	Placebo ($n = 29$) no. failing (%)	Total ($n = 60$) no. failing (%)
Composite ($P = 0.011$)	16 (51.6)	24 (82.8)	40 (66.7)
Individual parameters			
EDSS ($P = 0.205$)	11 (35.5)	15 (51.7)	26 (43.3)
AI ($P = 0.951$)	12 (38.7)	11 (37.9)	23 (38.3)
9HPT ($P = 0.007$)	5 (16.1)	14 (48.3)	19 (31.7)
BBT ($P = 0.068$)	4 (12.9)	10 (34.5)	14 (23.3)
Parameters of first failure			
EDSS	1 (3.2)	4 (13.8)	5 (8.3)
AI	4 (12.9)	2 (6.9)	6 (10.0)
9HPT	2 (6.5)	9 (31.0)	11 (18.3)
BBT	1 (3.2)	2 (6.9)	3 (5.0)
EDSS, AI	5 (16.1)	3 (10.3)	8 (13.3)
EDSS, 9HPT	0	1 (3.4)	1 (1.7)
AI, 9HPT	1 (3.2)	1 (3.4)	2 (3.3)
9HPT, BBT	1 (3.2)	0	1 (1.7)
EDSS, 9HPT, BBT	1 (3.2)	0	1 (1.7)
AI, 9HPT, BBT	0	1 (3.4)	1 (1.7)
EDSS, AI, 9HPT, BBT	0	1 (3.4)	1 (1.7)

EDSS: Expanded Disability Status Scale; AI: Ambulation Index; 9HPT: 9-Hole Peg Test; BBT: Box and Block Test.

[a]Composite outcome is defined as sustained treatment failure on EDSS, AI, 9HPT or BBT.

Table 12.4. Sustained treatment failure by treatment group separately for baseline EDSS strata[a] (reprinted with permission from Goodkin et al. *Annals of Neurology* 1995;37:30–41)

Failure parameter	EDSS < 6.0 ($n = 19$)		EDSS ≥ 6.0 ($n = 41$)	
	Methotrexate ($n = 9$) no. failing (%)	Placebo ($n = 10$) no. failing (%)	Methotrexate ($n = 22$) no. failing (%)	Placebo ($n = 19$) no. failing (%)
Composite ($P^b = 0.350/0/046$)	5 (55.6)	8 (80.0)	11 (50.0)	16 (84.2)
Individual parameters				
EDSS ($P = 0.656/0.309$)	4 (44.4)	6 (60.0)	7 (31.8)	9 (47.4)
AI ($P = 0.650/0.707$)	4 (44.4)	3 (30.0)	8 (36.4)	8 (42.1)
9HPT ($P = 0.628/0.017$)	2 (22.2)	4 (40.0)	3 (13.6)	10.(52.6)
BBT ($P = 0.999/0.037$)	1 (11.1)	1 (10.0)	3 (13.6)	9 (47.4)

[a]Composite outcome is defined as sustained treatment failure on EDSS, AI, 9HPT or BBT. (See Table 12.3 footnote for explanation of abbreviations.)

[b]First *P*-value given is for EDSS <6.0; second is for EDSS ≥6.0.

groups was highly significant ($P < 0.001$). Significant differences in sustained treatment failure distributions favoring MTX were also evident for the 9HPT ($P = 0.006$) and BBT ($P = 0.035$) components of the composite outcome measure. A trend favoring MTX treatment was evident for the EDSS component of the composite outcome measure but this did not reach statistical significance ($P = 0.157$). No significant difference between treatment group was observed with the AI ($P = 0.925$).

Table 12.4 (above) lists the rates for sustained treatment failure for the two strata used in randomization: EDSS < 6.0 ($n = 19$) and EDSS ≥ 6.0 ($n = 41$). A

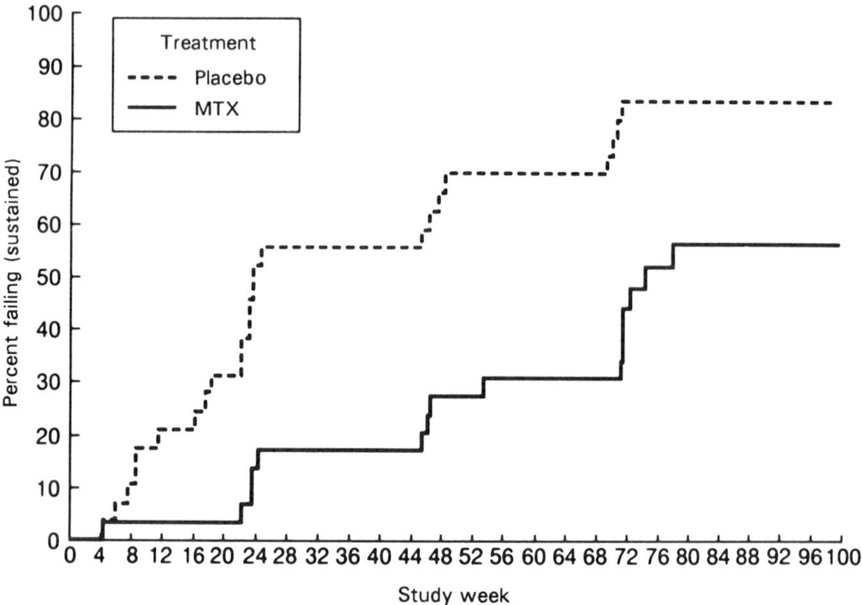

Figure 12.2. The curves demonstrate the probability of sustained treatment failure by study week. Details regarding the required duration and magnitude of change using the composite outcome measure are provided in the text. (Reprinted with permission from Goodkin et al. *Annals of Neurology* 1995;37:30–41.)

significant reduction in sustained treatment failure rate favoring MTX treatment was evident in the EDSS stratum ≥6.0 using the composite outcome measure ($P = 0.046$) and the 9HPT ($P = 0.017$) and the BBT ($P = 0.037$). A trend favoring MTX treatment was also evident for the EDSS but this did not reach statistical significance ($P = 0.309$). No significant difference was evident between treatment groups using the AI component of the composite ($P = 0.707$). Although no significant differences in sustained treatment failure rates between treatment groups were observed in the EDSS <6.0 stratum, the sample size was small ($n = 19$) and the power to detect significant differences was limited.

The possibility that the primary or the secondary progressive clinical course influenced sustained treatment failure rates in each of the treatment groups was also considered. Primary progressive MS was defined as a progressive course since disease onset and secondary progressive MS was defined as a relapsing–remitting disease onset with a subsequent chronic progressive course. Forty-two of the 60 patients entered into this study had secondary progressive MS. A statistically significant MTX treatment effect on the rates of sustained treatment failure measured with the composite outcome variable was found for secondary progressive patients ($P = 0.005$) but not for primary progressive patients ($P = 0.630$) (Table 12.5). Again, the power to detect differences between groups in the primary disease group was limited due to a small sample size ($n = 18$).

The results of the Cox proportional hazard modeling (Table 12.6) indicated

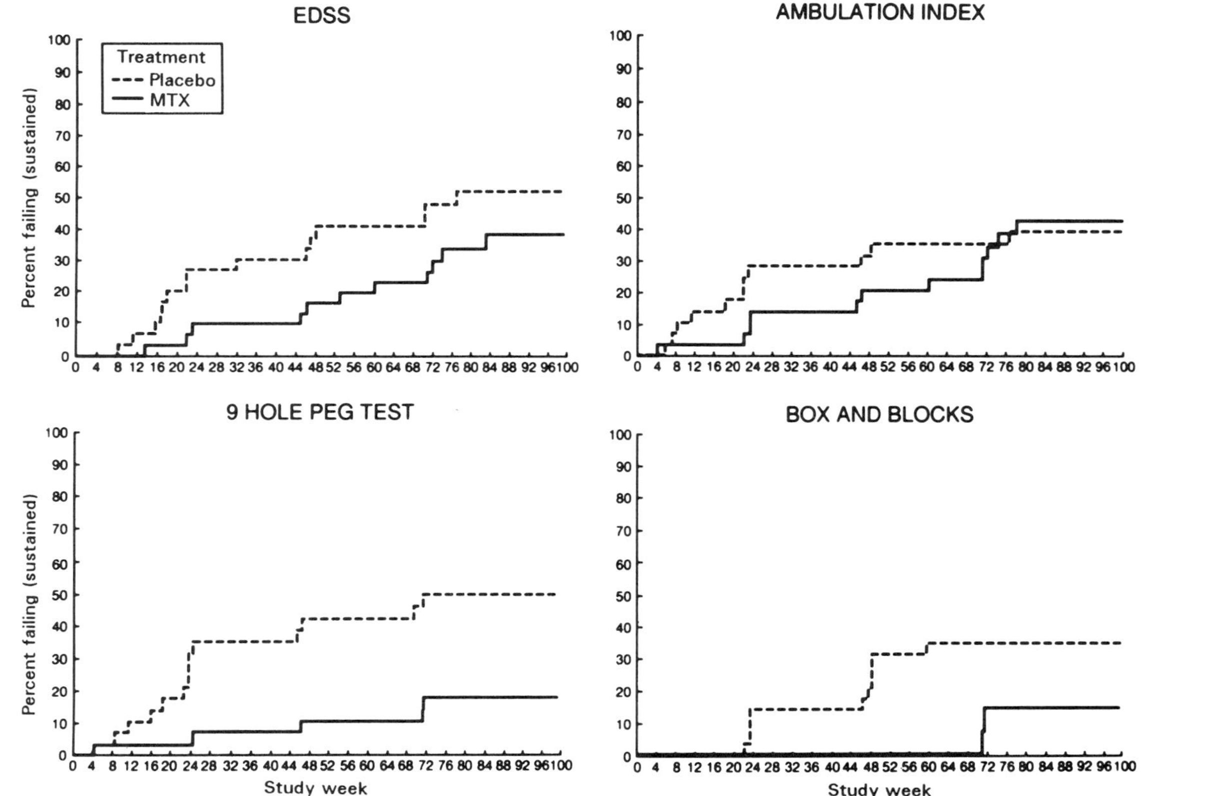

Figure 12.3. The curves demonstrate the probability of sustained treatment failure by each of the components of the composite outcome measure by study week. Details regarding the required duration and magnitude of change for each component are provided in the text. (Reprinted with permission from Goodkin et al. Annals of Neurology 1995;37:30–41.)

Table 12.5. Sustained treatment failure by treatment group separately by clinical course[a] (reprinted with permission from Goodkin et al. *Annals of Neurology* 1995;37:30–41)

Failure parameter	Primary ($n = 18$)		Secondary ($n = 42$)	
	Methotrexate ($n = 7$) no. failing (%)	Placebo ($n = 11$) no. failing (%)	Methotrexate ($n = 24$) no. failing (%)	Placebo ($n = 18$) no. failing (%)
Composite (P^b = 0.630/0.005)	3 (42.9)	7 (63.6)	13 (54.2)	17 (94 4)
Individual parameters				
EDSS (P = 0.999/0.108)	1 (14.3)	3 (27.3)	10 (41.7)	12 (66.7)
AI (P = 0.245/0.245)	3 (42.9)	1 (9.1)	9 (37.5)	10 (55.6)
9HPT (P = 0.245/0.008)	0	3 (27.3)	5 (20.8)	11 (61.1)
BBT (P = 0.497/0.084)	0	2 (18.2)	4 (16.7)	8 (44.4)

[a]Composite outcome is defined as sustained treatment failure on EDSS, AI, 9HPT or BBT. (See Table 12.3 footnote for explanation of abbreviations.)
[b]First P-value given is for EDSS <6.0; second is for EDSS ≥6.0.

Table 12.6. Results of Cox proportional hazard regression modeling sustained failure on composite outcome (reprinted with permission from Goodkin et al. *Annals of Neurology* 1995;37:30–41)

Parameter[a]	Coefficient (SE)	P-value	Hazard ratio (HR)	95% CI for HR
Treatment status: placebo	1.39 (0.35)	<0.001	4.02	2.20–7.97
Disease course: secondary	1.02 (0.39)	0.009	2.76	1.29–5.96

SE: Standard error; CI: Confidence interval.
[a]Cox model was implemented in a stepwise fashion. Factors eligible for inclusion in the model were treatment group, disease course, gender, Expanded Disability Status Scale, add-on status,age and disease duration.

that treatment group was the strongest predictive factor ($P < 0.001$) of sustained treatment failure on the composite outcome when treatment group, gender, disease type (primary or secondary progressive), baseline EDSS stratum, "add-on" study status, age and disease duration were considered. Patients on placebo were 4.02 times (95% CI 2.02–7.97) more likely to fail than patients on MTX. After accounting for treatment group, only secondary progressive disease status was significantly predictive of sustained treatment failure ($P = 0.009$).

Four MTX patients experienced five exacerbations and five placebo patients experienced seven exacerbations prior to reaching sustained treatment failure status. Although a trend favoring MTX treatment was evident, time to first exacerbation did not differ significantly between treatment groups (Log-rank test P-value = 0.395). Ten MTX patients and ten placebo patients were treated with oral prednisone prior to reaching sustained treatment failure status. No patient received intravenous methylprednisolone before reaching sustained treatment failure status.

Neuropsychologic Measures. A total of 40 patients had complete baseline and year 2 data for the five key neuropsychologic outcome variables. Baseline scores for the MTX and placebo groups on the five neuropsychologic variables selected

Table 12.7. Effects of methotrexate on neuropsychologic test performance

Measure	Baseline performance (mean ± SD)	2-year change (mean ± SD)	F (1,36)
Boston Naming Test (pro-rated total)			0.60
MTX	54.8 ± 4.9	1.6 ± 4.0	
Placebo	53.2 ± 7.1	0.4 ± 3.6	
WAIS-R Block Design (raw score)			1.88
MTX	25.9 ± 6.1	0.9 ± 0.52	
Placebo	24.4 ± 9.3	-0.3 ± 6.2	
PASAT-2" total			11.73*
MTX	30.5 ± 9.6	8.0 ± 8.1	
Placebo	30.6 ± 13.3	1.0 ± 7.0	
CVLT Long-Delay Free Recall			0.75
MTX	9.8 ± 4.0	0.4 ± 2.5	
Placebo	8.1 ± 4.1	-0.3 ± 2.8	
WCST Perseverative Responses			0.27
MTX	11.1 ± 11.1	-2.7 ± 8.2	
Placebo	18.7 ± 18.8	-0.5 ± 10.7	

A multivariate analysis of covariance (MANCOVA) for all five dependent variables, with age and education as covariates, was performed first to assess overall treatment effects across cognitive domains ($F(5,32) = 2.28$, $P = 0.07$). Next, analyses of covariance (ANCOVAs) were performed separately for each dependent variable, again using age and education as covariates. The last column in the table refers to F-values for each of these ANCOVAs. Only the ANCOVA for the PASAT was statistically significant.
*$P = 0.002$

for the primary neuropsychologic outcome analysis are shown in Table 12.7. There were no statistically significant differences between the two groups at baseline on any of these variables ($P > 0.10$). The overall MANCOVA approached, but did not quite achieve, statistical significance due to the small sample size ($P = 0.07$). Inspection of mean changes for the two groups on each of the dependent variables revealed that treatment effects were evident primarily on one measure, the PASAT-2" ($P = 0.002$). The performance of the MTX group also improved relative to that of the placebo group on the other four neuropsychologic measures, although changes on these measures were generally modest (<0.33 SD for the MTX group and <0.15 SD for the placebo group).

In order to examine when these treatment group differences were evident, changes in the PASAT-2" performance of patients in the add-on study were examined at weeks 6, 12, 18 and 24, and years 1 and 2. Box plots of change in scores at 6 weeks, 24 weeks, 1 year and 2 years are shown in Figure 12.4. As is evident in this figure, the performance of the two groups started to diverge as early as 6 weeks into treatment, with the greatest between-group difference evident at 6 months to 1 year. Changes in the PASAT-2" performance of the MTX and placebo group were significantly different at each of the six time points ($P < 0.03$).

Imaging Measures. The availability of annual Gd+ MRI scans is shown in Table 12.8. Of the 60 study participants, 53 had at least one scan available. One placebo patient could not be scanned because of a cardiac pacemaker, one MTX patient was too large to fit into the scanner and two MTX patients were non-compliant.

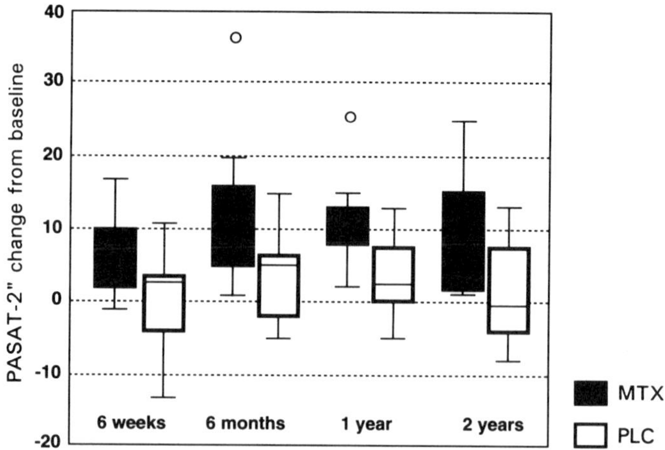

Figure 12.4. Change in PASAT-2" scores at weeks 6 and 24, and at years 1 and 2. A treatment effect is evident at each time point (individual t-tests, $P < 0.03$). MTX: methotrexate; PLC: placebo.

Table 12.8. MRI availability by treatment group

Availability[a]	MTX	Placebo
Baseline only	4	5
Week 52 only	3	0
Baseline, week 52	11	8
Baseline, week 104	1	6
Baseline, weeks 52, 104	9	9
Total	28	28

[a]Four patients had no MRI data: MTX, dropout; MTX, too large for scanner; MTX, non-compliant; placebo, metallic implant.

Baseline scans from three additional patients were technically unsatisfactory. Thirty seven patients (20 MTX, 17 placebo) had baseline and week 52 scans, and 25 patients (10 MTX, 15 placebo) had baseline and week 104 scans. Forty-four patients (21 MTX, 23 placebo) had at least two scans. The declining number of scans at weeks 52 and 104 reflected the unwillingness or inability of patients to comply with annual MRI examinations.

The median number of T2W lesions across patients was 47, with a range of 4–145. The highest number of lesions on one scan was 201 and the lowest number was four. The T2W-TLA was comparable for the two treatment groups at baseline with medians and interquartile ranges of 16.4 (7.8–30.5) and 26.6 (9.1–42.2) for the MTX and placebo groups respectively. There were 4/25 (16%) patients in the MTX group and 9/28 (32%) patients in the placebo group who evidenced at least one enhancing lesion at baseline.

Descriptive information on the percentage change and absolute change from baseline T2W-TLA is given in Table 12.9 for patients with data available at 52 and 104 weeks. There were no significant treatment differences at either time period on either measure. A comparison restricted to patients with secondary progressive disease course (20 MTX and 17 placebo patients with more than one

Table 12.9. Percentage change and absolute change from baseline T2W total lesion area by treatment group

Study week	Treatment group	No.	Change from baseline median (inter-quartile range)
Absolute change			
52 ($P = 0.46$)[a]	MTX	20	1.7 (−2.6–13.5)
	Placebo	17	0.1 (−5.2–9.1)
104 ($P = 0.60$)[a]	MTX	10	8.1 (0.8–10.8)
	Placebo	15	9.4 (−2.3–32.9)
Percentage change			
52 ($P = 0.39$)[a]	MTX	20	27.3 (−1.88–66.8)
	Placebo	17	1.9 (−21.2–22.6)
104 ($P = 0.99$)[a]	MTX	10	38.3 (5.7–66.3)
	Placebo	15	53.9 (−6.8–79.0)

[a]*P*-values from Wilcoxon rank sum test.

MRI) also failed to reveal significant treatment group differences (data not shown).

In general there was not much Gd+ in the patients who completed annual Gd+ MRI examinations. Only four of the MTX and nine of the placebo patients had some enhancement at baseline. Of these patients, all of the four MTX, and five of the nine placebo patients had enhancement of only one lesion. One patient in the placebo group had enhancement of 17 lesions. There were no statistically significant differences between treatment groups in the percentage of patients with enhancement at 52 or 104 weeks. At 52 weeks 4/23 (17%) patients in the MTX group and 1/17 (6)% in the placebo group had enhancement, and at 104 weeks, 1/10 (10%) patient in the MTX group and 4/15 (27%) in the placebo group had enhancement. There was no clear pattern of change in enhancement across the treatment period for either of the two treatment groups.

Table 12.10. Absolute and percentage change in T2W total lesion area, number and percentage change in enlarging and new T2W lesions by study group for add-on study patients. Additional details are provided in Figures 12.5–12.7. Results given are from the GEE approach to repeated measure regression.

MRI outcome	Treatment group		Study week	
	β^a (SE)	*P*-value	β^b (SE)	*P*-value
T2W total lesion area[c]				
Absolute change	7.97 (3.53)	0.032	0.27 (0.08)	0.004
Percentage change	12.73 (13.46)	0.352	1.41 (0.67)	0.044
Enlarging lesions[d]				
No.	2.77 (1.51)	0.077	0.16 (0.05)	0.003
Percentage change	0.98 (1.07)	0.369	0.15 (0.10)	0.144
New lesions[d]				
No.	5.16 (4.09)	0.218	−0.03 (0.12)	0.804
Percentage change	0.82 (2.06)	0.693	0.01 (0.15)	0.942

[a]Represents the average increase in MRI outcome for the placebo group compared with the MTX group.
[b]Represents the average increase in MRI outcome for each sequential scan.
[c]Reference scan is the baseline scan. Correlation structure between observations on the same person was modeled as exchangeable (i.e. the same for each pair of observations).
[d]Reference scan is the previous scan. Correlation structure between observations on the same person was modeled as autoreggressive.

Of the 35 patients enrolled in the add-on study, 31 (16 MTX and 15 placebo) completed scans at baseline, 6, 12, 18 and 24 weeks. One MTX patient completed scans at study weeks 0 and 6, one placebo patient at weeks 0, 6, 18 and 24, and one MTX patient at weeks 0, 6, 12 and 18. One MTX patient was non-compliant and had no scans. Missing scans were due to patient non-compliance or unanticipated technical problems. The median of the average number of lesions per scan was 52 lesions, with the average ranging from six to 132 lesions. The highest number of lesions on one scan was 151, and the lowest number of lesions was two.

The following T2W-lesion outcomes were explored: the absolute difference and percentage change in TLA from baseline; the number and percentage of enlarging lesions from the previous scan; and the number and percentage of new lesions from the previous scan. These results are provided in Table 12.10 (page

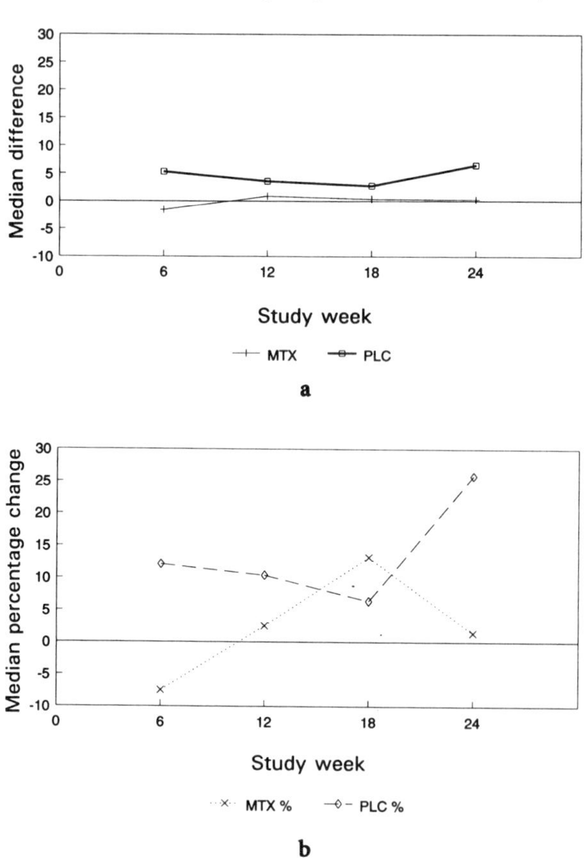

Figure 12.5. (a) Median absolute difference and (b) percentage change in T2W-TLA from baseline by treatment group for add-on study patients. An MTX treatment effect is seen with absolute difference from baseline ($P = 0.03$) but not when expressed as percentage change from baseline ($P = 0.35$).

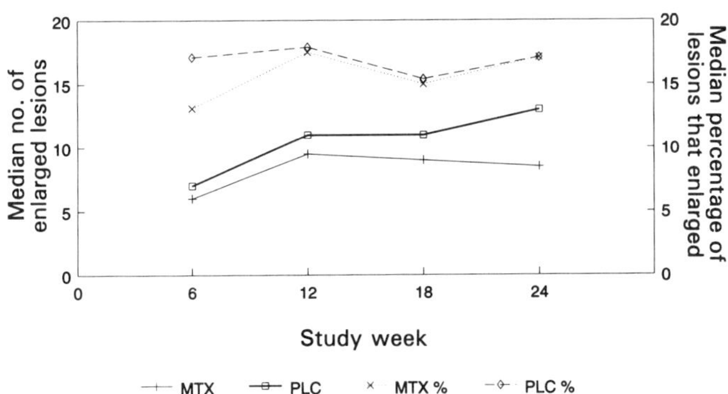

Figure 12.6. Median change in number and percentage of enlarging lesions from baseline by treatment group for add-on study patients. A marginal MTX treatment effect is seen in the number of enlarging lesions by study week ($P = 0.084$) but not in the percentage of enlarging lesions ($P = 0.37$).

271) and the median changes by treatment group are plotted in Figures 12.5–12.7. The absolute difference in each of these outcomes was considerably less variable than the percentage changes. The absolute difference and percentage change in T2W-TLA increased by study week and the absolute difference in TLA showed a treatment effect ($P = 0.03$) favoring MTX. This treatment group difference in absolute increase in T2W-TLA was not statistically significant ($P = 0.35$) when expressed in terms of the percentage change from baseline T2W-TLA. The number of enlarging lesions increased significantly ($P = 0.004$) by study week, and a marginal treatment effect ($P = 0.08$) favoring MTX was seen with this measure. These effects were not statistically significant when expressed as the percentage of enlarging lesions by treatment group ($P = 0.37$). There were no significant differences in the number or percentage of new T2W lesions by study group or study week.

Gadolinium enhancement was evident in 18 (nine MTX, nine placebo) of 31 patients who had all 6-weekly scans for 6 months. Nine MTX patients had enhancement on a total of 20 scans (four at baseline) and 48 lesions. Four of these lesions showed persistent or recurrent enhancement and the remainder were new enhancing T1W lesions. Nine placebo patients had enhancement on a total of 27 scans (seven at baseline) and 73 lesions. Only six of these lesions were persistent or recurrent enhancement. There was no detectable difference in enhancement or enhancement pattern between the two treatment groups (data not shown).

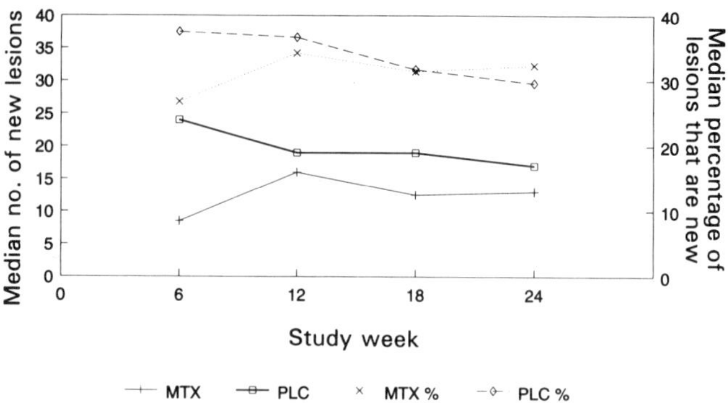

Figure 12.7. Median change in number and percentage of new T2W lesions by treatment group for add-on study patients. No significant treatment effect is observed. PLC: placebo.

Integrity of the Blind

The treating physician was forced to break the treatment code for three patients (MTX = 2, placebo = 1) who required temporary cessation of therapy or dosage adjustment. The code was also broken for three matched patients in the comparison treatment group, who were then treated similarly in order to preserve the blind. Patients were not informed of treatment assignments in these instances and the examining physician was never informed of any medication adjustment. The treatment code was not broken in any other instance. An assessment of the blind was administered at the end of the treatment period for all patients. The examining physician, study nurse and patients were asked individually to make the following choices of treatment assignment during the study: MTX, placebo or "I do not know". Thirty-two per cent of the MTX and 28% of the placebo patients correctly guessed their assignment. The study nurse was only able to assign treatment for two patients. One was assigned correctly and one was not. The examining physician was able to assign treatment on one patient and that was done incorrectly.

Global Opinion of Patient Outcome

At the time treatment was terminated for each patient, study participants, the study nurse and the examining physician rendered a global opinion about whether the patient's clinical status was better, the same or worse, than when that patient entered the study. No significant differences in clinical status distributions between the MTX and placebo groups were detected by this measure. Sixty-eight per cent of both the MTX and the placebo patients thought they were worse than at study entry.

Adverse Events

Adverse experiences observed in the patients participating in this study included upper respiratory infection, urinary tract infection, nausea, headache, fever, mucocutaneous herpes, sore muscles, backache, indigestion and diarrhea. Adverse experiences were similarly distributed in the MTX and placebo treatment groups. Twenty-seven MTX patients reported 113 adverse experiences and 26 placebo patients reported 103 adverse experiences. No patient discontinued medication as a direct result of side effects attributable to MTX. Side effects requiring temporary or permanent cessation of therapy occurred in three patients. One MTX patient required temporary cessation of therapy due to diarrhea, which was attributed to the use of an antibiotic prescribed for a urinary tract infection. Therapy was restarted without further problem. A second patient, who was given placebo, was observed to have leukopenia, thrombocytopenia and SGOT abnormalities on three successive laboratory tests. The drug was temporarily discontinued until it was subsequently determined that this elevation was caused by the administration of isoniazid for a positive intermediate strength PPD skin test found at study entry. Isoniazid was discontinued and the drug (placebo) was subsequently restarted without problem after laboratory results returned to normal. A third patient, who was taking MTX, was found to have intermittently elevated SGOT levels that were less than twice the upper limit of the normal range. This patient had a temporary weekly dose reduction from 7.5 mg to 5.0 mg. It was subsequently determined that this patient was taking aspirin. The elevated SGOT levels were no longer evident after aspirin was discontinued and the drug dose was increased to 7.5 mg without further adverse event.

Post-hoc Analyses

The chi-square test was used to investigate the relative independence of the four parameters that comprised the composite outcome measure. Changes in the EDSS and AI were significantly related ($P < 0.001$) as were changes on the 9HPT and BBT ($P < 0.001$). However, changes on measures weighted to ambulation (i.e the EDSS and AI) were not significantly related to changes on the tests of upper extremity function ($P = 0.241$). This observation enabled the investigators to reanalyze the data using a disjunctive composite outcome consisting only of the EDSS and 9HPT. There was a total of 34 sustained treatment failures using this approach; 13 in the MTX group and 21 in the placebo group ($P = 0.017$). Of the 34 failures, 15 were detected by the EDSS alone, eight by the 9HPT alone, and 11 by both the EDSS and 9HPT. Kaplan–Meier treatment failure estimates indicated a significantly worse sustained treatment failure distribution for placebo-treated patients using this simplified disjunctive composite ($P < 0.005$).

An alternative method of analyzing the four outcome parameters as multiple endpoints was pursued in the following manner:

1. The log-rank scores for sustained treatment failure were determined for each of the four components;

2. Each of the scores were ranked separately over the combined sample (treated and untreated);
3. The four ranks were summed for each subject;
4. A *t*-test was performed on the rank sum scores (O'Brien 1984; Popcock et al. 1987).

The results of the *t*-test are consistent with, although not as strong as, the results of the primary analysis and indicate that the MTX group had a better sustained treatment failure rate than the placebo group ($P = 0.07$).

Implications of the Phase II Study of Weekly Low Dose Methotrexate

1. It is anticipated that there will be considerable interest in the potential clinical use of MTX in patients with chronic progressive MS on the basis of this study, since there was an evident treatment effect on measures of upper extremity function, neuropsychologic testing and serial Gd+ MRI scans. The difference in outcome between treatment groups was apparent within 6 months of initiating therapy and was sustained for 2 years. The results of this study appear to be valid, since the formal assessment documented effective blinding of study subjects and the personnel who scored the subjects for outcome and the two arms of the study were well matched. With respect to the latter, we considered the possibility that the slightly disproportionate number of males and patients with primary progressive MS assigned to the placebo group biased this study in favor of a treatment effect for MTX. This was considered unlikely since a gender-related treatment effect was not observed in the neuropsychologic testing or Gd+ MRI outcomes used in this study. Since MTX is widely available, relatively inexpensive, and unassociated with severe adverse effects, we suspect it will achieve significant use in chronic progressive MS patients. We believe that treatment decisions should be individualized and made on the basis of careful deliberations by patients and their neurologists.
2. This study has implications for the methods of measuring treatment outcome in chronic progressive MS patients. The clinical benefits observed with MTX treatment were defined as sustained change in any one of the components of the composite outcome measure (Goodkin et al. 1992a). This approach differs from earlier studies that have relied exclusively upon the EDSS as the primary outcome measure in clinical trials. The investigators chose this approach because it is widely recognized that the EDSS is primarily determined by ambulatory status and is insensitive for detecting change in neurologic impairment in the context of clinical trials. These investigators previously suggested that a composite outcome measure including the EDSS and a test of upper extremity function could improve the ability to detect change in neurologic functional status because: performance on the 9HPT or BBT was below the tenth percentile performance level for age and sex matched controls in 78% of MS patients whose EDSS scores were greater than 3.5; and deterioration of greater than 20% from baseline performance on either of these upper

extremity function tests could confidently be attributed to change in functional status rather than test performance variability (Goodkin et al. 1988). The post-hoc analysis of data derived from this study demonstrated that prespecified change in the EDSS and tests of upper extremity function were not related. A similar result was found in relapsing-remitting MS patients with lower EDSS scores followed prospectively in a natural history study (Rudick et al. 1995). These results suggest that a disjunctive composite of the EDSS and 9HPT can increase the sensitivity of the EDSS, or other measures that predominantly measure gait, for detecting change in chronic progressive MS patients who have EDSS scores of 3.0–6.5 at study entry.

3. Although valid treatment group differences were detected, the question remains about how clinically significant is the observed benefit. The patients' global opinions of treatment outcome might be interpreted to suggest that this change in upper limb performance has no clinical significance. However, it should be recognized that a patient's global opinion fails to clarify the degree or character of worsening in each treatment group. Thus, patients in both treatment groups could perceive themselves as globally worse even if a clinically significant benefit in upper extremity function was present only in patients on active therapy. This study was not designed to determine if the observed change in upper extremity functional performance is clinically meaningful. Similarly, the clinical significance of change on other outcome measures that are widely used in MS clinical trials (e.g. EDSS) has also not been established. The issue of clinical relevance of change in functional or imaging assessments is at present a matter of clinical judgment. In the investigator's opinion, the observed change in 9HPT performance is clinically significant and we believe that low dose weekly oral MTX offers a relatively non-toxic treatment option for patients with chronic progressive MS.
4. The results from a number of the secondary outcomes were consistent in showing a modest benefit in favor of MTX. This demonstrates the value of additional outcomes beyond the primary outcome, and further supports the validity of the result in this study. The treatment effect measured by neuropsychologic testing was most significant on the PASAT-2", a test of auditory information processing. Treatment effects on other neuropsychologic measures were in the predicted direction, but not statistically significant. It is not clear at this point whether MTX has global neuropsychologic benefits and the PASAT-2" is simply the most sensitive measure of these, or whether MTX has selective effects on information processing, but not other cognitive functions. It is noteworthy that the PASAT-2" was the only measure in the principal neuropsychologic outcome analysis that was administered frequently for the first 6 months as part of the add-on study. It is unclear whether this difference in the frequency with which measures were administered may have played a role in the outcome. Analyses of between-group differences on other information processing measures (such as the SDMT) and other measures administered frequently as part of in the add-on study (such as the BSRT and the 10/36 SRT) are currently under way and should aid the interpretation of this finding. Although some may question the robustness of the neuropsychologic effects of MTX, it is worth noting that changes in PASAT-2"

performance coincide with the time course of treatment effects on measures of upper extremity function and Gd+ MRI in this study. We are currently examining the concordance between upper extremity, neuropsychologic and MRI measures, in order to determine whether they identify similar groups of treatment responders, or whether they are relatively independent indicators of treatment outcome, and thus, might be used to construct a more sensitive composite outcome measure.

The Gd+ MRI results from this study are also consistent with the neurologic and neuropsychologic evidence of a modest MTX treatment effect. Although the treatment effect measured by serial Gd+ MRI was also modest and confined to those imaging measures with the least variability (absolute increase in T2W-TLA), it is noteworthy that any treatment group differences were evident with MRI, since this study was designed only to explore the use of MRI activity as a secondary outcome measure. Specifically, the preplanned analyses of imaging data were not powered to detect treatment group differences based upon TLA, or gadolinium-enhanced or unenhanced MRI activity. The treatment group difference in change from baseline T2W-TLA at 1 and 2 years was 17% in placebo versus interferon beta-1b treated patients (Paty et al. 1993; and see Chapter 11). In order for us to detect a 17% difference in median group change of T2W-TLA between MTX and placebo treated patients at a single time point (e.g. 2 years), given the variability in our sample, with 80% power, and an alpha level of 0.05, a total of 476 patients (238 patients per treatment group) would have been needed. Only 32% (9/28) of the placebo patients in our study who had scans at baseline had enhancing lesions on their baseline MRI. In order to detect a change from 32% to 16% at one time point (e.g. 6 months), with 80% power, an alpha level of 0.05, and assuming no correlation between the two measurements, 109 patients per treatment group would be needed. If correlations of 0.2 and 0.4 are assumed for the repeat observations, then 87 and 63 patients per group would be required, respectivcly.

We have considered the possibility that the observed treatment effect measured by imaging parameters was a reflection of the inequality of baseline T2W-TLA and percentage of baseline scans with Gd+ activity. Specifically, since the placebo-treated group had on average slightly greater baseline TLA and percentage of scans with Gd+ activity, it might be argued that the placebo group was at greater risk to experience subsequent MRI activity and progression of functional impairment than the methotrexate-treated patients. Although quantitative brain MRI lesion load predicts the clinical course of patients with clinically isolated syndromes suggestive of MS (Filippi et al 1994) and serial brain MRI scans demonstrate more activity in patients with relapsing–remitting and secondary progressive MS than patients with benign disease or primary progressive MS (Filippi et al. 1995; Kidd 1994), baseline mean T2W-TLA at study entry did not predict the differences in the proportion of relapsing–remitting and benign MS patients who subsequently experienced clinical relapses or developed new and enlarging lesions on monthly neurologic examinations and Gd+ MRI scans for 6 months (Kidd et al. 1994). Thus, it remains uncertain whether the modest baseline differences in T2W-TLA or Gd+ T1W lesions in MTX and placebo patients have relevance in terms of predicting future MRI activity, change in neuropsychologic testing, or change in the components of the clinically-based composite outcome used in this study.

5. Our findings are relevant to other clinical investigators who wish to use Gd+ MRI activity as a primary or secondary outcome measure in future controlled clinical trials involving patients with chronic progressive MS. Although Gd+ MRI detects disease-related activity in relapsing-remitting MS patients 5–10 times more frequently than clinically-based outcome measures, our data strongly suggest that this is not the case in patients with primary or secondary chronic progressive disease who have experienced less than two clinical exacerbations in the preceding 2 years and no clinical exacerbations within the preceding 8 months. Other investigators have observed that MRI activity may be less frequent in patients whose clinical course is progressive from onset without exacerbations, or begins with an exacerbation and is followed by insidious progression unassociated with frequent exacerbations, than in patients whose clinical course is characterized by frequent relapses (Filippi et al. 1995; McFarland et al. 1992). The combined weight of these observations emphasizes the importance of considering the frequency and recency of clinical exacerbations when designing a clinical trial involving patients with secondary progressive and primary progressive MS. A run-in phase, as proposed by McFarland (1992), particularly in clinical trials designed to detect treatment group differences in Gd+ activity in patients with secondary progressive MS, can be used to advantage to limit study entry to patients who have new gadolinium-enhancing lesions. This will help to assure that sample size estimates that are based upon a reduction in gadolinium-enhanced lesion frequency are adequately powered to detect the projected treatment group differences.
6. In summary, the clinical, neuropsychologic testing, and Gd+ MRI data from our study each support the notion that low dose, weekly, oral MTX offers a new, relatively non-toxic treatment option for patients with chronic progressive MS. This study also provides data that are relevant to the design of future clinical trials involving patients with chronic progressive MS. Gd+ MRI activity and T2W-TLA are not likely to offer any advantage over the clinically-based composite outcome measure used in this study for determining the sample sizes necessary to detect treatment group differences in therapeutic trials that involve patients with chronic progressive MS who have study-entry EDSS scores of 3.0–6.5 and have experienced fewer than two clinical exacerbations in the 2 years preceding study entry.

Adverse Reactions with Methotrexate in Diseases Other than Multiple Sclerosis

Considerable experience with MTX-induced adverse reactions has also been gained from patients with RA. When administered orally at a dose of 7.5 mg each week, adverse reactions in these patients are usually mild and do not result in discontinuation of therapy (Goodman and Polisson 1994). Minor reactions include gastrointestinal discomfort, nausea, muscositis, headache, rash, fatigue, alopecia and minor infections. Major toxicity is relatively uncommon in patients with RA who have received the same low-dose of oral MTX for extended periods of time (Goodman and Polisson 1994). Major toxicity in patients with RA consists principally of pulmonary disease, liver dysfunction and bone marrow suppression.

Although hepatotoxicity is potentially a major adverse effect, early reports of severe hepatic fibrosis, cirrhosis and even death in patients with psoriasis who were treated with daily MTX in moderate to high doses have not been substantiated in long-term, prospective studies of patients with RA treated with low dose, weekly MTX. Prior to 1993, there were only six well described cases of patients with RA who developed cirrhosis or symptomatic liver disease while taking the drug (Goodman and Polisson 1994). A subsequent survey of 16 699 patients with RA, who received the drug for more than 5 years, reported the crude 5-year frequency of approximately 1/1000 (Walker et al. 1993). It remains uncertain whether alcohol consumption predisposes to hepatic complications in the absence of known liver disease (Kremer et al. 1989; Whiting et al. 1991). Until this question is resolved, patients receiving methotrexate should be cautioned repeatedly to avoid the consumption of alcohol. We are unaware of any report documenting biopsy-proven progression from normal liver, or mild fibrosis, to cirrhisis in otherwise healthy patients with RA who were treated with MTX.

Severe hematologic adverse events are uncommon, although mild cytopenia has been reported in 10%–24% of patients with RA receiving long-term, low-dose oral MTX (Goodman and Polisson 1994). Risk appears to be increased in patients with a prior hematologic disorder, Felty's syndrome, renal insufficiency or red blood macrocytosis, or in those to whom trimethaprim-sulfamethoxazole or non-steroidal anti-inflammatory medications are administered.

Interstitial pneumonitis, a potentially fatal pulmonary complication of MTX therapy in patients with RA, is rare. Typical clinical manifestations of MTX-induced pneumonitis include progressive or acute dyspnea and dry cough, often associated with malaise, chills, myalgia and fever. Chest radiography may be normal, but it more commonly reveals a diffuse interstitial, reticulonodular or alveolar infiltrate with a predilicition for the lung bases and midlung fields. This adverse effect is believed to be idiosyncratic since the exact pathogenesis of MTX-induced pneumonitis is unknown and as yet no risk factors have been established.

MTX is a potent abortifacient and numerous examples of teratogenic effects have been reported. Its use should be avoided in men and women of child-bearing potential unless appropriate contraceptive measures are followed.

The potential carcinogenicity of low dose MTX has been identified by case reports only and several large studies have not shown any excess risk of cancer in patients taking MTX for psoriasis or trophoblastic tumors (Rustin et al. 1983; Stern et al. 1982). Extrapolating the risk of cancer in patients taking MTX for disorders other than RA or MS is probably not yet justified. Although the true risk in such individuals must be determined by careful epidemiologic studies, present information suggests that the probability of developing a malignancy from MTX exposure is small.

Drug Interactions

Vinca alkaloids, daunorubicin and cytarabine increase the cellular uptake of MTX, while penicillin, hydroxyurea, mercaptopurine, neomycin, kanamycin, corticosteroids, bleomycin and asparaginase decrease cellular uptake. The clinical significance of these interactions is uncertain. MTX may be displaced from plasma albumin by sulfonamides, salicylates, tetracyclines, chloramphenicol and phenytoin. The resulting increase in the free concentration of MTX may potentiate the drug's toxicity. In addition, salicylates and probenecid may compete with MTX for renal tubular secretion. Caution should be exercised if these drugs are given concomitantly, since the reduced rate of excretion may result in elevated plasma levels of MTX and more frequent or more severe adverse reactions (Bennett 1992).

Therapeutic Potential

Although approved for use in RA, psoriasis, certain forms of leukemia and trophoblastic tumors, MTX is not approved by the United States Food and Drug Administration for use in patients with MS. However, unlabeled or unapproved use of medications is common in the United States. Although low dose, weekly, oral MTX is not approved for use in such patients, the observed treatment effect, modest toxicity, ready availability and limited cost make it likely that many patients with this chronic progressive disease will seek and gain access to this therapy. Treatment decisions under these circumstances should be individualized and, optimally, should follow consultation with a physician who is experienced in the care of patients with MS and is thoroughly familiar with the administration procedures, pharmacokinetics, potential drug interactions and adverse effects known to occur with this drug. Additional clinical trials using higher doses of oral and parenteral MTX are currently planned or under way. The results of these trials should help to better define the therapeutic potential of MTX in patients with MS.

Acknowledgements

Supported in part by grants from the National Multiple Sclerosis Society (Dr Goodkin RG-4126-A-2 and RG-2109-A/B). Coded drug and placebo tablets were supplied by the American Cyanimid Company, Pearl River, New York.

APPENDIX

Pyramidal Functions

0. Normal.
1. Abnormal signs without weakness.
2. Mild weakness (motor strength 4/5 in one extremity or 4+/5 in more than one extremity).
3. Moderate paraparesis or hemiparesis (4/5 or 4–/5), or severe monoparesis (≤3/5).
4. Severe triparesis, paraparesis or hemiparesis (≤3/5); moderate quadriparesis (4/5 or 4–/5); or monoplegia.
5. Paraplegia, hemiplegia, or severe quadriparesis (≤3/5).
6. Quadriplegia.
7. Untestable.
8. Unknown.

Cerebellar Functions

Note: Test finger to nose, heel/knee/shin, rapid alternating movements, and gait. This is a test of cerebellar function and not of weakness. If one or more limbs cannot be tested for any reason, score only the remaining limbs.

0. Normal. (No evidence of cerebellar dysfunction: this score may be used if one or more limbs are unco-ordinated due to weakness, apraxia or sensory loss.)
1. Abnormal signs without interference in routine function.
2. Mild ataxia. (Limb ataxia in any or all limbs or gait ataxia that is adequate to interfere with routine function.)
3. Moderate ataxia. (Moderate ataxia of one or more limbs or gait that requires some physical or mechanical adaptation to complete a targeted activity. Examples include the requirement to hold a wall or a companion's arm to hop or tandem walk, or to use a buttonhole device to fasten buttons. The adaptation permits the activity to be completed.)
4. Severe ataxia. (This score is applied when there is ataxia of 1 or more limbs or gait. Patients with a severe ataxia cannot complete a targeted activity, even with mechanical or human assistance, even though the activity may be initiated.)
5. Unable to perform co-ordinated limb movements or gait. (This score is only used when routine activities in one or more limbs or gait cannot even be initiated because ataxia is so severe that injury will result.)
6. Untestable. (This score will be applied most commonly when motor strength is 3/5 or less in all four limbs.)
7. Unknown.

Brainstem Functions

0. Normal.
1. Signs only. There is no interference with function. (Use this score for unsustained nystagmus.)
2. Mild impairment. (Use this score for sustained conjugate nystagmus, dysconjugate eye movements without associated nystagmus (incomplete internuclear ophthalmoplegia (INO)), or paresis of one or more extraocular muscles innervated by neurones originating in the brainstem.)
3. Moderate impairment. (Use this score for dysconjugate nystagmus (complete INO), paralysis of one or more extraocular muscles innervated by neurons originating in the brainstem, or when speech is affected due to brainstem dysfunction but remains intelligible.)
4. Severe impairment. (Use this score when speech is impaired by brainstem dysfunction and is marginally intelligible.)
5. Inability to swallow or speak due to brainstem dysfunction.
6. Untestable.
7. Unknown.

Sensory Functions

0. Normal.
1. Mild impairment. There is a loss of vibration, pain or temperature, or position sense involving the toes or fingers of one or more limb.
2. Moderate impairment. There is a loss of vibration, pain or temperature, or position sense up to the ankle or wrist in one or more limbs.
3. Severe impairment. There is a loss of vibration, pain or temperature, or position sense up to the knee or elbow in one or more limbs.
4. Loss of the above described sensory function(s) proximal to the knee or elbow in one limb.
5. Loss of the above described sensory function(s) in more than one limb
6. Untestable.
7. Unknown.

Bowel and Bladder Functions

Ask about both bladder and bowel functions during the past 2 weeks. Score the worst as follows. Place an "X" after bladder score if the patient performs intermittent self-catheterization.

Bladder

0. Normal.
1. Bladder symptoms but not incontinence.

2. Incontinence less than twice per week.
3. Incontinence two or more times per week, but not daily.
4. Daily incontinence.
5. Indwelling catheter.
6. Grade 5 bladder function plus grade 5 bowel function.
7. Untestable. (Use this score if change in function is due to change in medication or presence of infection.)
8. Unknown.

Bowel

0. Normal.
1. Mild or intermittent constipation but no incontinence.
2. Severe and continuous constipation but no incontinence.
3. Incontinence less than twice per week.
4. Incontinence two or more times per week, but not daily.
5. Daily incontinence.
6. Grade 5 bowel function plus grade 5 bladder function.
7. Untestable. (Use this score if change in function appears to be due to a change in medication or the presence of infection.)
8. Undetermined.

Visual Functions

Note: All visual acuities (VA) are best corrected.

0. VA better than 20/30 and no sign of optic nerve disease.
1. VA equal to or better than 20/30 with signs of optic nerve disease (e.g. afferent pupil defect).
2. Worst eye with maximal corrected VA 20/40–20/50.
3. Worst eye with maximal corrected VA 20/70.
4. Worst eye with maximal corrected VA 20/100–20/200.
5. Worst eye with maximal corrected VA worse than 20/200 and maximal VA of better eye better than 20/60.
6. Grade 5 plus maximal VA in better eye worse than 20/60.
7. Untstable.
8. Unknown.

Mental Functions

Note: This score is not used in the calculation of EDSS scores when neuropsychologic testing is performed as part of a controlled clinical trial.

0. Normal.

1. Mood alteration only.
2. Mild decrease in mentation.
3. Moderate decrease in mentation.
4. Marked decrease in mentation.
5. Dementia or chronic brain syndrome.
6. Untestable.
7. Unknown.

References

Alarcon GS, Schrohenloher RE, Bartolucci AA, Ward JR, Williams HJ, Koopman WJ (1990) Suppression of rheumatoid factor production by methotrexate in patients with rheumatoid arthritis. Evidence for differential influences of therapy and clinical status on IgM and IgA rheumatoid factor expression. Arthritis Rheum 33:1156–1161

Bannwarth B, Labat L, Moride Y, Schaeverbeke T (1994) Methotrexate in rheumatoid arthritis: an update. Drugs 25:25–50

Beatty WW, Paul RH, Wilbanks SL, Hames KA, Blanco CR, Goodkin DE (1995). Identifying multiple sclerosis patients with mild or global cognitive impairment using the Screening Examination for Cognitive Impairment (SEFCI). Neurology 45:718–723

Bennett DR (Ed) (1992) Antineoplastic agents: antimetabolites. In: Drug evaluations annual. The American Medical Association Division of Drugs and Toxicology, Chicago, IL, pp 1897–1900

Calabrese LH, Taylor JV, Wilke WS, Segal AM, Clough JD (1988) Methotrexate (MTX) immunoregulatory T-cell subsets and rheumatoid arthritis: is MTX an immunomodulator? Arthritis Rheum 31(Suppl 1):C20

Cox DR (1922) Regression models and life tables. J R Stat Soc 85:87–94

Crilly A, McInness IB, McDonald AG et al (1995) Interleukin 6 (IL-6) and soluble IL-2 receptor levels in patients with rheumatoid arthritis treated with low dose oral methotrexate. J Rheumatol 22:224–226

Currier RD, Haerer AF, Maydrech EF (1993) Low dose oral methotrexate treatment of multiple sclerosis. Neurology 12:1268–1271

Filippi M, Horsfield MA, Morrissey SP et al. (1994) Quantitative brain MRI lesion load predicts the course of clinically isolated syndromes suggestive of multiple sclerosis. Neurology 44:635–641

Filippi M, Campi A, Martinelli V et al. (1995) A brain MRI study of different types of chronic–progressive multiple sclerosis. Acta Neurol Scand 91:231–233

Fisher RA (1922) On the interpretation of the chi-square from contingency tables and the calculation of *P*. J R Stat Soc 85:87–94

Folstein MF, Folstein SE, McHugh PR (1975) Mini-mental state: a practical method for grading the cognitive state of patients for the clinician. J Psychiatr Res 12:189–198

Goodkin DE, Hertzgaard D, Seminary J (1988) Upper extremity function in multiple sclerosis: improving assessment sensitivity with box-and-block and nine-hole-peg-tests. Arch Phys Med Rehabil 69:850–854

Goodkin DE, Hertsgaard D, Rudick RA (1989) Exacerbation rates and adherence to disease type in a prospectively followed-up population with multiple sclerosis: implications for clinical trials. Arch Neurol 46:261–264

Goodkin DE, Rudick RA, VanderBrug Medendorp S et al. (1992a) Low-dose (7.5 mg) oral methotrexate for chronic progressive multiple sclerosis: design of a randomized, placebo-controlled trial with sample size benefits from a composite outcome variable including preliminary data on toxicity. Online J Curr Clin Trials Sep 25 (Doc No 19)

Goodkin DE, Ross JS, VanderBrug Medendorp S, Konecsni J, Rudick RA (1992b) MRI lesion enlargement in multiple sclerosis: disease-related activity, chance occurrence, or measurement artifact? Arch Neurol 49:261–264

Goodkin DE, Cookfair D, Wende K et al. (1992c) Inter- and intrarater scoring agreement using grades 1.0–3.5 of the Kurtzke expanded disability status scale (EDSS). Neurology 42:859–863

Goodkin DE, Rudick RA, VanderBrug Medendorp S et al. (1995) Low-dose (7.5 mg) oral methotrexate reduces the rate of progression in chronic progressive multiple sclerosis. Ann Neurol 37:30–41

Goodman TA, Polisson RP (1994) Methotrexate: adverse reactions and major toxicities. Rheum Dis Clin North Am 20:513–528

Goto M, Miyamoto T, Nishioka K, Uchida S (1987) T cytotoxic and helper cells are markedly increased and T suppressor and inducer cells are markedly decreased in rheumatoid synovial fluids. Arthritis Rheum 30:737–743

Grosflam J, Weinblatt ME (1991) Methotrexate: mechanism of action, pharmacokinetics, clinical indications, and toxicity. Curr Opin Rheumatol 3:363–368

Hafler DA, Weiner HL (1989) MS: a CNS and systemic autoimmune disease. Immunol Today 10:104–107

Hauser SL, Dawson DM, Lehrich JR et al. (1983) Intensive immunosuppression in progressive multiple sclerosis: 1. Clinical results of a multicenter, randomized, double-blind, placebo-controlled trial. Neurology 43:655–661

Hine RJ, Everson MP, Hardon JM et al. (1990) Methotrexate therapy in rheumatoid arthritis patients diminishes lectin-induced mono-nuclear cell proliferation. Rheumatol Int 10:165–169

Jolivet J, Cowan KH, Curt GA, Clendeninn NJ, Chabuer BA (1983) The pharmacology and clinical use of methotrexate. N Engl J Med 309:1094–1104

Kaplan EL, Meier P (1937) Nonparametric estimation from incomplete observations. J Am Stat Assoc 32:675–701

Kidd D, Thompson AJ, Kendall BE, Miller DH, McDonald WI (1994) Benign form of multiple sclerosis: MRI evidence for less frequent and less inflammatory disease activity. J Neurol Neurosurg Psychiatry 57:1070–1072

Kremer JM, Lee RG, Tolman KG (1989) Liver histology in rheumatoid arthritis patients receiving long-term methotrexate therapy. A prospective study with baseline and sequential biopsy sample. Arthritis Rheum 32:121–127

Kurtzke JF (1983) Rating neurologic impairment in multiple sclerosis: an expanded disability scale (EDSS). Neurology 33:1444–1452

Lezak MD (1995) Neuropsychological assessment, 3d edn. Oxford University Press, New York

Liang K-Y, Seger SL (1986) Longitudinal data analysis using generalized linear models. Biometrika 73:12–22

Lisak RP, Heinz RG, Keis MW, Alvord EC (1970) Dissociation of antibody production from disease suppression in the inhibition of allergic encephalomyelitis by myelin basic protein. J Immunol 104:1435–1446

Mahler ME, Davis RJ, Benson DF (1989) Screening multiple sclerosis patients for cognitive impairment. In: Jensen K, Knudsen L, Stenager E, Grant I (eds) Mental disorders, cognitive deficits, and their treatment in multiple sclerosis. Libbey, London, pp 11–14 (Current Problems in Neurology, vol 10)

McFarland HF, Frank JA, Albert PS et al. (1992) Using gadolinium-enhanced magnetic resonance imaging lesions to monitor disease activity in multiple sclerosis. Ann Neurol 32:758–766

Morgan SL, Baggott JE, Vaughn WH et al. (1990) The effect of folic acid supplementation on the toxicity of low-dose methotrexate in patients with rheumatoid arthritis. Arthritis Rheum 33:9–18

Neumann JW, Ziegler DK (1972) Therapeutic trial of immunosuppressive agents in multiple sclerosis. Neurology 22:1268–1271

Nielsen HJ, Hammer JH (1992) Possible role of histamine in pathogenesis of autoimmune diseases: implications for immunotherapy with histamine-2 receptor antagonists. Med Hypotheses 39:349–355

Nielson HJ, Nielson H, Georgsen J (1991) Ranitidine for improvement of treatment resistant psoriasis. Arch Dermatol 127:270

O'Brien PC (1984) Procedures for comparing samples with multiple endpoints. Biometrics 40:1079–1087

Olsson T (1992) Immunology of multiple sclerosis. Curr Opin Neurol Neurosurg 5:5195–5202

Paty DW, Li DKB, the UBC MS/MRI Study Group and the IFNB Multiple Sclerosis Study Group (1993) Interferon beta-1b is effective in relapsing-remitting multiple sclerosis: II. MRI analysis results of a multicenter, randomized, double-blind, placebo-controlled trial. Neurology 43:662–667

Peto R, Peto J (1972) Asymptotically efficient rank invariant test procedures. J R Stat Soc [A] 135:185–198

Peyser JM, Rao SM, LaRocca NG, Kaplan E (1990) Guidelines for neuropsychological research in multiple sclerosis. Arch Neurol 47:94–97

Popcock SJ, Geller NL, Tsiatis AA (1987) The analysis of multiple endpoints in clinical trials. Biometrics 43:487–498

Poser CM, Paty DW, Scheinber L et al. (1983) New diagnostic criteria for multiple sclerosis: guide-

lines for research protocols. Ann Neurol 13:227–231
Reynolds WJ, Perra M, Yoon SJ, Klein NM (1985) Evaluation of clinical and prognostic significance of T-cell regulatory subsets in rheumatoid arthritis. J Rheumatol 12:49–56
Rose CD, Fawcett PT, Gibney K, Doughty RA, Singsen BH (1994). Serial measurements of soluble interleukin 2 receptor levels (sIL2-R) in children with juvenile rheumatoid arthritis treated with oral methotrexate. Ann Rheum Dis 53:471–474
Rudick RA, Goodkin DE (eds) (1992) Treatment of multiple sclerosis: trial design, results and future perspectives. Springer-Verlag, London
Rudick RA, Medendorp SV, Namey M, Boyle S, Fischer J (1995) Multiple sclerosis progression in a natural history study: predictive value of cerebrospinal fluid free kappa light chains. Multiple Sclerosis. 1:150–155
Rustin GJS, Rustin F, Dent J, Booth M, Salt TS, Bagshawe KD (1983) No increase in second tumors after methotrexate chemotherapy for gestational trophoblastic tumors. N Engl J Med 308:473–476
Segal R, Yaron M, Tartakovsky B (1990) Methotrexate: mechanism of action in rheumatoid arthritis. Semin Arthritis Rheum 20:190–200
Sperling RI, Benincaso AI, Anderson RJ, Coblyn JS, Austen KF, Weinblatt ME (1992) Acute and chronic suppression of leukotriene B_4 synthesis ex vivo in neutrophils from patients with rheumatoid arthritis beginning treatment with methotrexate. Arthritis Rheum 35:376–384
Stern RS, Sierler S, Parrish JA (1982) Methotrexate use for psoriasis and the risk of noncutaneous or cutaneous malignancy. Cancer 50:869–872
Walker AM, Funch D, Dreyer NA et al. (1993) Determinants of serious liver disease among patients receiving low-dose methotrexate for rheumatoid arthritis. Arthritis Rheum 36:329–335
Weinblatt ME, Coblyn JS, Fox DA et al. (1985) Efficacy of low-dose methotrexate in rheumatoid arthritis. N Engl J Med 312:818–822
Weinblatt ME, Weissman BN, Holdsworth DE et al. (1992) Long-term prospective study of methotrexate in the treatment of rheumatoid arthritis: 84-month update. Arthritis Rheum 35:129–137
Whiting-O'Keefe QE, Fye KH, Sack KD (1991) Methotrexate and histologic hepatic abnormalities: a meta-analysis. Am J Med 90:711–716
Wilcoxon F (1945) Individual comparisons by ranking methods. Biometrics Bull 1:80–83

13 Treatment of Multiple Sclerosis with Copolymer 1

Kenneth P. Johnson and M.B. Bornstein*

Background

Multiple sclerosis (MS) is an immunopathic disease that is characterized pathologically by focal areas of inflammation and demyelination in the central nervous system white matter. As the immunologic nature of MS has become better defined, it has been possible to consider rational therapies to be tested in a scientifically rigorous fashion in well defined populations of MS patients (Chapters 2 and 3). One such treatment is copolymer 1, which has now been tested in a small preliminary open study, two well controlled pilot trials and, recently, a large multicenter Phase III investigation. Each of these trials has provided significant information about the clinical value of copolymer 1 and has clarified the excellent patient tolerance of the therapy. This chapter will review the structure and findings of these four sequential clinical trials.

The synthetic polypeptide copolymer 1 (Copaxone®) is prepared from L-alanine, L-glutamic acid, L-lysine and L-tyrosine and is one of a series of compounds prepared at the Weizmann Institute in Israel, which, alone or in combination with various lipids, might simulate the ability of myelin basic protein (MBP) to induce or suppress experimental allergic encephalomyelitis (EAE) (Arnon 1981; Arnon and Teitelbaum 1980; Keith el al. 1979; Lando et al. 1979; Teitelbaum et al. 1971, 1973, 1974; Webb et al. 1973, 1976). None of the series was encephalitogenic (i.e. capable of inducing EAE), but some, particularly copolymer 1, did suppress EAE in animals challenged with either whole white matter or MBP in complete Freund's adjuvant. The laboratory investigations showing the effectiveness of copolymer 1 in preventing or decreasing the severity of EAE involved mice, rats, guinea-pigs, rabbits, monkeys, chimpanzees and baboons, and are of particular interest to MS clinical trials (Arnon 1981; Arnon and Teitelbaum 1980; Keith et al. 1979; Teitelbaum et al. 1971, 1973, 1974; Webb et al. 1973, 1976). In addition, extensive laboratory studies failed to demonstrate any toxicologic or other undesirable side reactions in experimental animals exposed to copolymer 1 under a variety of testing situations (A. Meshorer, personal communication). Finally, Abramsky et al. (1977) first evaluated copolymer 1 for

*Dr Bornstein died in September 1995. His contributions to advances in the treatment of multiple sclerosis were important, and we ask the reader to join us by pausing to remember him. (Eds.)

its effect on three patients with acute disseminated encephalomyelitis (ADE) and four with advanced MS. The three ADE patients reportedly recovered rapidly and completely. The MS patients may have demonstrated slight improvements. There were no significant undesirable side reactions in those first clinical studies. Subsequent clinical trials have included a preliminary trial, two pilot trials (one involving relapsing-remitting (RR) patients and the second, secondary progressive (SP) patients), and a Phase III multicenter trial, which enrolled 251 RR patients into a double-blind, placebo-controlled study. All have shown significant therapeutic effects or substantial trends in benefiting various phases of MS.

Mechanism of Action

The therapeutic effect of copolymer 1 on EAE and MS is thought to involve inhibition of the immune response to MBP and possibly other myelin antigens. Copolymer 1 has been shown to inhibit cell-mediated immune responses to MBP and prevent EAE in several species of animals, including non-human primates (Arnon 1981; Arnon and Teitelbaum 1980). Published investigations of cellular and humoral immune responses in vitro and in EAE suggests that copolymer 1 has at least partial cross-reactivity with MBP (Teitelbaum et al. 1991). Two principle mechanisms are proposed: induction of antigen-specific suppressor cells and interference with T-cell activation by competition with MBP for the major histocompatibility complex class II binding site responsible for antigen presentation. Evidence for the second mechanism is considerably stronger since it has been repeatedly demonstrated in both murine and human T-cell lines, including some derived from patients with MS (Teitelbaum et al. 1992; Fridkis-Hareli et al. 1994; Racke et al. 1992).

Efficacy

Preliminary Trial

The preliminary trial involved 16 patients, four RR and 12 secondary progressive (SP), and was conducted as an open study (Bornstein et al. 1982) (Table 13.1). The investigator was aware that all patients were being treated with copolymer 1. The initial dosage schedule, chosen on the basis of studies with laboratory animals at the Weizmann Institute was 5 mg/ml in sterile saline solution, administered intramuscularly five times a week for the first 3 weeks, three times a week for the next 3 weeks, twice a week for the next 3 weeks, and, finally, once a week for the balance of a 6-month period.

At entry, patients were examined by the evaluating neurologist, samples of peripheral blood and cerebrospinal fluid were obtained, and copolymer 1 injections were started. The patients were followed on an outpatient basis and their neurologic status re-evaluated at various times during the course of the trial.

Table 13.1. Results of preliminary trial of copolymer 1 in 16 patients with multiple sclerosis (based on Bornstein et al. 1982)

	Age range (years)	Treatment duration (years)	Result
Relapsing–remitting			
2 patients	30–39	0.5–2.0	No effect
2 patients	27–32	2.0	Relapses stopped
Secondary progressive			
9 patients	25–46	0.5–3.0	No effect
3 patients	34–49	0.5–2.0	Arrested progression

The specific aims were to determine:

1. Did copolymer 1 produce any significant or undesirable side reactions?
2. Did it produce any useful benefit?
3. Could a dosage schedule be established for further (pilot) trials?

During this early study of copolymer 1, some patients demonstrated improvements in various neurologic functions, such as improved bladder control or increased strength. Later, when the dosage was reduced, as originally planned, these early improvements disappeared and most patients returned to their previous neurologic status or continued their progressive course. To determine whether the previously observed effect was drug-related, the dosage was then gradually increased. After the first 18 months, those patients still in the trial were receiving 20 mg/day in 1 ml of saline.

The patients occasionally reported transient slight pain, discomfort, itching, swelling or redness at the injections sites. No systemic or general reactions were noted or reported. Two of the four RR patients withdrew from the study at the time of an acute attack, one of whom later restarted therapy. The other 14 patients remained in the study for at least 6 months as originally planned. Of the total group of 16 patients, 11 demonstrated no apparent benefit in that they either had relapses during the course of the study or continued their progressive course while five demonstrated definite improvement such as the cessation of relapses or improved balance, strength and gait.

Laboratory examinations included a complete blood count (CBC), routine urinalysis and culture, blood chemistry analysis (sequential multiple analysis (SMA) 6 and 12), VDRL (test for syphilis), cerebrospinal fluid protein, glucose and cells. Except for an occasional and transient eosinophilia (reaching 16% in one instance), no significant abnormalities were noted. Lymphoblast transformation in response to phytohemagglutinin, MBP and copolymer 1 was not observed.

Following these preliminary results, the evaluation of copolymer 1 was extended to rigorous double-blind, randomized, placebo-controlled pilot trials.

Over 50 other patients have been treated with copolymer 1 in early open studies: 13 for less than 1 year, 25 for 1–3 years, six for 3–5 years, three for 5–10 years, and three for over 11 years. No patient in this group has demonstrated any significant or undesirable local or systemic reactions or late sequelae.

Pilot Trial of Patients with Relapsing–Remitting Multiple Sclerosis

The objectives of the pilot trial of the RR patients were: to determine the proportion of patients who were free of attacks in the copolymer 1 and the placebo groups; to provide a comparison of the degree of disability developed over 2 years of participation in the trial; and to characterize significant or undesirable side effects.

Methods

The trial was approved by the Committee on Clinical Investigations of the Albert Einstein College of Medicine and by the Federal Food and Drug Administration (FDA).

Preparation and Characterization of Copolymer 1

Copolymer 1 was first prepared at the Weizmann Institute of Science, Rehovot, Israel, and later by the Bio-Yeda Company in Rehovot. All batches were analyzed for their amino acid composition, molecular weight, cross-reactivity with MBP, and suppression of EAE in guinea-pigs.

Copolymer 1 was dissolved in bacteriostatic saline at a concentration of 20 mg/ml. Sterile, single-dose vials containing 1 ml of bacteriostatic saline alone or the copolymer 1 solution were stored at –20°C. Patients received a monthly supply of 32 vials of the appropriate solution. The preparation and distribution of vials and patient compliance were monitored by a clinical assistant.

Patient Recruitment and Enrollment

Enrolled patients had definite MS (Poser et al. 1983), were 20–35 years of age, had at least two well documented relapses in the 2 years before entry, with a score no higher than 6 (ambulatory with unilateral assistance) on the Disability Status Scale (DSS) (Kurtzke 1955) and were emotionally stable as determined by psychosocial evaluation.

Questionnaires from 932 volunteers were reviewed; 140 were evaluated in neurologic and psychosocial examination, and 90 of these were excluded for various reasons. Fifty patients were accepted into the trial.

Study Design and Data Collection

Study patients were evaluated, then matched according to sex, relapse rate per year, and degree of disability as measured by the DSS in three strata: 0–2, 3–4, and 5–6. The random assignment of the first patient of a pair determined the assignment of both. The patient was enrolled after instruction in the method of self-injection and the completion of a consent form. Nine patients who had a relapse after screening were enrolled after their condition had become stable.

Patients were evaluated at 1 month and then every 3 months for 2 years. At each visit, a blinded neurologist, unaware of the patient's treatment group, completed a neurologic examination and DSS evaluation. The patient's description of local or generalized side effects and changes in neurologic status were reported to the unblinded clinical assistant.

Patients were re-evaluated when they reported new symptoms or a worsening of pre-existing symptoms that persisted for 48 hours or more. The neurologist verified relapses on the basis of study criteria. An event was counted as a relapse only when the patient's symptoms were accompanied by observed objective changes on the neurologic examination involving an increase of at least one point in one of the Functional Systems Scores (FSS) or the DSS. Sensory symptoms unaccompanied by objective findings or transient neurologic worsening were excluded. Patients experiencing an acute relapse were evaluated at frequent intervals until a stable neurologic baseline was re-established. Seventy-four per cent of 62 relapses in the placebo group and 75% of the 16 relapses in the copolymer 1 group were treated with steroids. Symptomatic medications, such as cholinergic and spasmolytic drugs, were permitted.

Laboratory Tests

Routine urinalyses, blood chemistry (SMA 20) determinations, and complete blood counts were performed at entry and every 3 months thereafter.

Statistical Methods

A rigorous statistical analysis program was developed prior to unblinding the trial. Details of the analytic package can be found in the final report of the trial (Bornstein et al. 1987).

Study Population

Fifty patients were enrolled: 48 in 24 matched pairs, and two unmatched patients, with one of each pair randomly assigned to each study group. Table 13.2 shows the baseline characteristics of the study population and of the 48 patients included in the analyses. The distributions of these characteristics were similar in the two treatment arms.

To guard against bias that might be introduced by dropouts, an attempt was made to include all the randomized patients in the analyses. Seven patients did not complete 2 years. Of these, two patients in the placebo group were dropped for psychologic reasons and were excluded from all the analyses because of unusable data. The partial data obtained from the other five patients were included. One patient taking copolymer 1 withdrew during a relapse after 2 months of

Table 13.2. Pilot RR trial: baseline characteristics of the study enrollees (based on Bornstein et al. 1987)

Characteristic	Treatment Group	
	Placebo	Copolymer 1
No. entered	23	25
Average age (years)	31.1	30.0
Average duration of disease (years)	6.4	4.9
Sex		
Male	10	11
Female	13	14
Race/ethnic group		
White	23	23
Black or Hispanic	0	2
Disability score (Kurtzke scale)		
0–2	10	13
3–4	7	5
5–6	6	7
Average disability score (DSS)	3.1	2.9
Prior relapse rate (over 2-year period)	3.9	3.8

treatment, then had a second relapse shortly after stopping medication. Both events were counted as study relapses.

Results

The final matched analysis of the principal endpoint (proportion of relapse-free patients) included 22 pairs. An unmatched analysis permitted the inclusion of an additional four patients, two who were unmatched and two who had been matched to two patients who were subsequently excluded (Figure 13.1). Analyses of relapses are reported both as matched and unmatched. Subsequent analyses were performed on an unmatched basis.

Relapses During the 2-Year Study Period

In the 22 matched pairs, there were 12 discordant pairs: two patients in the placebo group had no relapses, whereas their matches on the copolymer 1 group did; 10 patients in the copolymer 1 group had no relapses, whereas their matches in the placebo group did. The remaining ten pairs had concordant results. The difference in discordant pairs between treatment groups was significant ($P = 0.039$). An unmatched analysis of the presence or absence of relapses was also significant ($P = 0.045$).

Figure 13.1 shows the occurrence and time of relapses in each patient during the trial. Over the 2 years, there were 62 relapses among 23 patients in the placebo group (average, 2.7) and 16 in the copolymer 1 group (average 0.6). The effect of treatment was also examined according to the entry DSS score. In the 0–2 stratum, there were 27 relapses over 2 years among ten placebo-treated patients (average 2.7) and four relapses among 13 copolymer 1-treated patients

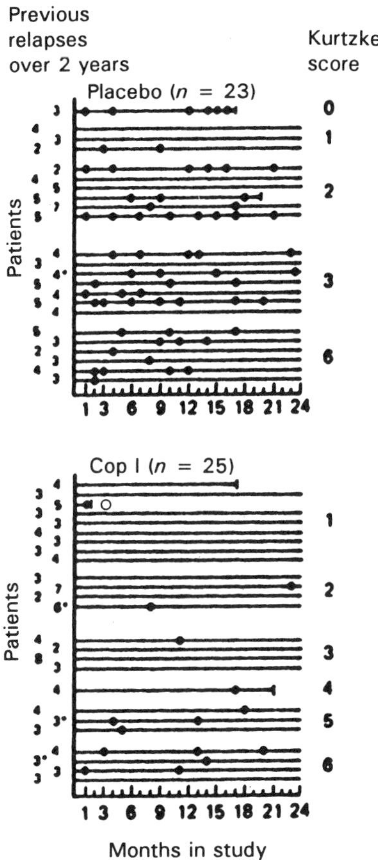

Figure 13.1. Relapses occurring during the 2 years of the RR trial. Each line represents a patient, and each circle a relapse. Patients are grouped according to their Kurtzke score on entry. The number of pretrial relapses are indicated to the left. Discontinued lines represent patients who withdrew before completion. The open circle indicates a relapse occurring after withdrawal that was included as a study event. Patients who were not included in the matched pair analyses are indicated by an asterisk. (Reprinted by permission of *The New England Journal of Medicine*: Bornstein et al. A pilot trial of COP I in exacerbating-remitting multiple sclerosis. 1987;317:408–414, Massachusetts Medical Society)

(average 0.3). In the 3–6 stratum, there were 35 relapses among 13 placebo-treated patients (average 2.7) and 12 relapses among 12 copolymer 1-treated patients (average 1.0).

The distribution of relapses for all 48 patients is shown in Table 13.3. Of the 25 patients in the copolymer 1 group, 14 (56%) were free of relapses, compared with six (26%) of the 23 patients in the placebo group. By contrast, 12 patients in the placebo group (52%) had three or more relapses, compared with one in the copolymer 1 group (4%). Patients were grouped according to whether they had

Table 13.3. Pilot RR trial: relapses according to treatment group (based on Bornstein et al. 1987)

No. relapses /patient	Placebo (no.) (%)	Copolymer 1 (no.) (%)
0	6 (26.1)	14 (56.0)
1	3 (13.1)	7 (28.0)
2	2 (8.7)	3 (12.0)
3	5 (21.8)	1 (4.0)
4	2 (8.7)	0 (0.0)
5	1 (4.3)	0 (0.0)
6	2 (8.7)	0 (0.0)
7	1 (4.3)	0 (0.0)
8	1 (4.3)	0 (0.0)
Total	23 (100.0)	25 (100.0)

no relapses, one to two, or three or more. The difference between these groups was significant at $P < 0.001$.

Multiple logistic regression analyses were performed on the effect of covariates, including treatment, sex, duration of disease, prior relapse rate, DSS score at entry and interactions of these variables. Only the treatment group and DSS score at entry had a significant effect. The multiple logistic-regression analyses showed that treatment with copolymer 1 independently increased the likelihood that a patient would be free of relapses ($P = 0.036$), as did a lower disability score of entry ($P = 0.003$). An estimate of relative risk with adjustment for sex, disability score at entry and previous relapse rate showed the risk of relapses to be 4.6 times greater for placebo than copolymer 1.

Change in Disability Status

Eleven patients in the placebo group (48%) and five patients in the copolymer 1 group (20%) had disease progression over the 2-year period. The difference between treatment groups in the proportion who remained stable or improved was of borderline significance ($P = 0.064$).

The distribution of the changes in DSS score according to treatment group for each baseline DSS score subgroup was of interest. In the 0–2 subgroup, copolymer 1 had a significant beneficial effect on disability status: 84.6% of patients receiving copolymer 1 were stable or improved, compared with 30% in the placebo group ($P = 0.012$). The average change in DSS score favored copolymer 1 by 1.7 units (there was an average worsening of 1.2 with placebo and an improvement of 0.5 with copolymer 1). In the DSS 3–6 subgroup, the proportions of patients whose conditions were stable, improved and worse were comparable in both treatment groups.

The effect of the previously identified covariates on the comparison of worsening versus disease stability or improvement was evaluated with the use of multiple logistic-regression analyses, which demonstrated a beneficial effect of copolymer 1 on disability status ($P = 0.033$). A patient taking placebo was four times more likely to have progression of disease than a patient taking copolymer 1, after adjustment for sex, DSS score at entry and previous relapse rate.

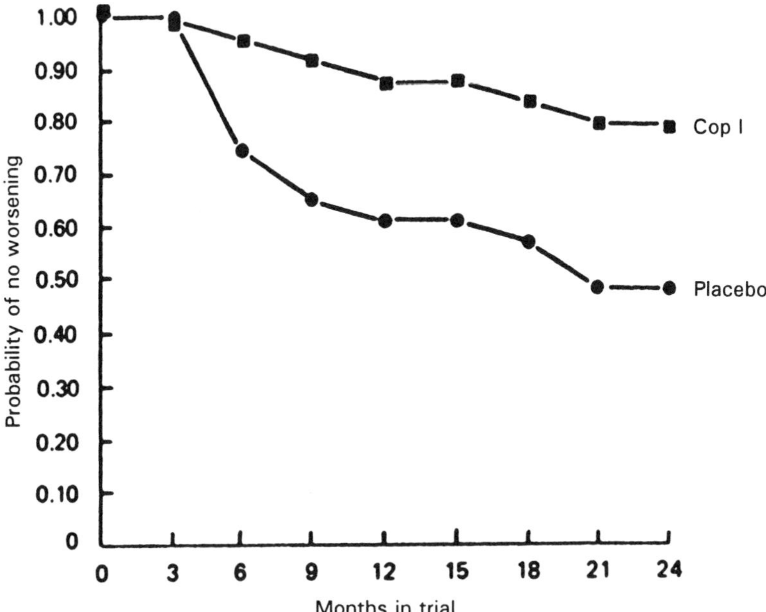

Figure 13.2. Curves representing the probability of no worsening from the baseline Kurtzke score in RR trial. Worsening was determined when first observed, but was counted only if it continued for 3 months. (Reprinted by permission of *The New England Journal of Medicine*: Bornstein et al. A pilot trial of COP I in exacerbating-remitting multiple sclerosis. 1987;317:408–414, Massachusetts Medical Society)

Figure 13.2 (above) is a survival curve showing the length of time before progression defined as an increase of at least 1 unit in the DSS score maintained for at least 3 months. Over the 2-year period, the curves were significantly different ($P = 0.05$), with the placebo group having progression sooner than the copolymer 1 group. Of the patients receiving placebo, 50% had progressed by the end of 18 months, whereas only 20% of those receiving copolymer 1 showed progression by the end of 24 months, when there was a significant difference ($P < 0.005$) favoring copolymer 1 therapy.

Laboratory Studies and Side Effects

The human leukocyte antigen characteristics of the 48 patients were unrelated to the effects of treatment. Urinalysis and blood examinations revealed no apparent changes in the function of the liver, spleen, kidney, bone marrow, gastrointestinal tract, heart or lungs.

More patients taking copolymer 1 reported reactions at the injection site. Soreness was reported during at least half the visits in 32% of the copolymer 1 group compared with 9% of the placebo group; itching was reported in 40% compared with 4%; swelling in 56% compared with none; and redness in 40% compared with 9%.

Two patients had a patterned, transient reaction to copolymer 1, which began immediately after an injection and consisted of a flush, sweating, palpitations, a feeling of tightness around the chest, difficulty with breathing, and associated anxiety. It lasted from 5 to 15 minutes and passed with no residual difficulties. In one patient, the reaction occurred three times in 21 months, and in the other, twice in 17 months. Experimental therapy was discontinued in both patients, who remained under observation for the balance of the trial. The remaining patients were alerted to the possibility of such reactions, informed of precautionary measures, and given a kit containing epinephrine and antihistamine tablets.

After the trial was completed, one of the two patients who had a reaction volunteered to take copolymer 1 in an unblinded manner. This patient reported a hypersensitivity reaction that included urticaria, itching and marked discomfort, which was controlled with epinephrine and steroids.

Blinding

After the trial, the effectiveness of the blinding was evaluated. Of 18 patients in the placebo group, 14 (78%) guessed correctly, as did 15 (68%) of 22 in the copolymer 1 group. The blinded neurologist correctly identified 70% of those taking placebo and 78% of those taking copolymer 1. He based his evaluation on the clinical status of the patient, as did the majority of the patients (68% of the copolymer 1 group and 61% of the placebo group). Approximately 20% of the patients based their guesses on the occurrence or absence of side effects. This suggests that the ability to guess treatment assignment correctly was influenced by the effect of treatment rather than by side effects.

The results of this trial were reported in 1987 (Bornstein et al. 1987).

Trial of Patients with Secondary Progressive Multiple Sclerosis

A second double-blind, randomized, placebo-controlled pilot trial was conducted on the SP MS patients (Bornstein et al. 1991).

Methods

The trial involved a coordinating center (Albert Einstein College of Medicine of Yeshiva University in the Bronx (Einstein), New York), and Baylor College of Medicine (Baylor) (Texas Medical Center in Houston, Texas). It was approved by the Internal Review Boards at both institutions and by the Federal FDA.

Patient Recruitment, Enrollment and Pretrial Observation

Patients were screened between December 1981 and October 1985. The entry criteria were:

1. A definite diagnosis of MS (Poser et al. 1983);
2. Evidence of a SP course for at least 18 months;
3. No more than two relapses in the previous 24 months;
4. 20–60 years of age;
5. Disability between 2.0 and 6.5 on the Kurtzke Expanded Disability Status Scale (EDSS) (Kurtzke 1983);
6. Emotionally stable as determined by psychosocial evaluation.

The EDSS was used to measure degree of neurologic dysfunction at entry and during the study.

Over 2000 patients were screened and 370 were evaluated neurologically and psychosocially. From these, 169 eligible patients were selected and gave informed consent. They were entered into the pretrial observation period, during which the study neurologist examined the patients for evidence of progression every 3 months for a minimum of 6 and a maximum of 15 months. Criteria for randomization to the treatment phase was demonstration of progression in any one of the following ways:

1. A worsening of 2.0 points in one of the functional systems' scores (FSS);
2. A worsening of 1.0 point in two unrelated functional systems;
3. A worsening of 2.0 points on the Ambulation Index (Hauser et al. 1983);
4. A worsening of 1.0 point on the EDSS.

Patients who progressed during this 6–15-month period and maintained the progression for at least 3 months were eligible for entry. In addition, patients must not have progressed beyond 6.5 on the EDSS or have experienced more than one relapse during the pretrial observation period. One hundred and six patients showed progression and were accepted into the treatment phase.

Study Design and Data Collection

The accepted patients signed a consent form and were randomized to either the copolymer 1 or the placebo treatment arm. They were instructed in the method of self-injection of medication on a twice-daily basis. The study was conducted in a double-blind manner. Only the statistician and the clinical assistant who distributed the medication at Albert Einstein College of Medicine were aware of patient assignments.

The principal endpoint was the time to reach a confirmed progression, defined as a worsening of 1 unit over the baseline EDSS for those patients with an entry EDSS of 5.0 or greater, or a worsening of 1.5 units for those with an entry EDSS less than 5.0 and maintained for at least 3 months. Each patient completed participation in the study when a confirmed progression was reached, or when the patient had been 2 years on study in the absence of a confirmed progression. Other endpoints included: time to unconfirmed progression; time to progression of 0.5 unit in the EDSS score; change in the EDSS score from baseline; and study neurologist's overall evaluation of patient's neurologic status.

The study design included planned subgroup analyses by strata of baseline EDSS scores of <5.0 or >5.5, and by center. Survival curves were calculated with life-table methods for the length of time before the endpoint under study, such as confirmed progression, was reached (Anderson et al. 1980).

The blinded neurologist performed a complete neurologic examination, and determined the FSS, EDSS, Ambulation Index and Incapacity Scale scores at entry and at each subsequent 3-month routine visit. Side effects and problems with injections or compliance were discussed only with the clinical assistant. Another blinded neurologist was available to examine patients with severe or unusual side effects. At no time during the trial did it become necessary for this neurologist to request a code break.

Some patients experienced acute relapses for which steroid therapy was permitted. Symptomatic medications, such as cholinergic and spasmolytic drugs, were also permitted. Blood and urine samples were obtained upon entry and at each visit. Routine urinalyses, blood chemistry (SMA 20) determinations, and CBCs were performed.

Study Population

One hundred and six patients were randomized into the trial: 55 at Einstein and 51 at Baylor. There were no significant differences between treatment arms for age, sex, race or baseline EDSS score. Eighty-six (81.1%) completed the study requirements. The remaining 20 patients (18.9%), ten on copolymer 1 and ten on placebo) withdrew: five for side effects, three at the time of demonstrating progression but prior to confirmation, and 12 for various other reasons.

Each early withdrawal was reviewed prior to the code break. It was determined that three of the withdrawals should be counted as confirmed progressions. One (placebo) stopped taking treatment after progression had been noted, but prior to a 3-month confirmation; one (copolymer 1) did not maintain progression at exit from the study, but demonstrated progression 3 months later and one (copolymer 1) progressed and was confirmed by the blinded neurologist via telephone information. The 20 early withdrawals were counted as follows: 17 patients (eight on copolymer one and 9 on placebo) who did not meet progression criteria were censored at the time of withdrawal and three patients (two on copolymer 1 and one on placebo) were counted as confirmed progression at the time of withdrawal.

Results

Time to Confirmed Progression

There were 23 confirmed progressions, 9 (17.6%) in the copolymer 1 treatment arm and 14 (25.5%) in the placebo arm. As previously stated, there were 20 early withdrawals from the trial: three of these patients were counted as confirmed progressions.

Figure 13.3 shows the probability of progression for each treatment arm. At 9 months, the placebo curve crossed the copolymer 1 curve and showed more

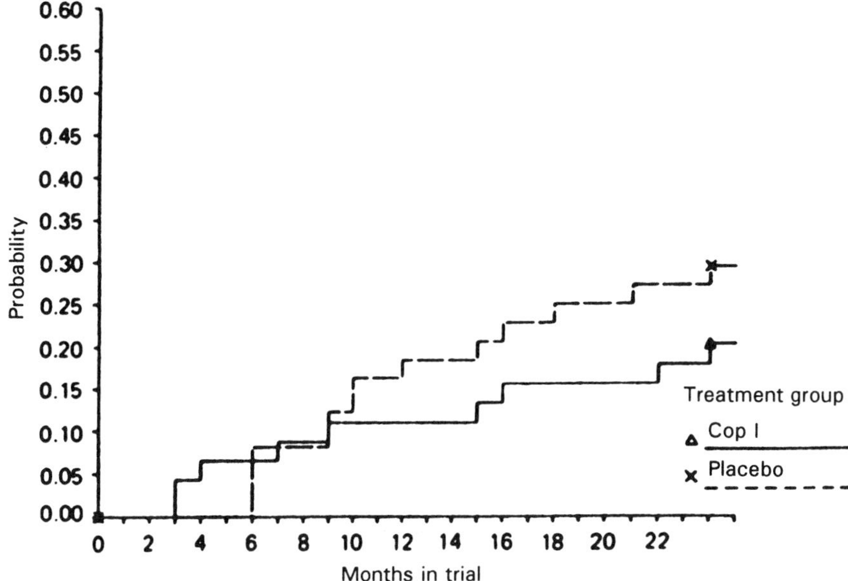

Figure 13.3. SP trial. Probability of progressing to confirmed progression. (Reprinted by permission of *Neurology*: Bornstein et al. A placebo-controlled, double-blind, randomized, two-center, pilot trial of Cop I in chronic progressive multiple sclerosis. 1991;41:533–539)

progression for the remainder of the trial.

The difference in the survival curves at the time points of 12 and 24 months were evaluated using a one-sided confidence limit. At 12 months, there was an 11.0% probability of progressing for copolymer 1 patients as compared with 18.5% for placebo patients ($P = 0.086$).

A proportional hazards model was used to examine the influence of other factors: treatment arm, age and baseline EDSS score, and their interactions on time to progression. The results were not statistically different.

Subgroup Analysis by Center

The disability data were also analyzed by center. For Einstein, the time to progression was significantly different at 24 months with a 21.4% chance of progression in the copolymer 1-treated arm and a 38.5% chance of progressing in the placebo arm ($P = 0.041$). For Baylor, patients in each treatment arm had a 19.0% chance of progressing by 24 months.

For the copolymer 1 group, the centers reported similar percentages of patients with confirmed progression, 18.5% (5/27) at Einstein and 16.7% (4/24) at Baylor. For the placebo group, the percentages for patients with confirmed progression at Einstein was 35.7% (10/28) which is more than twice that at Baylor, 14.8% (4/27). Comparing the placebo effect at the two centers, the probability of progressing at 24 months for Einstein was significantly higher than Baylor (38.5% versus 19.0%) ($P = 0.046$, 2-tail).

Change in EDSS Score

The change from baseline EDSS score was evaluated for patients who completed 24 months on trial. For those 20 patients who dropped out, the change was calculated for their period on study. For the copolymer 1-treatment arm, 19.6% of the patients improved, 37.3% remained stable and 43.1% worsened; on the placebo arm 14.5% improved, 34.6% were stable and 50.9% worsened (Figure 13.4). Since the patients were expected to continue to worsen over the 24 months in trial, both stabilization and improvement in EDSS scores are considered beneficial effects. Combining these categories, 56.9% of the copolymer 1 treatment arm were stable or improved compared with 49.1% of the placebo. This difference is not statistically significant but does show a trend in favor of copolymer 1.

Laboratory Studies and Side Effects

Routine evaluation of urine and blood showed no changes in the function of the liver, spleen, lymph nodes, kidney, bone marrow, gastrointestinal tract, heart or lungs in either group.

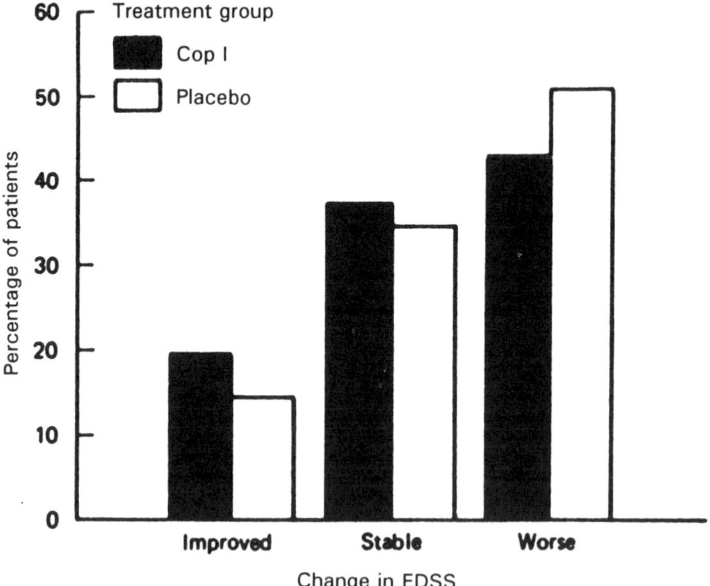

Figure 13.4. SP trial. Changes in EDSS score from baseline by treatment group. (Reprinted by permission of *Neurology*: Bornstein et al. A placebo-controlled, double-blind, randomized, two-center, pilot trial of Cop I in chronic progressive multiple sclerosis. 1991;41:533–539)

A higher percentage of copolymer 1 patients ($P = 0.001$) reported soreness (83% versus 47%), itching (61% versus 17%), swelling (80% versus 23%) and redness (85% versus 30%) at the injection site.

Twelve copolymer 1- and three placebo-treated patients reported transient self-limiting systemic reactions, which included a flush, palpitations, difficulty with breathing and anxiety. Two copolymer 1 and one placebo patient reported the full complement of symptoms; the remaining ten copolymer 1 and two placebo patients reported only a few of these symptoms. The reactions were transient, lasting from a few seconds to about 1 hour, the median time being 2.5 minutes (mean 12.4 minutes). One patient reported an allergic (urticarial) response to copolymer 1.

Blinding

To preserve the blinding, the evaluating neurologists and the patients avoided discussing side effects, which were reported to the clinical co-ordinators. A non-blinded neurologist was available to evaluate and treat any serious side effects or reactions that might be drug-related.

The effectiveness of the blinding was evaluated after the study. The rate of correct guesses for the remaining 88 patients responding was about the same in each treatment arm, with about half of the patients (56.2% copolymer 1 and 53.6% placebo) making the correct assessment.

Phase III Multicenter Trial in Relapsing–Remitting Multiple Sclerosis Patients

Between 1987 and 1991, the copolymer 1 project was transferred from the Weizmann Institute to the commercial firm, Teva Pharmaceuticals Limited of Petah Tiqva, Israel. Considerable effort was made to refine the manufacturing process to insure availability of a highly standardized preparation that could be used in a Phase III clinical trial. This process was successfully completed in 1991 when a standardized form of copolymer 1 with an average molecular weight of 4700–13 000 Da was made available in quantities sufficient for clinical investigation.

To conduct a pivotal Phase III investigation, 11 universities were recruited in the USA, all of which had previously established excellent records for performing clinical research in MS. They included: the University of California, Los Angeles; the University of Maryland, Baltimore; the University of Pennsylvania, Philadelphia; the University of New Mexico, Albuquerque; the University of Rochester, Rochester; the University of Southern California, Los Angeles; the University of Texas, Houston; the University of Utah, Salt Lake City; Wayne State University, Detroit; the University of Wisconsin, Madison; and Yale University, New Haven. The trial was under the direction of Dr Kenneth P. Johnson, Project Director. It was supported by Teva Pharmaceuticals Limited, Petah Tiqva, Israel, with additional funding from the Federal FDA Orphan Drug Program and the

National Multiple Sclerosis Society. A data management group, the National Medical Research Corporation of Hartford, Connecticut, was selected to distribute the drug and to monitor the course of the trial. The study was conducted according to a protocol approved by the FDA. The results of this 2-year trial have been reported by Johnson etal. (1995).

Conduct of the Trial

The study was designed to compare the patient tolerance and therapeutic effect of daily subcutaneous injections of copolymer 1 20 mg versus placebo over 24 months, with the MS relapse rate as the primary outcome variable. The study was designed and the patients were recruited to confirm the conclusions of the previous pilot RR trial (Bornstein et al. 1987). A detailed training session was held for both neurologists and co-ordinators. The entire protocol, the precise definition of a relapse (per protocol) and a careful discussion of the EDSS were undertaken. The trial began in October 1991. During the course of the trial, investigator meetings were convened at approximately 6-month intervals to clarify any difference in protocol interpretation. The Project Director, members of the data management group and the sponsor made visits as needed to individual sites.

For the purposes of this trial, an MS relapse was defined as the appearance or reappearance of a neurologic abnormality, which persisted for at least 48 hours and was preceded by clinical stability for at least 30 days. Relapses had to consist of new or recurrent objective changes on the neurologic examination. Symptoms associated with fever were excluded and changes in bowel/bladder or cognitive functions were not considered relapses for this trial. Secondary endpoints included the proportion of relapse-free patients, time to first relapse following onset of therapy, proportion of patients with sustained disease progression (defined as an increase of at least 1 full step on the EDSS (Kurtzke 1983), which persisted for at least 3 months), and mean change in EDSS and the ambulation index between the treatment groups from baseline to conclusion.

The patient population consisted of both men and women between the ages of 18 and 45 with clinically definite MS or laboratory-supported definite MS (Poser et al. 1983). All patients were ambulatory, with EDSS scores ranging from 0 to 5.0 and a history of at least two well defined and documented relapses in the 2 years prior to entry. All were neurologically stable and had been off corticosteroid therapy for at least 30 days prior to onset. No enrolled patient had previously received copolymer 1 or immunosuppressive therapy, including total lymphoid irradiation. Other exclusion criteria included pregnancy, insulin-dependent diabetes mellitus, a positive HIV or HTLV-1 serology or the need for constant use of aspirin or non-steroidal anti-inflammatory drugs. Women were required to use an adequate method of contraception.

Patients were carefully instructed in the method of subcutaneous self-injection and received a 1-month's supply of study medication. Patients returned to the study site monthly to receive medication and report side effects. At 3-monthly intervals, the patients underwent a complete neurologic evaluation following a two-neurologist protocol. An examining neurologist evaluated only objective neurologic signs without discussing symptoms or side effects. A treating neurologist evaluated both symptoms and adverse events and was responsible for providing corticosteroid therapy at the time of a confirmed relapse. A nurse co-ordinator was in frequent contact with each patient. Both of the neurologists and the nurse co-ordinator were blinded to the patients' study medications. A single protocol for corticosteroid therapy consisting of three daily doses of methylprednisolone 1000 mg given intravenously, followed by an oral taper of prednisone was used at all investigative sites.

At the time of new symptoms or a suspected relapse, patients were instructed to call their center immediately, where they were evaluated within 7 days. Once an MS relapse was documented, patients were treated as medically indicated.

In addition to a chest radiograph and an electrocardiogram prior to onset of therapy, the patients were evaluated by urinalysis, immunologic studies, a serum chemistry panel and copolymer 1 antibody assays at 3-month intervals. An independent safety monitoring committee met quarterly to review all adverse events and laboratory determinations. The Safety Committee was also blinded throughout the course of the trial. The protocol was approved by the institutional review board of each participating university and all patients gave written informed consent.

The final data set was evaluated using several cohort definitions. The intention to treat analysis of all randomized patients was considered to be of primary importance. Other evaluated cohorts excluded patients who did not complete 6 months of treatment, patients who failed to complete 2 years (730 days) of treatment, and patients who missed over 5% of consecutive study medication dosages or 10% of total dosages during the study. There was strong internal consistency of statistically significant findings and trends among the various evaluated cohorts. Therefore, only the results of the most rigorous intention to treat analysis are presented here.

The proportions of withdrawals were compared using the Cochran–Mantel–Haenszel test. Time to withdrawal was analyzed using the log-rank test. For demographic and medical history characteristics, two-sample *t*-tests were used for continuous variables and exact probability tests for discrete variables.

Mean relapse rate was analyzed using analysis of covariance, with tests for study drug-by-center interaction and including a priori defined covariates: sex, duration of disease (years), prior 2-year relapse rate, and baseline Kurtzke EDSS. Proportions of relapse-free patients were tested using logistic regression incorporating the same covariate effects. Time to first relapse was evaluated using Weibull regression. The proportion of progression-free patients was analyzed using logistic regression.

Changes from baseline for Kurtzke EDSS and ambulation index were assessed using repeated measures analysis of covariance. Analyses of the change from baseline to 24 months were also conducted. Categorical repeated measures and 24-month endpoint analyses were performed on Kurtzke EDSS change from baseline, classified as "improved" (reduction of at least one step) "worsened" (increase of at least one step) or "no change".

Results

Beginning in October 1991, 284 patients were screened and 251 were randomized to the two treatment groups by May 1992. The two groups were well matched for age, sex, duration of disease, mean relapse rate in the prior 2 years, EDSS and Ambulation Index. A majority of participants were women (73%) and Caucasian (94%). The mean age was 34 years. For those in the copolymer 1 group, 51 were in the 0–2, 57 in the 2–4 and 17 in the >4 EDSS range. The placebo group consisted of 68 in the 0–2, 46 in the 2–4 and 12 in the >4 EDSS range.

During the course of the trial, 19 patients (15.2%) withdrew from the copolymer 1 group and 17 (13.5%) from the placebo group. The proportion of patients who withdrew and the time to withdrawal were statistically similar over the duration of the trial for both groups. Three patients in the copolymer 1 group withdrew when they became pregnant and one stopped medication because of disease progression. Two patients in the placebo group failed to comply with the protocol. Two copolymer 1 patients withdrew for serious adverse events: one after 50 days on treatment developed immediate flushing, chest tightness, dyspnea, nausea and vomiting (see below), which lasted for over 90 minutes after the injection, and one, after 131 days on treatment, developed generalized lymph node enlargement. Lymph node biopsy from that patient revealed only chronic inflammatory change. Three other patients receiving copolymer 1 and one patient on placebo withdrew because of transient self-limiting systemic reactions, which were brief and not considered serious.

During 2 years of dosing, the copolymer 1 group experienced 161 confirmed relapses, while the placebo group experienced 210 relapses (Table 13.4). The mean relapse rate over 24 months for the copolymer 1 group was 1.19 and for the placebo group, 1.68, a reduction for the copolymer 1 group of 29%, which was statistically significant ($P = 0.007$). The annualized relapse rate was 0.59 for the copolymer 1 and 0.84 for those receiving placebo. The secondary endpoints related to the relapse rate; the proportion of relapse-free patients and the median time to first relapse both favored copolymer 1 treatment but did not reach statistical significance. When the patient population was divided into those with no relapses, one or two relapses, or three or more relapses, there was a clear advantage for copolymer 1 therapy ($P = 0.023$).

The disability outcome for the two groups is shown in Table 13.5. Based on the EDSS, copolymer 1 had a significant effect on neurologic disability (Figure 13.5). Over 2 years, more copolymer 1-treated patients showed neurologic improvement whereas more placebo-treated patients worsened ($P = 0.037$). However, there was no demonstrable difference in the proportion of patients in either group who were free of sustained disease progression: 78.4% of the copolymer 1-treated group versus 75.4% of those receiving placebo. The mean Ambulation Index was almost identical between the two groups after 2 years of therapy.

Table 13.4. Phase III trial: relapse experience of copolymer 1 and placebo groups (based on Johnson et al. 1995)

	Copolymer 1 (*n* = 125)	Placebo (*n* = 126)	Reduction vs placebo (%)	*P*-value
Primary endpoints				
Relapse rate over 24 months (covariate adjusted mean)	1.19	1.68	–29	0.007
Annualized relapse rate	0.59	0.84		
Observed relapses over 24 months	161	210		
Secondary endpoints				
Percentage of relapse-free patients	33.6	27.0		0.098
Median time to first relapse (days)	287	198		0.097
No. relapses/patient				
0	42	34		0.023
1–2	60	55		
≥3	23	37		

Table 13.5. Phase III trial: disability experience measures by EDSS and Ambulatory Index of copolymer 1 and placebo groups (based on Johnson et al. 1995)

	Copolymer 1	Placebo	*P*-value
Percentage of patients with a change in disability between baseline and conclusion			
Improved (EDSS decrease ≥1)	24.8	15.2	
No change	54.4	56.0	0.037*
Worse (EDSS increase ≥1)	20.8	28.8	
Mean (±SD) EDSS change from baseline	–0.05 ± 1.13	0.21 ± 0.99	0.023**
Percentage of progression-free patients	78.4	75.4	NS
Mean (±SD) Ambulation Index	0.27 ± 0.94	0.28 ± 0.93	NS

NS: Not significantly different.
*Categorical repeated measures.
**Repeated measures analysis of covariance.

Twenty-seven patients recruited at the University of Pennsylvania underwent frequent gadolinium-enhanced cranial MRI using an advanced protocol and analysis package. Preliminary information indicates a trend towards benefit with copolymer 1, especially in relation to the appearance of enhanced lesions, however, final interpretation of this small substudy must await publication of the results. The small number participating at the University of Pennsylvania makes it highly unlikely that statistically significant differences between groups will be verified.

The safety profile observed in this trial indicated that treatment with copolymer 1 was very benign. No differences in vital signs were noted between groups and there were no laboratory differences observed between the two treatment groups. The most frequent adverse event was a localized injection site reaction consisting of mild erythema and induration, which occasionally persisted for several days. It occurred at least once during 730 days of injections in 90% of the copolymer 1-treated group and in 60% of those receiving placebo. At no time was skin necrosis observed. The other adverse event that had been recognized in all earlier copolymer 1 therapeutic trials was a transient self-limiting systemic reaction (Table 13.6). It was sporadic and unpredictable, occurred immediately after an injection and was characterized by an inconsistent combination of flush-

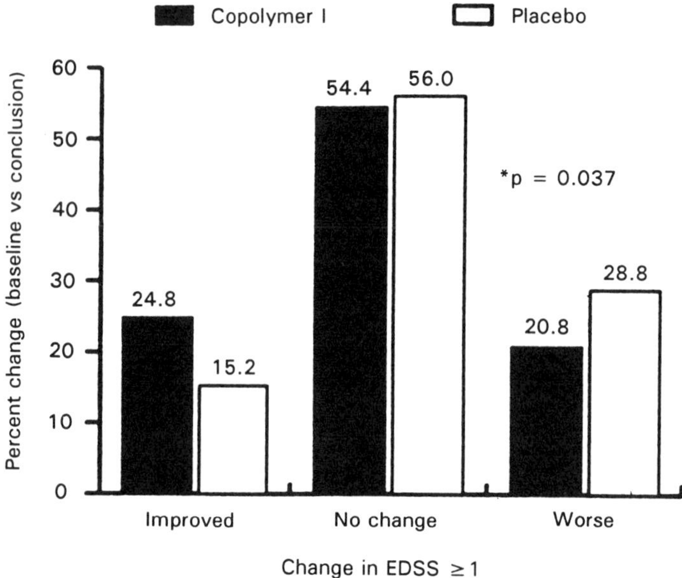

Figure 13.5. Phase III trial. Effects on neurologic disability of treatment group. (Reprinted by permission of *Neurology*: Johnson et al. Copolymer I reduces the relapse rate and improves disability in relapsing-remitting multiple sclerosis: results of a Phase III multicenter, double-blind, placebo-controlled trial. 1995;45:1268–1276)

Table 13.6. Incidence of transient self-limited systemic reactions (based on Johnson et al. 1995)

	Treatment group	
	Copolymer 1 ($n = 125$)	Placebo ($n = 126$)
Systemic reaction (%)	19 (15.2)	4 (3.2)
Primary symptoms		
Flushing without chest pain	6	2
Chest pain without flushing	6	2
Both chest pain and flushing	7	0
Secondary symptoms		
Palpitation	6	0
Anxiety	2	2
Dyspnea	16	2

ing and chest tightness, accompanied at times by shortness of breath, palpitations or anxiety. It lasted for between 30 seconds and 30 minutes and resolved spontaneously without sequelae. This reaction was reported at least once in 15% of copolymer 1-treated patients and in 3% of those receiving placebo. It rarely occurred more than once during the course of the trial but was experienced seven times by one patient over the course of 2 years. This reaction resulted in the discontinuation of therapy by four patients in the copolymer 1 group and by one in the placebo group. While not an abnormal occurrence, three women became pregnant during the course of the trial, all in the copolymer 1-treated group. One elected to have a therapeutic abortion and continue treatment, while two withdrew and delivered normal infants.

After 2 years of treatment, patients were offered the opportunity to remain on their study medication (copolymer 1 or placebo) in a blinded fashion for an additional period until all participants had concluded 2 years of treatment. Approximately 100 patients in each group elected to continue for an average of 5.5 additional months. Preliminary assessment of clinical activity related to both primary (relapse rate) and secondary (disability) outcome measures indicates that all those in the copolymer 1 group continued to improve with further therapy.

Serum was collected at 3-month intervals for determination of antibody levels to copolymer 1. A validated enzyme-linked immunosorbent assay (ELISA) copolymer 1 study showed that all patients exposed to copolymer 1 had developed binding antibody, whereas no placebo patient showed antibody at the conclusion of the study. A limited number of Israeli patients given copolymer 1 in an open label study developed ELISA binding antibody but showed no neutralizing activity to copolymer 1. The finding that the clinical effect was evident throughout the trial and appeared to improve during the study extension suggests that neutralizing activity did not develop. This issue continues to be analyzed.

Discussion

The extensive clinical investigation of copolymer 1 as a therapy for MS spanning the years from the late 1970s to 1994 consistently demonstrates two major themes: first that the treatment given at a dose of 20 mg by subcutaneous daily injection has a significant effect on reducing the MS relapse rate and reducing disability, and secondly, that it is quite safe and well tolerated when employed for prolonged periods of time.

A treatment that positively affects the MS relapse rate is of substantial importance. Relapses frequently cause significant, although short-term, neurologic disability and can be accompanied by increased fatigue and, in some patients, pain that is hard to control. Time is frequently lost from work and medical expenses are often increased. Patient anxiety and disruption of family life is common. A 30% reduction in relapses, as shown in the most recent copolymer 1 trial, is therefore of real benefit to the MS population.

Some recent prospective natural history studies of MS have clearly shown that there is a relationship between the early relapse rate and the risk of fixed disability within a finite period of time (Weinshanker et al. 1989) (and see Chapter 5). Therefore, there is the promise that medications that reduce the relapse rate will also affect the progression to permanent disability caused by MS. The combined experience with copolymer 1 therapy now available for analysis, shows either statistically significant evidence or strong trends for benefit in terms of neurologic disability. This has been shown in both RR and in SP MS. Future studies and long-term observation of patients on therapy will, it is hoped, strengthen the evidence concerning the therapeutic effect on neurologic disability.

The thought of embarking on a course of therapy measured in years or even decades, which requires frequent injections of a medication, is daunting for both therapists and for patients. Nevertheless, all current evidence suggests that prolonged therapy covering many months and almost certainly many years, will be required adequately to benefit from therapies such as copolymer 1 and beta interferons. There is little precedent in clinical medicine for this type of therapy, which does not immediately benefit the patient, but reduces the risk of relapses and perhaps fixed disability years later. In this unique situation, both therapists and patients must consider the safety profile of the medication. Substantial evidence collected from numerous trials indicates that copolymer 1 therapy is well tolerated during long-term continuous therapy. There are no flu-like symptoms, as commonly noted in patients starting beta interferon therapy, and there are no reported laboratory abnormalities. There have been no observed sequelae of therapy after years of treatment with copolymer 1. The side effects clearly related to copolymer 1 administration are injection site reactions, which tend to be relatively mild, and the transient reactions consisting of flushing, chest tightness and anxiety, which appear at rare and unpredictable intervals. None of these side effects have proven to be serious or life threatening, have serious consequences for the patient, or have, except in rare instances, required termination of the treatment plan.

The clear beneficiaries from the recent developments in MS therapy, which indeed herald a new era, are the patients and their treating neurologists. It is now necessary for therapists to become familiar with copolymer 1, beta interferon (Chapter 11) and other treatments under consideration, and to choose the therapy most suitable for each patient, based on the evidence available about mechanism of action, therapeutic effect and patient tolerance. Laboratory evidence even suggests the first two medications shown to alter the natural course of MS (beta interferon and copolymer 1) could be used concurrently, it is hoped, to provide greater therapeutic effect. Studies of MBP-sensitive lymphocytes show that cells react less to MBP when treated with both copolymer 1 and interferon beta 1b than to either medication alone (Milo and Panitch 1995). The concept of combined therapy must await proper clinical investigation however.

Acknowledgements

(Please also note acknowledgements in first edition of this text.) B. R. Brooks, University of Wisconsin, Madison; J. A. Cohen, University of Pennsylvania, Philadelphia; C. C. Ford, University of New Mexico, Albuquerque; J. Goldstein, Yale University, New Haven, Connecticut; R. P. Lisak, Wayne State University, Detroit, Michigan; L. W. Myers, University of California, Los Angeles; H. S. Panitch, University of Maryland, Baltimore; J. W. Rose, University of Utah, Salt Lake City; R. B. Schiffer, University of Rochester, Rochester, New York; T. Vollmer, Yale University; L. P. Weiner, University of Southern California, Los Angeles; J. S. Wolinsky, University of Texas, Houston; and the Copolymer 1 Multiple Sclerosis Study Group; Shaul Kadosh, Howard Hait, Yafit Stark, Irit Pinchasi, at Teva Pharmaceuticals Industries Limited; Nina Spiller, at the

National Medical Research Corporation; Stanley van den Noort, University of California, Irvine; Aaron Miller, Maimonides Medical Center, New York, New York; David Mellits, Johns Hopkins Hospital, Baltimore, Maryland; Stephen Reingold, National Multiple Sclerosis Society, New York, New York; Irving H. Gomolin, Gurwin Jewish Geriatric Center, New York, New York, Safety Committee Members.

The Phase III multicenter study was supported by the Federal Food and Drug Administration Orphan Drug Program No. FD-R000559-01, the National Multiple Sclerosis Society No. RD 2202-A-6, and Teva Pharmaceutical Industries, Limited, Petah Tiqva, Israel.

References

Abramsky O, Teitelbaum D, Arnon R (1977) Effect of a synthetic polypeptide (Cop 1) on patients with multiple sclerosis and acute disseminated encephalomyelitis: preliminary report. J Neurol Sci 31:433–438

Anderson S, Auguier A, Hauck W et al. (1980) Statistical methods for comparative studies. Wiley, New York, pp 199–214

Arnon R (1981) Experimental allergic encephalomyelitis: susceptibility and suppression. Immunol Rev 55:5–30

Arnon R, Teitelbaum D (1980) Desensitization of experimental allergic encephalomyelitis with synthetic peptide analogues. In: Davison AN, Cuzner ML (eds) The suppression of experimental allergic encephalomyelitis and multiple sclerosis. Academic Press, New York, pp 105–117

Bornstein MB, Miller A, Teitelbaum D, Arnon R et al. (1982) Multiple sclerosis: trial of a synthetic polypeptide. Ann Neurol 11:317–319

Bornstein MB, Miller A, Slagle S et al. (1987) A pilot trial of Cop 1 in exacerbating-remitting multiple sclerosis. N Engl J Med 317:408–414

Bornstein MB, Miller A, Slagle S et al. (1991) A placebo-controlled, double-blind, randomized, two-center, pilot trial of Cop 1 in chronic progressive multiple sclerosis. Neurology 41:533–539

Fridkis-Hareli M, Teitelbaum D, Gurevitch E et al. (1994) Direct binding of myelin basic protein and synthetic copolymer 1 to class II major histocompatibility complex molecules on living antigen presenting cells: specificity and promiscuity. Proc Natl Acad Sci USA 91:4872–4876

Hauser SL, Dawson DM, Lehrich JR et al. (1983) Intensive immunosuppression in progressive multiple sclerosis: a randomized three-arm study of high dose intravenous cyclophosphamide, plasma exchange, and ACTH. N Engl J Med 308:173–180

Johnson K, Brooks BR, Cohen JA et al. (1995) Copolymer 1 reduces the relapse rate and improves disability in relapsing-remitting multiple sclerosis: results of a Phase III multicenter, double-blind, placebo-controlled trial. Neurology 45:1268–1276

Keith AB, Arnon R, Teitelbaum D et al. (1979) The effect of Cop 1, a synthetic polypeptide on chronic relapsing experimental allergic encephalomyelitis in guinea pigs. J Neurol Sci 42:267–274

Kurtzke JF (1955) A new scale for evaluating disability in multiple sclerosis. Neurology 5: 580–583

Kurtzke JF (1983) Rating neurological impairment in multiple sclerosis: an expanded disability status scale (EDSS). Neurology 33:1444–1452

Lando Z, Teitelbaum D, Arnon R (1979) Effect of cyclophosphamide on suppressor cell activity in mice unresponsive to EAE. J Immunol 123:2156–2160

Milo R, Panitch H (1995) Additive effects of copolymer-1 and interferon beta-1b on the immune responses to myelin basic protein. J Neuroimmunol 61:185–193

Poser CM, Patty DW, Scheinberg L et al. (1983) New diagnostic criteria for multiple sclerosis: guidelines for research protocols. Ann Neurol 13:227–231

Racke MK, Martin R, McFarland H, Fritz RB (1992) Copolymer 1-induced inhibition of antigen-specific T-cell activation: interference with antigen presentation. J Neuroimmunol 37:75–84

Teitelbaum D, Meshorer A, Hirshfeld T et al. (1971) Suppression of experimental allergic encephalomyelitis by a synthetic polypeptide. Eur J Immunol 1:242–248

Teitelbaum D, Webb C, Meshorer A et al. (1973) Suppression by synthetic polypeptides of experimental allergic encephalomyelitis induced in guinea pigs and rabbits with bovine and human basic encephalitogen. Eur J Immunol 3:273–279

Teitelbaum D, Webb C, Bree M et al. (1974) Suppression of experimental allergic encephalomyelitis in rhesus monkeys by a synthetic basic copolymer. Clin Immunol Immunopathol 3:256–262

Teitelbaum D, Aharoni R, Sela M, Arnon R (1991) Cross-reactions and specificities of monoclonal antibodies against myelin basic protein and against the synthetic copolymer 1. Proc Natl Acad Sci USA 88:9528–9532

Teitelbaum D, Milo R, Arnon R, Sela M (1992) Synthetic copolymer 1 inhibits human T-cell lines specific for myelin basic protein. Proc Natl Acad Sci USA 89:137–141

Webb C, Teitelbaum D, Arnon R et al. (1973) In vivo and in vitro immunological cross-reactions between basic encephalitogen and synthetic basic polypeptides capable of suppressing experimental allergic encephalomyelitis. Eur J Immunol 3:279–286

Webb C, Teitelbaum D, Herz A et al. (1976) Molecular requirements involved in suppression of EAE by synthetic basic copolymers of amino acids. Immunochemistry 13:333–337

Weinshenker BG, Bass B, Rice G, Noseworthy J et al. (1989) The natural history of multiple sclerosis: a geographically based study: 2. Predictive value of the early clinical course. Brain 112:1419–1428

14 Treatment of Multiple Sclerosis with Cladribine

Jack C. Sipe, J.S. Romine, J. Zyroff, J. Koziol and E. Beutler

Background

Cladribine, also known as 2-chlorodeoxyadenosine (2-CdA) or Leustatin®, is an adenosine deaminase-resistant purine nucleoside that selectively targets lymphoid cells, with relatively low toxicity toward other tissues (Beutler 1992). The history of the development of cladribine begins with the discovery of a relationship between severe combined immunodeficiency disease (SCID) with severe lymphopenia and inherited deficiency of the enzyme adenosine deaminase (ADA). ADA deficiency was discovered serendipitously by Giblett et al. in 1972 while investigating the linkage of immunodeficiency to a variety of genetic markers. For many years the severe lymphopenia in SCID that results from complete ADA deficiency was not understood.

The answer to this problem was discovered in 1977 by Carson et al., who found that degradation of lymphocyte purine deoxyribonucleotides is entirely dependent on the activity of ADA. Carson proposed that the accumulation of deoxyribonucleotides in lymphocytes is related to high levels of lymphocyte deoxycytidine kinase which specifically predisposes these cells to accumulate lethal levels of these compounds. The prediction that ADA-deficient lymphocytes contained extraordinarily high levels of deoxyribonucleotides was soon verified. It has been postulated that DNA strand breaks in the presence of excess 2-CdA-ribonucleotides leads to NAD exhaustion and results in cell death of lymphocytes, or apoptosis (Carson et al. 1986).

This insight into the cause of selective lymphocyte depletion in ADA deficiency served as the starting point for a systematic search for an ADA-resistant purine nucleoside that could selectively kill lymphoid cells (Carson et al. 1979). Of the approximately 25 compounds synthesized by Carson and colleagues, 2-CdA, or cladribine, was found to have the most favorable therapeutic ratio (Carson et al. 1980, 1982, 1983). Phase I and II clinical studies were begun by Ernest Beutler in collaboration with Carson (1984). Patients with advanced lymphoid neoplasms, patients undergoing bone marrow transplantation, and patients with cutaneous T-cell lymphomas and chronic lymphocytic leukemia were treated with 2-CdA (Beutler et al. 1991; Kay et al. 1992; Piro 1992; Saven and

Piro 1993; Saven et al. 1991, 1992a, b, 1993a, b). Of all the neoplastic disorders, the best and most durable responses were seen in patients with hairy cell leukemia (Piro et al. 1992; Saven and Piro 1993). By 1993, a total of 350 patients with hairy cell leukemia had been treated at Scripps Clinic. Of 146 patients that had been followed sufficiently long for evaluation, 97% responded with an 86% complete and durable remission rate after a single treatment (Piro et al. 1990). Cladribine has also been used with some success in patients with certain autoimmune disorders, including Coombs' positive autoimmune hemolytic anemia and immune thrombocytopenia (Figueroa and McMillan 1993). Even now, the range of therapeutic possibilities for cladribine is being expanded into many different hematologic and autoimmune disorders (rheumatoid arthritis, inflammatory bowel disease). In March 1993, the drug was licensed for the treatment of hairy cell leukemia. In this chapter, the extension of cladribine treatment to multiple sclerosis (MS) will be reviewed.

Mechanisms of Action

Despite decades of research, the molecular or biochemical basis for MS remains unknown. In the absence of a known primary cause, there are many pieces of circumstantial evidence to indicate that the body's own immunocytes are directed or programmed to produce an autoimmune attack upon central nervous system (CNS) myelin to cause the symptoms of MS (Hughes 1992). The details of the pathogenesis of MS and the relationship to therapeutic strategies are discussed in Chapters 2 and 16 of this monograph.

Without a specific rationale for MS therapy, physicians have been forced to employ treatments designed to affect the disordered immune response that appears to mediate or cause the disease. In the past, immunosuppressive therapy has involved the use of many different types of drugs, often with serious side effects, and with only a few drugs showing mild efficacy in double-blind investigations (Jacobs et al. 1994).

With this background, we first proposed to test cladribine in patients with chronic progressive MS because of the selective lymphocyte depletion induced by the drug with relatively low toxicity toward other tissues. Our plan to use cladribine in this manner followed extensive experience with the use of the drug in leukemias, lymphomas and other autoimmune disorders.

One current hypothesis of the presumed autoimmune mechanisms in MS involves transvascular migration of the blood–brain barrier by activated T cells that pass into the CNS parenchyma and produce perivascular lymphocytic infiltration in MS plaques. The activated T cells may promote disease by direct damage to myelin and oligodendrocytes or by the activation of macrophages that contribute to demyelination. Because activated T cells, irrespective of their specificity, appear to play a major role in the pathogenesis of CNS demyelination in MS, we decided to test selective lymphocyte depletion by cell death or apoptosis induced by cladribine.

Clinical Pharmacokinetics

The structure of cladribine is shown in Figure 14.1. Except for the substitution of a chlorine atom for hydrogen at the 2-position of the purine ring, the structure is identical to deoxyadenosine. The chlorine substitution apparently confers resistance to ADA sufficient to prevent deamination of the adenine ring. The relative selectivity for lymphocyte killing was demonstrated in cell culture systems by Carson et al. (1983). The sensitivity of various cell lines in tissue culture bears a very close relationship to the ratio of cellular deoxycytidine kinase activity to deoxynucleotidase activity. Those cells with high levels of deoxycytidine kinase activity, such as lymphocytes and peripheral blood monocytes are very sensitive to CdA both in vitro and in vivo (Beutler 1994). In the bone marrow, stem cell precursors of the erythroid, monocyte and granulocyte series are affected at drug concentrations that are achieved in vivo (Petzer et al. 1991). Although cladribine is sometimes incorporated into DNA, this is not its only mechanism of action and, in the case of lymphocytes, cell death by apoptosis is the primary event. In contrast with other chemotherapeutic agents, cladribine has the ability to kill both resting and dividing T cells. The chief mechanism of action is thought to be the appearance of strand breaks that begin to accumulate in the DNA of lymphocytes as early as 4 hours after exposure to 2-CdA, presumably because of high levels of deoxynucleotides that interfere with DNA repair (Beutler 1994).

The pharmacokinetics of cladribine given by continuous intravenous infusion, and by subcutaneous and oral administration, have recently been described (Liliemark and Juliusson 1991; Liliemark et al. 1992). It is clinically effective by all three routes of administration. In humans, continuous intravenous infusion is consistent with a two-compartment model with alpha and beta half-lives of 35 ± 12 minutes and 6.7 ± 2.5 hours, respectively (Liliemark and Juliusson 1991). The area under the time versus concentration curves was nearly identical for 24-hour and 2-hour infusions, indicating that cladribine can be administered inter-

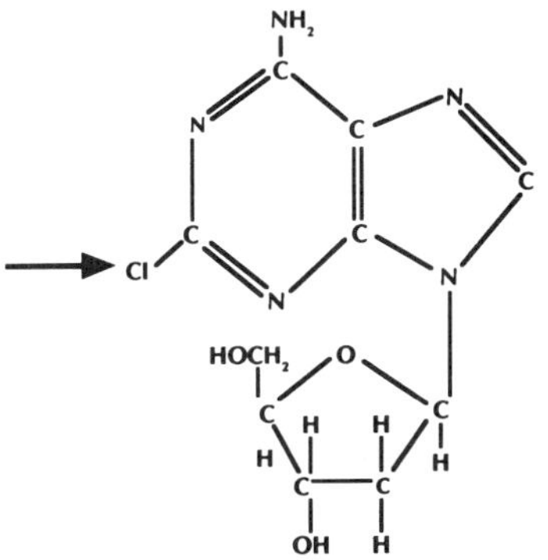

Cladribine
2 chloro 2-deoxyadenosine (2CdA)

Figure 14.1. The chemical structure of cladribine.

mittently with retained antiproliferative activity when compared with continuous infusion (Liliemark and Juliusson 1991).

The equivalent dose of oral drug is approximately twice that of the intravenous dose because of degradation of cladribine by gastric acid and intestinal enzymes. As a consequence, the bioavailability of cladribine by the oral route is more variable than when parenterally administered, probably because of differences in the amount of gastric acid present in individual patients, which may, for example, result in higher levels of cladribine in patients with achlorhydria.

More recently, it has been found that the bioavailability of subcutaneously administered cladribine is the same as by continuous intravenous infusion (Liliemark et al. 1992). The subcutaneous route of administration is less cumbersome for the patient than continuous intravenous infusion and it avoids the possibility of complications related to a surgically implanted subcutaneous venous access device or an indwelling intravenous catheter. For this reason, and because of the question of variable absorption of orally administered drug, we currently favor administration of cladribine by subcutaneous injection.

Current experimental treatment guidelines require normal renal and hepatic functions for patients treated with cladribine. Consequently, there are currently no data available on possible alteration of drug kinetics in patients with impaired hepatic or renal function since these patients have been excluded from clinical trials if: the serum creatinine is >133 μmol/l (>1.5 mg/dl), or if the calculated creatinine clearance falls below 80% of the age-adjusted normal value for the laboratory, or the serum SGOT, SGPT or hepatic alkaline phosphatase are elevated to twice the upper limit of normal or greater. Additional information on the pharmacokinetics, renal clearance, and cerebrospinal fluid concentration of cladribine has recently been described in children with acute leukemia (Kearns et al. 1994).

Efficacy

Two studies of cladribine treatment in patients with chronic progressive MS have been completed.

Study I

Study I, initiated in January 1990, was a Phase II, open-label study in which four patients were given, on a monthly basis, six doses of cladribine 0.087 mg/kg per day as a 7-day infusion by intravenous catheter. Examining neurologists, patients and nurses knew that the active drug was being administered to all patients. There was clear-cut evidence of improvement following treatment as manifested clinically by improvement in the Scripps Neurologic Rating Scale (SNRS) scores. Apart from the expected suppression of absolute lymphocyte counts and mild macrocytosis, there were no side effects or problems experienced by these four patients. Platelet counts remained within the normal range. Improvements in clinical status as measured by the SNRS remained stable for up to 2 years after treatment (see results discussed later). This small, uncontrolled pilot study indicated that 2-CdA could be safely administered to patients with chronic progressive MS. While the clinical response to treatment was encouraging, a larger placebo-controlled study was needed to evaluate further efficacy and toxicity.

Study II

The next study of cladribine treatment of chronic progressive MS was designed as a 2-year duration, Phase III, double-blind, placebo-controlled cross-over study. Data were to be analyzed at the end of the first year. If no conclusive difference was noted between the cladribine and placebo groups, patients were to be crossed over to opposite treatment arms and followed for a second year. The study began in January of 1992, and, after 1 year, highly beneficial results in favor of cladribine were observed. Because of these results the original protocol was modified for the second year (details to follow). For the sake of clarity, the first year of the original protocol will be referred to as Study II Part A. The results of this part of the study have recently been reported (Sipe et al. 1994a, b). The second year of Study II, after the protocol was modified, will be referred to as Study II Part B.

Study II Part A

The study was carried out in 51 patients with clinically definite or laboratory-supported definite chronic progressive MS with a duration of illness of at least 2 years. Forty-eight of the 51 patients were organized into 24 pairs matched by age, sex and disease severity (Kurtzke Extended Disability Status Scale (EDSS) ± 0.5). The statistician (JK) used a random number table to assign pair members to either the cladribine or placebo treatment arms. Both groups had central venous access devices surgically implanted. Patients on the cladribine arm were given monthly 7-day continuous infusions of 0.1 mg/kg per day cladribine (0.7 mg/kg course) for a total of four courses (total dose = 2.8 mg/kg cladribine). Patients on the placebo arm were given saline intravenously. Masking was double-blind; patients, neurologists, neuroradiologists and nurses had no knowledge of which medication a patient was receiving. Patients were examined monthly and two neurologic rating scale scores (EDSS and SNRS) were recorded. All analyses were undertaken on an intent-to-treat basis. Based on the results of Study I, we estimated that a sample size of 22 matched pairs of patients would be sufficient to detect a 15% improvement in the SNRS while on cladribine compared with no improvement while on placebo, with a statistical power of 0.90 using a one-sided *t*-test at an alpha level of 0.05. The site for all studies was Scripps Clinic and Research Foundation, a tertiary care center and ambulatory clinic with an associated research institute.

One patient for whom no suitable match was identified was started on the cladribine arm, but this individual moved out of town and left the study after 8 months on the protocol. Two patients, both randomly assigned to cladribine, were lost to follow-up at 2 and 3 months on study, respectively. One of these patients died of an unrelated illness, and the other moved out of the area. The loss of these two patients in the initial cladribine arm was not attributed to treatment, and we therefore recruited two additional patients appropriately matched by the blinded neurologists (JS and JR) and assigned by the statistician to cladribine as replacements. One patient receiving placebo withdrew from the study after 4 months on the protocol for reasons related to lack of stabilization of disease. This patient was not replaced. The analyses reported in Study I Part A are based on the experience of 24 matched pairs and exclude the three patients who were initially on cladribine but did not complete a full year of the study. Patients were allowed to continue on other medications to treat troublesome symptoms of MS, for example, baclofen (Lioresal®) for spasticity or oxybutynin (Ditropan®) for bladder dysfunction.

Study II Part B

As discussed earlier, the original protocol was modified after the first year (Part A) of Study II was completed. During the second year (Part B), blinding was maintained and patients were crossed over to the opposite treatment arm (i.e. patients treated with cladribine in the first year received placebo in the second year and vice versa). However, we elected to reduce the dose of cladribine to one-half of that given during the first year. The reason for this protocol modification was to determine if a beneficial therapeutic effect could be achieved and the frequency of side effects reduced at a lower dose. Therefore, a total dose of cladribine of 1.4 mg/kg was administered in divided doses so that the first monthly course consisted of 0.7 mg/kg cladribine, the second and third of 0.35 mg/kg cladribine, and the fourth, saline placebo.

Beginning in the second year, those patients who had received cladribine in the first year were given four infusions of saline placebo at monthly intervals. There were only a few deviations from the planned drug dosages. One patient received only two courses and two patients only three courses of cladribine because of thrombocytopenia. At the beginning of this phase of the study, five patients who were to have received placebo were given a single 0.7 mg/kg infusion of cladribine by error. Separate analysis showed that the response of these patients was not greater than others and the data of these patients have been retained.

During the second year, four additional patients were lost for reasons unrelated to the study and, accordingly, a 24-month or longer follow-up was possible in 21 of 24 patients who had received cladribine in the first year, and 22 of 24 patients who had received placebo in the first year.

Outcome Measures

The SNRS was designated as the primary outcome measurement. Secondary outcome parameters included the EDSS, and serial volumetric measurements of enhanced and unenhanced brain lesions as determined by magnetic resonance imaging (MRI) examinations. Cerebrospinal fluid was also collected for analysis at baseline, 6, 12, 18 and 24 months.

Data Analysis

Analysis of the neurologic scores and MRI measurements in Study II were undertaken with a split plot analysis of variance, the appropriate parametric statistical method for analysis for cross-over trials with a quantitated response (Jones and Kenward 1989). For patients who had completed at least 18 months of the study, the last available observations were carried forward. In the case of missing data, similar analyses were done in which these data were modeled under the representation that they were missing at random, and these analyses yielded no significant difference from those reported here. Kaplan–Meier curves were also used to compare neurologic rating scale measurements between the two treatment groups during the first year of the study (Koziol and Maxwell 1983). Two-sided *P*-values are reported in all data.

Results

Study I

The SNRS scores of the patients in the Phase II, open-label Study I are shown in Figure 14.2. There was evidence of improvement, as manifested by improvement in the SNRS scores following treatment. The improvement in these patients' clinical status as measured by the SNRS score remains stable for up to 2 years after treatment.

Study II–Part A

The results of the clinical performance scales in Study II Part A are shown in Figure 14.3 and have been reported previously (Sipe et al. 1994a, b). Both SNRS and EDSS systems showed progressive deterioration in patients randomized to placebo, while the average SNRS and EDSS scores of patients receiving cladribine improved modestly during the first year. Absolute changes in neurologic scores were favorable in SNRS ($P = 0.001$ at 12 months) and EDSS ($P = 0.013$ at 12 months) scoring systems. Patients were also analyzed for differences in EDSS and SNRS rating scores in matched pairs; in other words, placebo minus cladribine (Figure 14.4). This analysis showed continuous improvement over 12

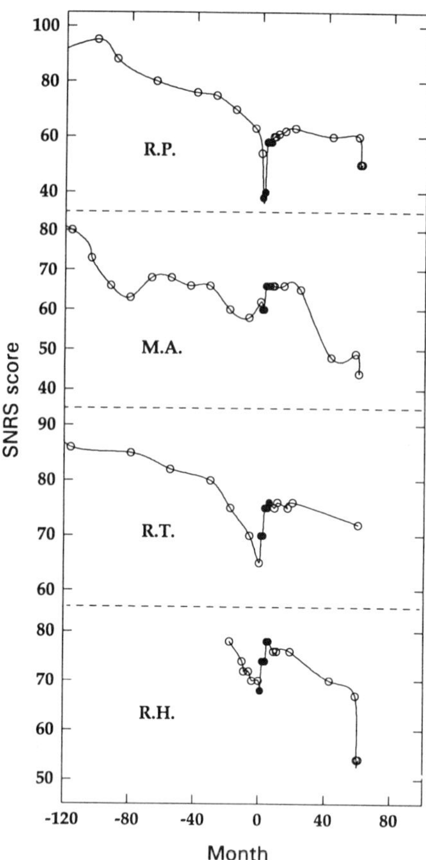

Figure 14.2. SNRS scores for four patients plotted over time. Open circles represent no treatment, filled circles indicate intravenous cladribine treatment.

months, with paired differences significantly greater than 0 (EDSS, $P < 0.004$; SNRS, $P < 0.001$). Non-parametric analysis of patients experiencing a change in EDSS scores of 1 point at 1 year was also undertaken. In the 23 patients receiving placebo who were evaluable at 12 months, the EDSS score in seven had progressed by at least 1 point, while the score had improved (decreased) in only one. Among the 24 patients receiving cladribine, the EDSS score of only one patient had worsened by at least 1 point, while the EDSS score improved (decreased) by at least 1 point in four patients. This analysis was significant at $P < 0.02$. Inter-rater and intra-rater reliability was tested with both examining neurologists (JS and JR) participating. Twenty patients (ten followed by each neurologist) were assessed independently by each examiner on the same day. Inter-rater agreement for SNRS was high with the weighted κ coefficient 0.976 for EDSS and 0.828 for SNRS. These data compared favorably with inter-rater agreements reported in other clinical trials of therapeutic agents in MS (Goodkin et al. 1992). Time to failure plots in the first year data analysis are shown in Figure 14.5. Failure was defined as an increase in the EDSS score of 1.0 or more, or a decrease in SNRS of

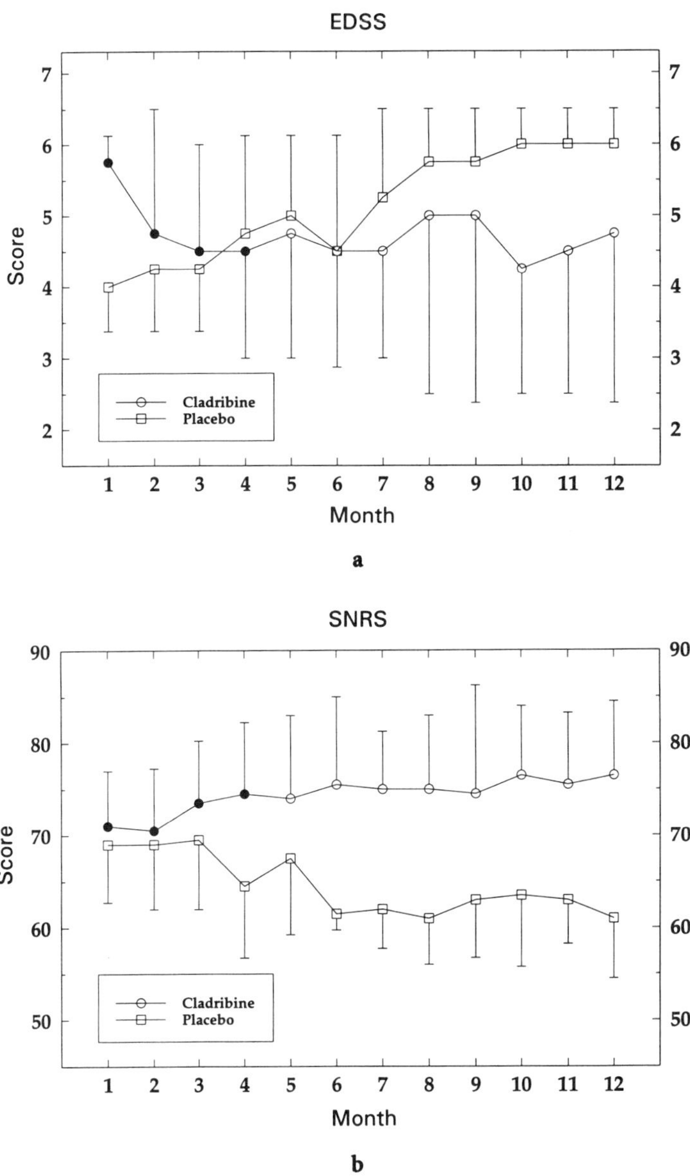

Figure 14.3. EDSS scores (a) and SNRS scores (b) of patients receiving cladribine or placebo in the first year of the randomized clinical trial. The four filled circles during the first 4 months of the study each represent the administration of cladribine at a dosage of 0.1 mg/kg body weight per day in a 7-day continuous intravenous infusion. Patients denoted by squares received infusions of saline during the first 4 months of the study. Medians and interquartile ranges are depicted.

10 points or more. Each of these statistics was highly significant (delta EDSS = 1.0, $P = 0.012$; delta SNRS = −10, $P = 0.004$) indicating that patients receiving cladribine fared better than those on placebo.

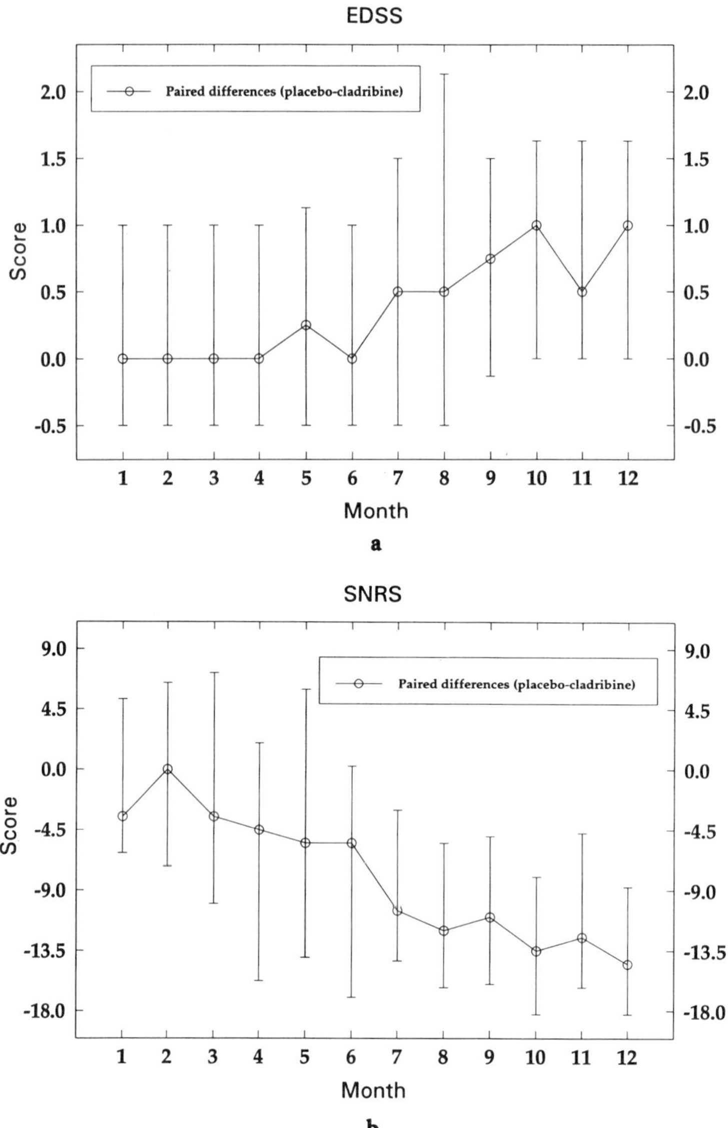

Figure 14.4. Paired differences (placebo during first year, cladribine during first year) in EDSS scores (a) and SNRS scores (b) during the initial year of the randomized clinical trial of cladribine in MS. Medians and interquartile ranges are depicted.

The MRI methods and data analysis of Study II Part A have been previously described (Sipe et al. 1994b). MRI scans performed on a 1.5T General Electric Signa Scanner included pre- and postcontrast scans. Images were obtained using conventional spin echo sequence with repetition times of 2500 ms and echo delay times of 30 ms and 90 ms. Sections were 4 mm thick with a 1 mm interslice gap.

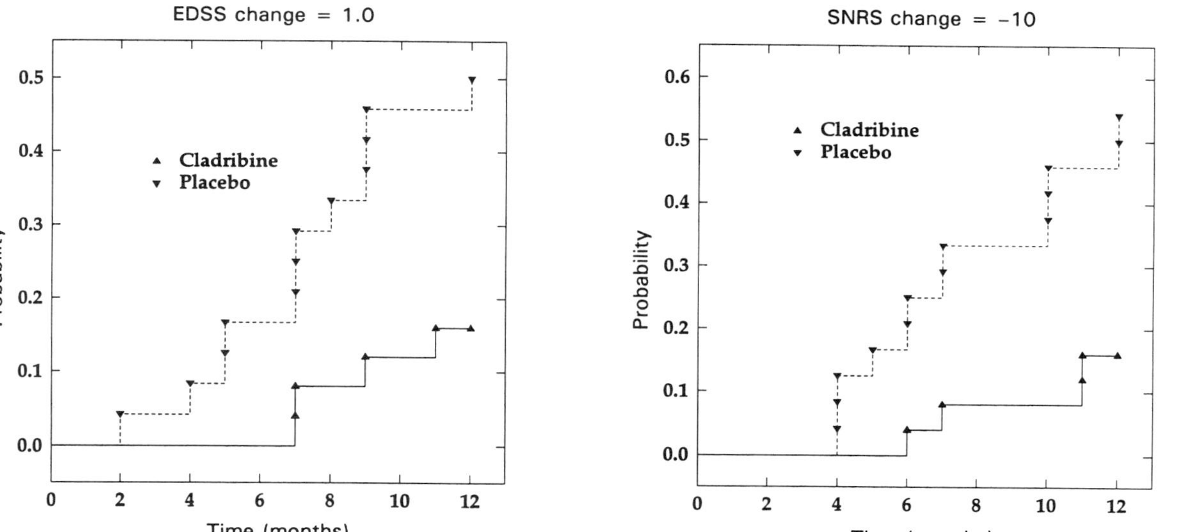

Figure 14.5. Time-to-failure plots over the first year of the clinical trial. For EDSS scores (a), failure is defined as an increase of 1 point or more relative to baseline for each patient; for SNRS scores (b), failure is defined as a decrease of 10 or more points relative to baseline.

Special attention was given by the neuroradiologist whose careful repositioning of patients guaranteed reproducible slice positions. Regions of demyelination on proton density-weighted scans and areas of contrast enhancement on T1-weighted scans were outlined by hand on film images by the neuroradiologist (JZ) who had no knowledge of the treatment protocol. All films were then duplicated by a technologist using the taped raw data and a computer work station (CEMAX, Santa Clara, CA). Pixel counts for each slice were converted into volumes by a volume-rendering software program. All the volumetric analyses were done by the same technologist. Analysis of the results of the MRI data showed no significance in either parametric or non-parametric analysis of variance based on the two-period cross-over design, and revealed no significant treatment effects on demyelinated (T2-weighted) lesions (data not shown). In contrast, the highly significant difference was seen in measurement of the enhancing volumes, a finding associated with the activity of demyelination (Table 14.1). For the purpose of this analysis, enhancing volumes were differentiated by designating the complete disappearance of enhancing volumes or their continued absence as "absent" and designating the emergence or continued presence of enhancing volumes as "present". Compared with placebo, only two individuals in the cladribine group had lesions present at 12 months, one with continuing enhancing lesions and one who developed new enhancing lesions where there had been none. The comparison between cladribine and placebo groups (Table 14.1) was favorable ($P < 0.001$, McNemar's test).

Study II Part B

Analysis of Study II Part B has shown the following results. EDSS and SNRS scores for each treatment group over 2 years are illustrated in Figure 14.6. Inspection of the curves suggests that the rates of improvement in patients after their cross-over at 12 months, with one-half dose of cladribine in patients who had first received placebo, shows the same general rate of improvement in both EDSS and SNRS scoring systems. Inspection also suggests that stabilization of disease produced by the lower dose of cladribine may be of shorter duration than that observed with the larger dose. Paired differences in EDSS and SNRS systems are shown in Figure 14.7. The analysis of variance, based on the two-period cross-over design with absolute changes in SNRS and EDSS as the endpoints, revealed no significant carryover effects between subjects or period effects within subjects. Highly significant treatment effects were seen expressed as the F statistic for assessing treatment effects, which were $F_{1,44} = 23.46$, $P < 0.001$ for SNRS, and $F_{1,44} = 10.19$, $P = 0.0026$ for EDSS.

Table 14.1. Numbers of patients with enhancing lesions on serial MRI brain scans

Time (months)	Initial placebo		Initial cladribine	
	Absent	Present	Absent	Present
6	13	11	18	6
12	12	12	22	2

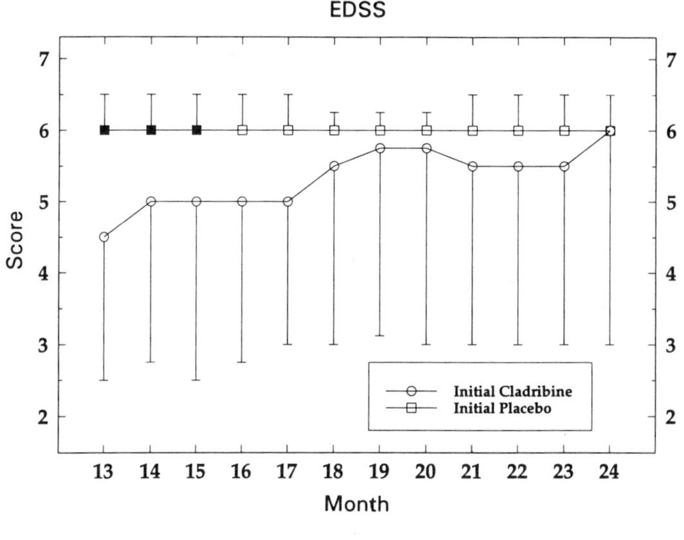

a

b

Figure 14.6. The EDSS scores (a) and SNRS scores (b) of patients receiving cladribine or placebo in the second year of the clinical trial. The patient group denoted by circles had received cladribine during the first year of the trial, and were crossed over to receive saline infusions at months 13, 14 and 15. The patient group denoted by squares had received saline infusions during the first year of the trial, and were crossed over to receive cladribine at months 13, 14 and 15. The filled square at month 13 represents the administration of cladribine 0.1 mg/kg body weight per day in a 7-day continuous intravenous infusion. The succeeding two filled squares represent the administration of cladribine 0.05 mg/kg body weight per day in a 7-day continuous intravenous infusion.

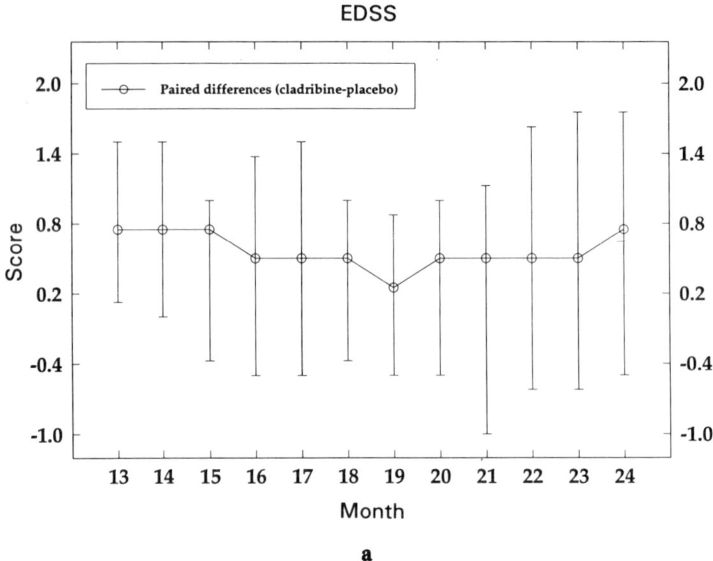

a

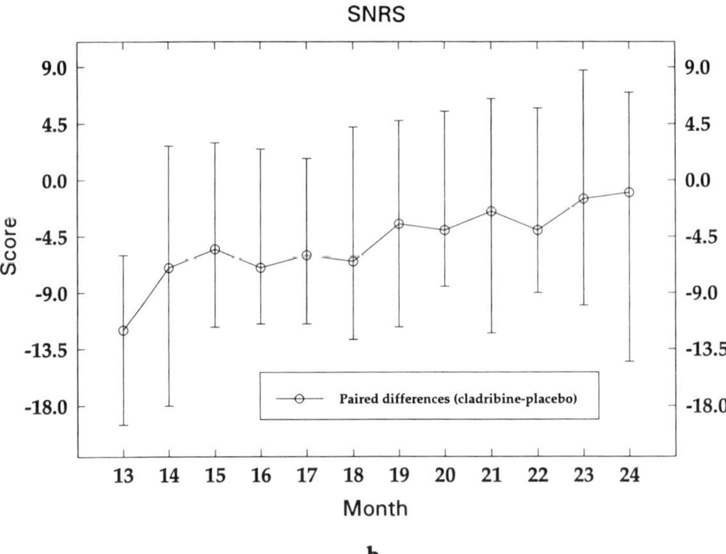

b

Figure 14.7. Paired differences (cladribine during second year, placebo during second year) in EDSS (a) and SNRS (b) scores during the second year of the randomized clinical trial of cladribine in MS. Pairing is as in Figure 14.4, but individuals who had received cladribine during the first year of the trial are here denoted as receiving placebo during the second year; similarly, individuals who had received placebo during the first year of the trial are here denoted as receiving cladribine during the second year. Medians and interquartile ranges are depicted.

Adverse Reactions

Monitoring for possible toxicity was carried out in Study II Parts A and B by unblinded investigators who had no role in the neurologic evaluation of patients or of MRI scans. The unblinded investigators regularly reviewed laboratory data but had direct patient contact with only four patients. Patients had no sensation of receiving cladribine and manifested no obviously apparent side effects or signs, such as nausea, fever, rash or hair loss. Three patients developed temporary marrow suppression with low platelet counts with one requiring hospitalization and treatment. Six patients in Study II Part A and two others developed mild herpes zoster. One patient died of acute fulminant hepatitis-B during the second month on cladribine, an event considered unlikely to be related to treatment.

The effect of cladribine on blood counts and marrow function in the above patients has been analyzed and previously reported (Beutler et al. 1994). All patients had normal blood counts at entry to the study. Subsequent laboratory results confirmed profound lymphocyte depletion in cladribine-treated patients compared with controls. There was only a minor reduction of granulocytes with cladribine compared with controls. CD4 cells showed severe depletion in cladribine-treated patients, while there was no change with placebo. Average platelet counts in cladribine patients declined to a nadir of about 150×10^9/l and gradually recovered to near normal levels after 12 months. After cladribine, hemoglobin levels declined moderately but there were no severe anemias compared with controls, except for one patient described below. Monocyte counts dropped rapidly in the first 7 days after cladribine infusion but rebounded to near normal levels within a month.

The single patient with marrow suppression severe enough to require hospitalization had been taking carbamazepine (Tegretol®) 1200 mg/day and phenytoin (Dilantin®) 550 mg/day for treatment of trigeminal neuralgia. Marrow suppression appeared in this patient after the fourth monthly course of cladribine. Several platelet and red cell transfusions were required as marrow function gradually recovered over 4–6 months. In this particular patient, the severity of marrow suppression and its persistence for several months after discontinuation of cladribine, underscore the powerful and long lasting effects of the drug. The above observations indicate that cladribine at this dose level can occasionally produce marrow suppression in hematologically normal patients, a possibility that may have previously been underestimated. However, it is noteworthy that no episodes of marrow suppression were observed with the reduced dose of cladribine used in Study II Part B.

The occurrence of mild herpes zoster has been the only other complication seen so far in these studies. No other opportunistic infections were encountered. One patient on placebo developed salmonella enteritis.

Additional observations on cladribine toxicity have been documented in earlier studies of patients with neoplastic disorders. With increasing dose level there is an increasing incidence of cytopenias, particularly thrombocytopenia, and severe marrow suppression with pancytopenia. When doses five to ten times the recommended dose for hairy cell leukemia were given as part of a marrow transplant preconditioning regimen, renal and central nervous system toxicity was encountered (Beutler 1994). Evidence of motor paralysis manifesting as paraparesis or quadriparesis was seen late in the course of marrow transplantation, usually several weeks after the conclusion of cladribine administration (Beutler et al. 1991). In a dose escalation study to determine the maximum tolerated dose of cladribine, two of 21 patients given 0.2 mg/kg per day experienced neurologic events with motor paralysis (Saven et al. 1993a). Severe motor weakness, possibly due to axonal peripheral nuuropathy, has been reported following the administration of cladribine at daily doses of 19–21 mg/m^2 per day for 5 consecutive days (Wong et al. 1994).

Because cladribine is incorporated into DNA, the theoretical long-term potential for complications or neoplasm must be considered. At the present time there have been no reports of new neoplasms associated with cladribine in more than 5000 patients receiving the drug worldwide. Table 14.2 summarizes all the

Table 14.2. Total adverse events in 125 MS patients treated with cladribine (1990 to June 1995)

Adverse event	Age/sex	Treated as part of study protocol	Cause	Total cladribine dose (mg/kg)	Related to cladribine (author's conclusion)
Deaths	40/F	Yes	Acute hepatic necrosis 2° to hepatitis-B infection	1.4	No
	43/F	Yes	Suicide	2.8	No
	31/F	Yes	Drowning in pool	2.8	No
	47/M	No	Respiratory failure 2° to quadraplegia from progressive MS	2.1	No
Marrow suppression	43/F	Yes	Cladribine[a]	2.8	Yes
	67/F	No	Cladribine[b]	2.1	Yes
Infections	41/F	Yes	Streptococcal pharyngitis	2.8	No
	43/F	Yes	Herpes zoster, mild segmental	2.8	Yes
	57/F	Yes	Herpes zoster, mild segmental	2.8	Yes
	39/M	Yes	Herpes zoster, mild segmental	2.8	Yes
	46/F	Yes	Herpes zoster, mild segmental	2.8	Yes
	51/F	Yes	Herpes zoster, mild segmental	2.8	Yes
	47/M	No	Herpes zoster, mild segmental	2.8	Yes
	50/F	Yes	Herpes zoster, mild segmental	2.8	Yes
	52/F	Yes	Herpes zoster, mild segmental	2.8	Yes
Thrombocytopenia	(4 patients)	Yes	Cladribine	2.8	Yes
Revision of Portacath	58/F	Yes	Defective Portacath	2.8	No
	43/F	Yes	Defective Portacath	2.8	No
	40/F	Yes	Defective Portacath	2.8	No
	40/F	Yes	Pneumothorax	2.8	No

[a]Previous treatment with Tegretol® and Dilantin®.
[b]Previous treatment with Leukeran®.

adverse events observed to date in association with the cladribine treatment of a total of 125 MS patients. Most of these patients were participants either in the completed studies described in this chapter or in ongoing studies. Only a few patients were treated outside a study protocol.

Drug Interactions

Drugs that produce marrow stem cell toxicity may have long-term effects that increase the likelihood of thrombocytopenia and marrow suppression with cladribine. The drugs most likely to be associated with marrow stem cell toxicity are chlorambucil (Leukeran®) and busulfan (Myleran®). Cyclophosphamide, methotrexate and azathioprine have less stem cell toxicity but they could still result in increased marrow sensitivity to cladribine. Cyclosporine is of less concern in this regard because it probably produces the least stem cell toxicity of any of the immunosuppressive drugs used in the treatment of MS.

During Study II Part A, the single patient who developed severe marrow suppression after cladribine treatment had been taking carbamazepine (Tegretol®) and phenytoin (Dilantin®) for trigeminal neuralgia. We believe it is possible that the folate antagonist effect of Dilantin® or the potential marrow suppressive effect of Tegretol® may have contributed to the increased marrow sensitivity of this patient to cladribine. A second patient, who had been previously treated with Leukeran®, and who was treated with cladribine outside the study protocol, also developed reversible marrow suppression. Therefore, it would seem advisable that any non-essential medication with a possible marrow suppressive effect should be discontinued at least 3 months prior to treatment with cladribine.

An increased incidence of opportunistic infection with *Listeria* has been reported in cancer patients treated with fludarabine (a purine nucleoside drug related to cladribine) and corticosteroids, possibly because of an additive immunosuppressive effect of the two drugs used together. Although the same problem has not been reported with cladribine, this observation would suggest that caution should be used in the concomitant use of highdose corticosteroids with cladribine, a situation that might arise during the course of experimental cladribine treatment of patients with relapsing–remitting MS.

Clinical Use

The evaluation of cladribine in the treatment of MS is not yet complete. At this time, it is not licensed for the treatment of MS and remains an experimental therapy best limited to the setting of research institutions and clinical trials.

Individual doses of cladribine are given in our institution only if the platelet count, granulocyte count and hemoglobin meet the criteria set forth below. If any of these criteria are not met, then the drug is withheld for that monthly treatment cycle and given the following month if the criteria are met at that time. The criteria for platelets specify a platelet count of 200 or higher, or the platelet count must be 150–200 × 10^9/l and represents more than 50% of the previous platelet count, or the platelet count must be 125–150 × 10^9/l and at least 80% of the prior count *unless* placebo was substituted for cladribine for the previous dose. In that event, the platelet count must be equal to or higher than the platelet count at the time that the last course of cladribine was given. The criterion for the granulocyte count is an absolute granulocyte count >100/µl. The criterion for the hemoglobin level is as follows: the hemoglobin has not declined more than 1.5 g/dl from the previous value, or 3 g/dl from the original baseline value. If any of these criteria are not met, cladribine is withheld.

Cladribine is discontinued if the patient develops a platelet count below 125 × 10^9/l, or a falling platelet count. An absolute granulocyte count <500/µl or hemoglobin <3 g/dl from the original baseline value are indications for discontinuation. Patients undergoing therapy are closely observed for signs of hematologic toxicity or opportunistic infection. Periodic assessment of complete blood counts is recommended, particularly during the first 4–8 weeks following each treatment. As with other potent chemotherapeutic agents, renal and hepatic function is also routinely monitored.

Cladribine produces no detectable local tissue reactions at subcutaneous injection sites, and it may be administered by nursing personnel either in the clinic or at home. The volume of injection per site is limited to 2 ml in order to minimize local bruising, subcutaneous hemorrhage and skin discoloration, which may occur with a larger injection volume. Consequently, the total daily dose may need to be divided into multiple injections for patients with higher body weight. Subcutaneous injections in our studies are given at sites in the anterior thigh and abdomen.

Therapeutic Potential

Currently, several clinical trials are in progress of cladribine as treatment for MS. A large Phase III multicenter American and Canadian trial of cladribine in chronic progressive MS was started in 1994. This study, using subcutaneous administration of cladribine, will seek to confirm the previously reported benefits (Study II Part A) of cladribine in chronic progressive MS (Sipe et al. 1994b). Six USA and Canadian centers are proceeding with the double-blinded, placebo-controlled protocol. If efficacy and safety are confirmed with the subcutaneous administration of cladribine, the drug could become available for general use in neurologic practice as an approved treatment for chronic progressive MS.

A trial of cladribine in 50 patients with relapsing–remitting MS is also presently under way at Scripps Clinic. Patients in this trial will be randomized to treatment with either six doses of cladribine given monthly at 0.07 mg/kg for 5 days by subcutaneous injection, or placebo (saline injection). Placebo doses will be substituted for cladribine in the event that blood counts fall below an acceptable level as determined by an algorithm for dose administration. Control patients will be randomly assigned to eight 5-day injections of sterile saline at monthly intervals. As in previous studies, patients, neurologists, nurses and neuroradiologists will be blinded throughout the study. The pharmacist will determine whether or not to administer cladribine, based on the algorithm applied for dose administration. No patients who are receiving ACTH, corticosteroids, beta interferon or immunosuppressive therapies will be included in the studies. In this study, cladribine is being compared with placebo and not to beta interferon because of the development of side effects in nearly all patients on beta interferon. For this reason, it would be very difficult to maintain a proper double-blinded study of beta interferon versus cladribine. Our primary objective is to evaluate the outcome of treatment of cladribine versus placebo in patients who have chosen not to take beta interferon or who have failed beta interferon therapy for relapsing-remitting MS.

Three outcome measurements will be followed in these study subjects: the frequency and severity of clinical relapses as judged by monthly or more frequent neurologic examinations; changes in the disability (EDSS) and performance (SNRS) neurologic rating scales; and the number and volume of active enhancing lesions ascertained from brain MRI scans. The study of patients with relapsing-remitting MS differs from our previous studies with cladribine in the following respects. First, a different form of MS, that of active relapsing-remitting disease, will be studied under this protocol. Secondly, the outcome criteria are different in that monthly MRI examinations will be performed to detect rapid changes in enhancing volumes. Thirdly, a different and somewhat smaller dose of cladribine will be used to minimize possible complications of thrombocytopenia and dermatomal herpes zoster. Lastly, cladribine will be given by subcutaneous injection rather than by intravenous infusion.

Finally, a study has also begun at Scripps Clinic to evaluate the retreatment of patients with chronic progressive MS whose disease has shown signs of resumption of worsening 1–2 years following cladribine therapy. Study subjects will be selected from those who have completed our previous studies of cladribine in chronic MS. Patients with definitely progressive symptoms will be considered for retreatment with a lower dose of cladribine. These patients will be randomized to five daily subcutaneous injections of cladribine 0.05 mg/kg day or placebo (saline) for six separate monthly courses, but a maximum of four of these will be active drug. Thus, in most patients, the final two courses will be placebo. This will allow most or all of the patients to receive the same total amount of drug should it be necessary to substitute placebo for drug on one or two occasions because of low blood counts. A primary endpoint for assessment of efficacy will be a comparison in changes in the SNRS scores and EDSS scores between the cladribine group and the placebo group during the first year of the protocol. Secondary endpoints include changes from baseline in MRI brain scan results. Because cladribine may produce cumulative marrow toxicity, these patients will be carefully monitored for signs of hematologic toxicity and marrow suppression. Dosing criteria for patients on this study remain the same as those on previous studies.

Clinical Outcome and Practical Considerations

Recently, it has become important to think about MS treatment results in terms of the outcome of treatment as assessed by the MS patient and family.

Many patients want to know if the final result of a long and sometimes risky and expensive treatment coincides with their and their families' expectations. In the case of cladribine, almost all of the patients from the placebo-controlled chronic progressive study have indicated that their expectations were met and in many cases exceeded. This is because the side effects and discomforts of cladribine treatment were essentially non-existent, except for eight patients who developed mild herpes zoster. In these patients, mild segmental zoster responded readily to treatment with acyclovir. In Study II Part A, there were four patients who experienced improvement in EDSS scores of 1 point or more at 1 year after treatment with cladribine.

Most of the other patients also either stabilized or improved; only one patient was worse by an EDSS score of 1 point or more. Many patients in Study II who had experienced a rapid decline while on placebo in Part A of the study also developed stabilization to slight improvement after receiving cladribine during Part B. A few patients who were using a cane for walking prior to cladribine were able to walk with greater stability and no longer needed the cane following treatment. In other instances, patients who had experienced sensory loss or pain noted significant improvement of sensory symptoms. Muscular power and strength improved and reflexes or Babinski signs normalized in some patients. However, symptoms of severe ataxia and dysarthria generally did not improve after treatment with cladribine.

Since cladribine therapy for MS is still undergoing evaluation, we are currently recommending that patients be treated with this agent only in research centers on approved protocols. Because it is a potent drug, there is significant potential for unwanted marrow suppression and possible serious complications including bleeding, anemia or opportunistic infection. Routine off-label use of cladribine in MS is therefore not currently recommended.

Summary

Cladribine is a new drug with properties of selective lymphocyte suppression that appears favorably to influence the clinical course of chronic MS. By selective targeting of both resting and dividing lymphocytes, cladribine may be able to destroy the activated immunocytes that produce CNS demyelination and thus produce a durable stabilization or improvement in most patients. Although the role of cladribine has not yet been fully defined, our hope is that this new drug will ultimately prove to be a useful therapeutic option for patients with all forms of active MS.

Acknowledgement

The authors acknowledge the outstanding work of Carolyn Koumaras, and the staff of the General Clinical Research Center. Supported by FDA grant FD-R-000280, NIH grants NS30218 and RR00833, The Sam and Rose Stein Charitable Trust Fund, and a grant from the R. W. Johnson Pharmaceutical Research Institute.

References

Beutler E (1992) Cladribine (2-chlorodeoxyadenosine). Lancet 340:952–956

Beutler E (1994) New chemotherapeutic agent: 2-chlorodeoxyadenosine. Semin Hematol 31:40–45

Beutler E, Piro LD, Saven A et al. (1991) 2-Chlorodeoxyadenosine (2-CdA): A potent chemotherapeutic and immunosuppressive nucleotide. Leuk Lymphoma 5:1–8

Beutler E, Koziol J, McMillan R, Sipe JC, Romine JS, Carrera CJ (1994) Marrow suppression produced by repeated doses of cladribine. Acta Haematol 91:10–15

Carson DA, Kaye J, Seegmiller JE (1977) Lymphospecific toxicity in adenosine deaminase deficiency and purine nucleoside phosphorylase deficiency: possible role of nucleoside kinase(s). Proc Natl Acad Sci USA 74:5677–5681

Carson DA, Kaye J, Matsumoto S, Seegmiller JE, Thompson L (1979) Biochemical basis for the enhanced toxicity of deoxyribonucleosides toward malignant human T cell lines. Proc Natl Acad Sci USA 76:2430–2433

Carson DA, Wasson DB, Kaye J et al. (1980) Deoxycytidine kinase-mediated toxicity of deoxyadenosine analogs toward malignant human lymphoblasts in vitro and toward murine L1210 leukemia in vivo. Proc Natl Acad Sci USA 77:6865–6869

Carson DA, Wasson DB, Lamon J et al. (1982) A potent new anti-lymphocyte agent: 2-chlorodeoxyadenosine [Abstract]. Blood 60(Suppl 1):161

Carson DA, Wasson DB, Taetle R, Yu A (1983) Specific toxicity of 2-chlorodeoxyadenosine toward resting and proliferating human lymphocytes. Blood 62:737–743

Carson DA, Wasson DB, Beutler E (1984) Antileukemic and immunosuppressive activity of 2-chloro-2′-deoxyadenosine. Proc Natl Acad Sci USA 81:2232–2236

Carson DA, Seto S, Wasson DB, Carrera CJ (1986) DNA strand breaks, NAD metabolism, and programmed cell death. Exp Cell Res 164:273–281

Figueroa M, McMillan R (1993) 2-Chlorodeoxyadenosine in the treatment of chronic refractory immune thrombocytopenia purpura [letter]. Blood 81:3484–3485

Giblett ER, Anderson JE, Cohen F et al. (1972) Adenosine deaminase deficiency in two patients with severely impaired cellular immunity. Lancet ii:1067–1069

Goodkin DE, Cookfair D, Wende K et al. (1992) Inter- and intrarater scoring agreement using grades 1.0 to 3.5 of the Kurtzke Expanded Disability Status Scale (EDSS). Neurology 42:859–863

Hughes RAC (1992) Pathogenesis of multiple sclerosis. J R Soc Med 85:373–375

Jacobs L, Goodkin DE, Rudick RA, Herndon R (1994) Advances in specific therapy for multiple sclerosis. Curr Opin Neurol 7:250–254

Jones B, Kenward MG (1989) Design and analysis of cross-over trials. Chapman and Hall, London

Kay AC, Saven A, Carrera CJ, Carson DA, Beutler E, Piro LD (1992) 2-Chlorodeoxyadenosine treatment of low-grade lymphomas. J Clin Oncol 10:371–377

Kearns CM, Blakely RL, Santana VM, Crom WR (1994) Pharmacokinetics of cladribine (2-chlorodeoxyadenosine) in children with acute leukemia. Cancer Res 54:1235–1239

Koziol JA, Maxwell DA (1983) A distribution-free test for paired growth curve analysis with application to an animal tumor immunotherapy experiment. Stat Med 1:83–89

Liliemark J, Juliusson G (1991) On the pharmacokinetics of 2-chloro-2-′deoxyadenosine in humans. Cancer Res 51:5570–5572

Liliemark J, Albertioni F, Hassan M, Pettersson B, Juliusson G (1992) On the bioavailability of oral and subcutaneous 2-chloro-2′-deoxyadenosine in humans: alternative routes of administration. J Clin Oncol 10:1514–1518

Petzer AL, Bilgeri R, Zilian U et al. (1991) Inhibitory effect of 2-chlorodeoxyadenosine on granulocytic, erythroid, and T-lymphocytic colony growth. Blood 78:2583–2587

Piro LD (1992) 2-Chlorodeoxyadenosine treatment of lymphoid malignancies. Blood 79:843–845

Piro LD, Carrera CJ, Carson DA, Beutler E (1990) Lasting remissions in hairy cell leukemia induced by a single infusion of 2-chlorodeoxyadenosine. N Engl J Med 322:1117–1121

Piro LD, Saven A, Ellison D, Thurston D, Carson DA, Beutler E (1992) Prolonged complete remissions following 2-chlorodeoxyadenosine (2-CdA) in hairy cell leukemia (HCL) [abstract]. Proc ASCO 11:259

Saven A, Piro LD (1993) Complete remissions in hairy cell leukemia with 2-chlorodeoxyadenosine after failure with 2′-deoxycoformycin. Ann Intern Med 119:278–283

Saven A, Carrera CJ, Carson DA, Beutler E, Piro LD (1991) 2-Chlorodeoxyadenosine treatment of refractory chronic lymphocytic leukemia. Leuk Lymphoma 5(Suppl):133–138

Saven A, Carrera CJ, Carson DA, Beutler E, Piro LD (1992a) 2-Chlorodeoxyadenosine: an active agent in the treatment of cutaneous T-cell lymphoma. Blood 80:587–592

Saven A, Figueroa ML, Piro LD, Beutler E (1992b) Complete hematological remissions in chronic myelogenous leukemia (CML) following 2-chlorodeoxyadenosine (2-CdA) [abstract]. Proc ASCO 11:261
Saven A, Kawasaki H, Carrera CJ et al. (1993a) 2-Chlorodeoxyadenosine dose escalation in nonhematologic malignancies. J Clin Oncol 11:671–678
Saven A, Lemon RH, Piro LD (1993b) 2-Chlorodeoxyadenosine for patients with B-cell chronic lymphocytic leukemia resistant to fludarabine [letter]. N Engl J Med 328:812–813
Sipe JC, Romine J, Zyroff J, Koziol J, McMillan R, Beutler E (1994a) Cladribine favorably alters the clinical course of progressive multiple sclerosis (MS) [abstract]. Neurology 44(Suppl 2):A357
Sipe JC, Romine JS, Koziol JA, McMillan R, Zyroff J, Beutler E (1994b) Cladribine in treatment of chronic progressive multiple sclerosis. Lancet 344:9–13
Wong ET, Vahdat L, Tunkel RS et al. (1994) Severe motor weakness from high-dose 2-chlorodeoxyadenosine [abstract] Ann Neurol 36:293

15 Ethical Considerations Raised by Clinical Trials

Richard Foa

Introduction

Many of the ethical issues raised by clinical trials in multiple sclerosis (MS) are no different from those that arise in clinical research in other diseases. They are the basic ethical problems of the conduct of research on human subjects, more specifically, the problems of research on ill and vulnerable human subjects.

Western society, having invested heavily in the promotion of medical progress through scientific research, must find a way to fulfill the countervailing obligation to protect its individual members. No individual can be required to participate in research, and we, as a society, have a higher obligation to protect the weaker among us. Yet, it is precisely the weaker who, by having diseases that are the objects of research, must become the subjects of research. The ill must volunteer or be conscripted. They often come to participate through a process that blends the two. This tension between two desirable ends, medical progress through science and the protection of the individual, creates the principal ethical conflict of clinical research.

The ethics of contemporary medical research have been strongly shaped by international codes of ethics and by revelations of violations of ethical standards in both the scientific literature and the popular press. The first of the modern codes is the Nuremberg Code, promulgated following the Second World War in response to Nazi medical experiments (Annas and Grodin 1992, Munson 1992). This code emphasizes the fundamental requirement for the informed voluntary consent of research participants. The Nuremberg Code was followed in 1964 by the World Medical Association's Declaration of Helsinki (Annas and Grodin 1992; Munson 1992). Revised in 1975, this "statement of principles" re-emphasized the importance of informed consent, giving shape to the content of consent documents as they are commonly written today. The Declaration of Helsinki also addressed the conflict between research and patient care, emphasizing the primacy of the doctor–patient relationship and the entitlement of all participants in research, including those in control groups, to the best current treatment.

Despite the clarity of these codes, they received scant attention from American researchers until the American medical community was jolted by revelations by Henry K. Beecher of unethical research conducted at several prestigious institutions, the Massachusetts General Hospital being prominent among them

(Rothman 1987). Beecher, then Dorr Professor of Research in Anesthesia, quickly sketched 22 examples. Skeptical that "a fully informed consent" could ever be obtained, he emphasized "the presence of a truly responsible investigator", one who is "intelligent, informed, conscientious, compassionate" as the most reliable safeguard of ethical experimentation (Beecher 1966).

More influential than Beecher's eye-opening article was the disclosure and public discussion in the early 1970s of the Tuskegee Syphilis Study (Kampmeier 1972, 1974). This study, started in 1932, was to examine the natural history of untreated latent syphilis and the cause of death in 875 black males in rural Macon County, Alabama. It included 399 untreated patients, 275 treated with variable amounts of neoarsphenamine, and 201 who were uninfected. Special attention was given to the development and consequences of syphilitic aortitis. Most alarming to most people was the fact that the study was continued for decades beyond the widespread availability of penicillin, but there was also shock and criticism regarding federal support for a study without a written protocol, that made no pretense of informed consent, that involved an uneducated minority population, and that yielded no information not known at the study's inception (Curran 1973).

In the last 20 years, with the explosive growth in medical research, there have continued to be periodic revelations of unethical research practices, past and present. As MS research moves into an era of the rapid expansion of clinical trials, combined with a shift towards increasing partnership with the biotechnology and pharmaceutical industries, the growing MS research community must pay renewed attention to the ethics of clinical trials. There must be broad rules governing their design and conduct.

A Code of Ethics

A brief and essential code of ethics for the conduct of MS clinical trials can be proposed, which is a distillation from earlier modern codes and experiences.

1. Substantial *new* information must be sought and the clinical trial must be capable of yielding that information. A poorly designed trial, a trial that cannot answer the question posed, an unfeasible trial or one undertaken by unqualified investigators is fundamentally unethical, even if it poses negligible risks to the participants. Furthermore, there must be agreement about the importance of the study question. It cannot merely be a personal interest of one investigator. With large clinical trials that receive public support, agreement should begin with peer approval among investigators, but should also include the interest and support of involved clinicians and affected patients. There must be monitoring of the research to make sure it remains true to its design and is not continued beyond the point that questions are answered or are found to be unanswerable.
2. The research must address a question that can only be answered through the use of human subjects. If the research question can be answered in the laboratory, by animal research, or through computer modeling, then a clinical

trial is inappropriate.

3. Benefits from the conduct of the trial must outweigh the harms. Benefits or harms can of course be looked at either in terms of society or individuals, so there must be a continuous balancing of individual and social interests. Trials inherently harmful to participants cannot be justified by appeal to some broader social benefit. Similarly, trials should not benefit only a few individuals at extraordinary expense to society.
4. There must be equity in the selection of research subjects. Clinical trials are often regarded as an opportunity by those who participate, since they mean access to new treatment or to leading clinicians. While keeping within the necessary requirements of trial design, there must be equal opportunity to participate in a trial according to gender, race and ethnic background. In some circumstances, ethically just selection of study participants may have the opposite implication. It may mean protection of specific individuals or groups from discriminatory inclusion in a trial if inclusion will identify a participant as a member of an undesirable group. It may also mean protection of particularly vulnerable individuals, the desperately ill or those unable to refuse, from being unfairly subjected to risks that others would not take.
5. Clinical research must be conducted with the informed consent of the participants. This is probably both the most frequently talked about and abused ethical requirement. The requirement to obtain informed consent represents the investigator's explicit recognition of the autonomy of the research subject. It should be an expression of the voluntary participation of the subject in the research and of a shared commitment with the investigator to the research goals. It should mean a process of communication and of shared decision making that continues throughout a clinical trial. It is a process in which the subject's choice receives utmost respect (Katz 1993). Informed consent does not mean merely obtaining a witnessed signature on a long and complex document before enrollment and randomization. In summary, the informed consent process should extend beyond a narrow legalistic requirement to share the minimum amount of information that protects the researcher and sponsoring institution from legal liability.

A Hypothetical Clinical Trial

To examine some ethical questions of specific relevance to contemporary clinical trials in MS, it is instructive to introduce a hypothetical new treatment and look at the problems that arise in the development of a Phase II/III clinical trial.

The hypothetical product is IMMUSTOP. It is a small polypeptide first studied by immunologists and biochemists interested in recovery from spinal cord injury. Those studies demonstrated no effect on axon regeneration but did show stimulation of myelin production. Further work showed an ability to inactivate T cells by competitively occupying cell surface receptors. IMMUSTOP has gone through Phase I trials with only a few minor toxicities. It is administered subcutaneously once a week. Possibilities for delivery transdermally or via a subcutaneous reservoir are being explored.

The original research received joint funding from the federal government, a large medical foundation and private groups. The drug was patented and the patent sold to a new biotechnology firm, Curecorp. Originally a limited partnership supported by venture capital, Curecorp is now publicly traded on the Nasdaq exchange.

The IMMUSTOP study is planned as a large multicenter clinical trial. The role and constitution of an external advisory committee has been a contentious issue. Curecorp, principal financial sponsor of the trial, would like a committee that is concerned about the ultimate financial success of the product. The principal investigator and author of the preliminary protocol would like a committee of scientific authorities that would give credibility and weight to the study, paying particular attention to enhancing public interest, opportunities to successfully enroll participants, and the importance of the anticipated outcome. These interests appear to dovetail but it can be predicted that there will be areas of potential conflict. Furthermore, there is corporate concern about the leakage of proprietary information about IMMUSTOP to unaffiliated scientists and clinicians.

Statisticians are relied upon to determine how large the study arms of the IMMUSTOP protocol must be and over what time interval the study must be conducted to produce significant results. Randomization of participants into different arms and double-blinding of subjects and investigators is presumed. Determining eligibility is a more complex matter. It has implications not only for the clarity and acceptability of the results but also for how convincingly they may be generalized to all patients.

The IMMUSTOP trial will, of course, have a "properly constituted" data and safety monitoring committee to look for early evidence of excessive toxicity or significant differences in outcome measures between groups. The committee will be empowered to terminate a treatment arm or the entire study should one study arm quickly prove unequivocally advantageous or disadvantageous.

In planning the trial, researchers and product managers are aware that there are simultaneous ongoing trials of interferon beta, copolymer 1, oral tolerization to myelin basic protein, and others that may have a significant impact on their trial. Only one of the competition, interferon beta-1b, has FDA approval and its imprimatur of effectiveness. A two-arm placebo-controlled trial would best show the efficacy of IMMUSTOP but it would exclude patients already on interferon beta, would prevent trial participants from using an "effective" treatment, and would preclude direct comparisons. The questions that they must answer are:

1. Is it ethical to do a placebo-controlled trial?
2. If this is done, how long can participants be excluded from using interferon beta or something else that might receive FDA approval during the trial?
3. If they set up a trial that compares IMMUSTOP and interferon beta, should their product be held to a higher standard of efficacy?
4. Will there be problems of recruitment and retention if participants in the IMMUSTOP trial are denied opportunities for other treatment?

Dr Willard is Assistant Professor of Neurology and Immunology and the MS specialist in his department. For him, the IMMUSTOP trial is an important opportunity to collaborate with colleagues in other centers and to secure the short-term financial stability of his MS clinic. It promises to raise his professional profile, please his chairman, and give him an opportunity to offer a promising new treatment to his patients. While these patients are "clinic" patients, they regard Dr Willard as their personal neurologist. Interferon beta has been unavailable to most for financial reasons.

Ethical Questions Relevant to the Conduct of a Clinical Trial

Monitoring the Trial

The conduct of clinical trials may be monitored by various committees. The functions and membership of these committees should be defined before the study is initiated. The structure and interaction of monitoring committees may vary according to the complexity and envisioned therapeutic and political impact of the clinical trial. For example, Spilker details three different models of how a data and safety monitoring committee might interact with other committees, investigators, clinical monitors and the study sponsor (Spilker 1991). However, in each of these models the data and safety monitoring committee is independent of the study sponsor, a design that ultimately enhances the credibility of the results of the study (Spilker 1991).

Ethical requirements in large multicenter MS trials may best be served by separating the functions of an external advisory committee from a data and safety monitoring committee. The functions and membership of these committees is discussed below and summarized in Table 15.1.

Table 15.1. Proposed monitoring committee structures and roles

Committee	Composition	Role
External advisory	Non-participating experts in MS	Determine need for study
	Head of data and safety monitoring committee	Insure adherence to code of ethics
	Advocate for MS patients and public interests	Endorse final conclusions
Data and safety monitoring	Independent expert statisticians	Interim data analysis
	Non-participating experts in MS clinical trials	Monitor beneficial trends
	Ethicist	Monitor harmful trends
		Recommend suspension of enrollment or termination of study

The External Advisory Committee

The existence of an external advisory committee is an acknowledgment that the proposed trial is undertaken to address an unmet *public* need, something that is beyond the financial interests of the sponsoring company and the academic interests of the investigators. The principal role of the committee is to identify that need and to insure that the trial is properly designed and conducted to address it. The external advisory committee may recommend termination of the study to the sponsor under previously agreed conditions.

This committee should include uninvolved experts in MS and in clinical trials whose impeccable credentials will contribute credibility to the trial's final conclusions. The head of the data and safety monitoring committee is an appropriate member of the external advisory committee because of that person's ability to provide timely efficacy and toxicity information that is relevant to study termination decisions. Committee membership should also include an advocate of the health care related interests of MS patients and the general public.

The Data and Safety Monitoring Committee

The role of the data and safety monitoring committee differs from the external advisory committee in that it focuses on the internal issues of trial conduct, data collection and data analysis while the trial is ongoing. This committee might report to the external advisory committee or to the study sponsor. By itself, however, it plays an important ethical role by also recommending early termination of a study in which there is unacceptable toxicity, or if treatment superiority is demonstrated sooner than expected according to predetermined statistical criteria (Wittes 1994). This is especially important if the endpoints are differences in therapeutic benefit between the treatment arms.

The committee should therefore be composed of individuals with the scientific and statistical expertise needed fully to understand and protect the trial and with the clinical and ethical sensitivity needed to protect trial participants. These individuals must be independent of sponsors and investigators.

The charge of this committee is not to be taken lightly. If the committee is too concerned with the statistical purity and validity of the data (the "integrity" of the study as planned), it may have the effect of prolonging ethically questionable practices. These could include the extended blinding of treating physicians and patients beyond a point when unblinding was originally promised or the extended use of an ineffective treatment or of a placebo.

Safety monitoring should be ethically unambiguous. If a particular treatment arm shows significantly greater toxicity than another, or if there is an unequivocally worse trend in terms of primary outcome measures, stopping the more dangerous arm ought to be an easy decision. For example, the first multicenter placebo-controlled trial of the efficacy of AZT for patients with AIDS or AIDS-related complex was terminated when only 27 of a total of 282 enrolled patients had completed the planned 24 weeks of treatment. This was because of 19 deaths and 45 new opportunistic infections in the placebo group, compared with one death and 27 new opportunistic infections in the treatment group (Fischl et al. 1987).

Decisions to terminate a study that are grounded in ethics are not always so straightforward. In a later study of the efficacy of AZT in asymptomatic HIV-positive patients whose CD4 lymphocyte counts were less than 500/μl, a decision to stop the trial as planned was made when more than twice as many patients receiving placebo developed AIDS than did patients receiving either high or low dose AZT. One primary objective of the trial, to determine whether AZT could delay the onset of AIDS was met. However, interruption meant loss of information about the long-term efficacy and safety of AZT and about the ultimate effect of treatment on survival (Volberding et al. 1990). Definitive information about the ultimate usefulness of AZT came only years later with the completion of the European Concorde Trial. An opportunity to answer these important questions was lost and there was arguably premature elation about the drug's effectiveness. This is not to suggest that the decision to stop this trial was in retrospect a wrong decision, but to emphasize that any decision to stop a trial may mean loss of valuable information. Adherence to good study design and thorough data analysis must be a part of a decision either to stop or to continue a clinical trial.

When an interim analysis of data shows a beneficial or harmful trend that has not yet reached statistical significance, the committee members, who remain masked to treatment assignment, must carefully monitor incoming data on that issue. While information regarding the trend may be withheld from investigators until an effect is established, the frequency of interim data analyses may need to be increased and decisions made about additional statistical analyses. If there is a trend toward a particularly bad outcome, such as increased disability or death, there must be a readiness to suspend enrollment pending further data or terminate the entire trial.

Relationships Between Investigators and Sponsors

The growing role of private industry in sponsorship of clinical research raises difficult questions about who controls the data, when or how it will be released, and whether this will be in a manner intended solely to influence the market strength of the sponsoring company. Although the business interests of the sponsor are legitimate and should be respected, these interests ultimately should not interfere with timely and accurate reporting of efficacy and toxicity data. Final data analysis and publication of principal results are traditionally the privilege and the responsibility of financially disinterested investigators. Similarly, there is a consensus that principal investigators and individuals financially tied to the sponsor of a trial should not sit on data and safety monitoring committees (Whitaker et al. 1995).

Inevitably, a large clinical trial will gather vast amounts of information that is not used to answer the principal study questions. Access to this information is important because it may hold answers to other questions that become more relevant after the study's primary outcomes are known. Such data might be pooled with data from other studies. They might include information of importance to small subgroups or individual patients, or might form the basis for new hypotheses and future treatment strategies. Because of these issues, mechanisms should be established to assure that data of importance to patients, other investigators, and to the public at large are made available to those who can utilize that information to help to answer additional relevant questions.

Blinding, Randomization, and Recruitment

Even strategies such as double-blinding and randomization, the pillars of the modern clinical trial, represent ethical choices. Randomization divides the study population into haves and have-nots, and winners and losers. Patients, propelled by a lack of satisfactory treatment options, generally enroll in studies with the hope of being randomized to the new treatment arm. No treatment, or older and less than satisfactory treatments, are always available without subjecting oneself to the demands of a protocol. So it is the chance of being given something new that enlivens trials for both patients and researchers.

The hope for an improvement or cure creates the first and foremost ethical obligation concerning randomization; the fact of randomization and the differences between treatment arms must be fully revealed to potential participants at the outset. This may result in loss of research subjects since many patients are willing to try something new and experimental but are unwilling to sacrifice themselves if given a one in two or one in three chance of receiving a placebo or conventional treatment.

Blinding is essential because investigators generally have the same positive bias in favor of the new treatment as their subjects (Noseworthy et al. 1994). This carries the risk that patients receiving experimental therapy will receive favored treatment if they can be identified. Blinding also highlights the conflict between the investigator's obligations as a treating physician and as a research scientist. While blinding is essential to science, it is wrong for a physician to provide an unknown treatment to a patient. A division of roles within a protocol between a "treating physician" with a primary obligation to the patient and an "examining physician" with a primary obligation to the protocol does not resolve this conflict. In reality, both are investigators with a strong commitment to the study. This division may only impose extra burdens upon participants who are then subjected to duplicate examinations. Ideally, a patient should continue to receive treatment from a physician uninvolved in the study.

Large trials with relevance to all MS patients or all patients with a particular major disease pattern (exacerbating–remitting, chronic progressive, etc.) should be designed to enroll patients in a fashion that reflects the demographic pattern of the illness. Such trials should therefore include rich and poor, people of different racial and ethnic backgrounds, and a proportionate number of men. Future large studies that fail to achieve proportionate participation of men and women and of members of different racial and ethnic groups may find that their conclusions are not well accepted by groups under-represented in the study.

Placebos

Two-arm or multiarm clinical trials are grounded in the concept of equipoise (Freedman 1987). There must be genuine uncertainty about the relative merits of the different treatment arms. Ethical use of placebos requires that the researcher does not have prior proof that the treatment under study is superior to a placebo under the circumstances of the trial. If proof of greater efficacy is available then it is unethical to randomize patients to a placebo group (Rothman and Michaels 1994). If there is evidence that a drug is superior to a placebo in terms of benefit A but there is equipoise with respect to benefit B, a placebo-controlled trial focusing on B may be ethical, particularly if that drug has side effects, risks or costs that mitigate against its universal use to achieve A. In contemplating enrollment in such a study, a patient concerned about outcome B may be randomized to the study drug or the placebo. A patient concerned about outcome A should not be recruited. For example, since the multicenter study of interferon beta-1b did not show a significant effect on long-term disability (IFNB Study Group 1993), a study looking at this parameter may have a placebo control. A study looking at exacerbation rates, however, should be a comparison with interferon beta (Goodkin and Kanoti 1994).

Whether or not a patient can be excluded through randomization from receiving a treatment of known benefit is a closely related question. This question arises when considering a comparison between a new treatment and one of proven efficacy. Subjects who may be randomized to a group not receiving standard treatment must be told of the risks of their choice. For example, if a trial is designed to compare a new treatment and interferon beta, investigators must have reason to believe that the new product is as good as or better than interferon beta in limiting exacerbations, *and* they must tell potential study participants that they might lose the benefits of interferon if randomized to the group receiving the newer treatment.

If during a lengthy clinical trial a new treatment becomes available that would benefit trial participants, they must be informed. If the new treatment is sufficiently different in purpose or character from the therapy under study that it can be given without significantly altering the ongoing protocol, it should be made available. If the new treatment might substitute for the therapy under study or interact in such a way to require alteration of the trial, then patients who might benefit should have the option of withdrawing in order to receive the new therapy. In this event, there should be a written addendum to the consent document. This will assure that patients who choose to continue in the study, or to leave, will make their decision on the basis of uniformly presented information about the new treatment.

Conflicts Between Care and Research

In our hypothetical case, Dr Willard is caught in a position of conflict between his responsibilities as a treating physician and as an investigator. He has an obligation to promote the individual well-being of each of his patients, but he has a commitment to the pursuit of knowledge for the benefit of MS patients generally. He must appreciate that patients who he recruits to the study are to some extent risking their immediate well-being for the benefit of others. While they might benefit from an effective new therapy, it is possible that they will encounter a harmful effect, or perhaps they will have no effect and that participation will delay the receipt of something better.

Dr Willard may rationalize recruiting for participation in the new trial as a way to provide treatment that his patients could otherwise not afford. For example, a two-arm study comparing IMMUSTOP with beta interferon would give some patients the opportunity to try interferon while the others receive a treatment hoped to be equal or better. Given their dependence upon him as their physician, his interest in the clinical trial and the rewards to him for enrolling participants may have a coercive effect upon his eligible patients. Whether real or imagined, they will feel a threat to the continuity of their care or sense a loss of interest on Dr Willard's part if they do not enroll. It is therefore essential that they be assured of his continuing attention and the ongoing availability of a full range of standard treatments if they refuse. Furthermore, they must be fully aware of treatment options other than the trial when they are recruited.

Informed Consent

It is at the level of the physician–patient relationship that the issues of informed consent come to life. Obtaining valid informed consent is not a matter of having someone sign a detailed Committee on Human Research or Institutional Review Board approved document that enumerates all risks and absolves research institutions of further responsibility. Rather, it is a process of communication that, built largely upon trust, may transform the physician–patient relationship into a research partnership. The understanding between researcher and subject is not based on the sharing of a fixed amount of information. Indeed, the amount of shared information may vary greatly from one participant to the next. Some may desire little and others a lot. All participants must, however, have some basic understanding of the intent of the study, its duration, its risks and what they may gain or lose by enrolling.

The research partnership that begins with the process of informed consent must continue throughout the trial. In return for the continuing participation of a patient, investigators have an ongoing obligation to disclose significant beneficial or harmful results as they are proven. New information from concurrent trials that may have relevance to a particular patient must also be shared. Research subjects must have freedom to quit without prejudicing future care.

The inclusion of cognitively impaired patients in clinical trials depends on the ability of these patients to understand the proposed research, and to distinguish between the consequences of study participation and the care to which they are otherwise entitled. Patients with cognitive impairment are a special group because of the severe impact of their illness; they are an important group to include in clinical trials. With our increasing awareness of the prevalence of MS-related dementia, it is unlikely that large clinical trials, particularly those looking at progressive or advanced illness, can or should exclude patients with dementia. In fact, the incidence and progression of dementia are likely to become important parameters in future trials that focus on disability.

Some may question the possibility of valid informed consent in studies that include patients with dementia, but this requires a fairly narrow understanding of the nature of the proposed research and its immediate implications for the subject's illness. Informed consent, again, does not necessarily require detailed understanding of the research nor does it require that patients be broadly competent to manage all aspects of their personal affairs. To include such patients will require a more careful balancing of the conflicting roles of physician and scientist. The medical care of the patient must take precedence, even if at the expense of scientific rigor.

With all participants, consent must be implicitly, if not explicitly, renewed throughout the trial. A signature on a detailed legalistic document that is filed and forgotten does not constitute morally valid consent.

Other Issues

There are additional ethical issues not raised by our hypothetical case. The following seem of particular relevance to modern clinical trials.

Qualifications of Clinical Investigators

Trials undertaken by unqualified investigators that cannot answer important questions because of poor design, execution or data analysis are unethical from the start. The Clinical Research Subcommittee of the Scientific Issues Committee of the American Academy of Neurology (1995) recently expressed concern about the future of clinical research because universities provide not only inadequate training in requisite methodologies but also inadequate support and encouragement from residency through faculty levels. As MS research moves into an unprecedented era of large clinical trials, it is critically important that established investigators and research teams promote the training of a new generation of clinical scientists.

Investigator and University Conflicts of Interest

Conflicts of interest jeopardize the credibility, if not the validity, of research when university-based investigators have a financial interest in the product or process tested. Similar problems arise when a university or other non-profit-making institution has a financial stake in a product studied in their own laboratories or clinics (Emanuel and Steiner 1995). While it is customary to call for disclosure of financial interest, such disclosure only reveals the conflict without pointing to a resolution. Disqualification from a clinical trial of those with a financial stake is an obvious but sometimes impractical solution. Some type of external monitoring is therefore needed. When there is a multicenter trial, expertise is not concentrated in one institution, so those with a financial interest can be excluded.

Investigators may also have early access to information about promising treatments and opportunities to invest in the companies developing those products. Given such an opportunity, researchers should either refrain from investing or withdraw from subsequent research on those products.

Concurrent Trials Competing for the Same Study Population

Interferon beta-1b is clearly only the first of several drugs that reduce the exacerbation rate in relapsing-remitting MS. As companies rush to procure the inclusion of competing products into Phase III trials, there will be increasing competition for the limited number of qualified study centers and for patients with an appropriate level of disease. Inevitably, individual centers will be trying to enroll patients simultaneously in competing studies and there will be unscientific incentives to enroll preferentially in one study over another. While some investigators may be biased in favor of one protocol based on their interpretation of preclinical or Phase I study results, inducements to enroll patients may take the form of direct financial support per participant, greater background support for the participating center from one study sponsor, or political considerations. When there are two competing studies in one center, to avoid biased enrollment potential participants must be told of both opportunities and there must be some standardization of the way study opportunities are presented. Where possible, there should be separation of study sites and a division between investigators conducting each trial within a single department.

Pharmaceutical Company Patient Registries

Registration of patients by Berlex for initial treatment with Betaseron® has given this pharmaceutical company direct access to a large group of MS patients, together with information about their individual illnesses and demographics. Such a database has never before existed. Patient identities and details of illness were previously only known and kept confidentially by those patients' physicians. In university-based research, confidential personal information about participants is protected by rules requiring removal of all information that identifies participants. While patient identities must be known and given to federal reviewers if requested, this information is not otherwise available to study sponsors, data analysts or the target audience. Patient lists owned by a single company, however, create enormous opportunities directly to recruit patients for future research by that company and for direct marketing, thus circumventing ongoing doctor–patient relationships. The potential commercial advantage from such a registry makes it likely that other companies will have the incentive to create similar registries as new, competing products reach Phase III testing. Patient lists may ultimately be sold to people interested only in marketing other products to selected subgroups. Patient registries should be resisted or rules written limiting their use.

Large Computer Databases

The development of large computer databases on MS create enormous opportunities for the rapid combination and comparison of data on a worldwide basis (Confavreaux and Paty 1995). While acknowledging the need to protect confidentiality, the authors give paramount importance to "preservation of the user's independence". With a need for commercial sponsorship to create such networks, there again must be concern about the potential for misuse of confidential information for private, commercial ends. There must be mechanisms to limit user access to information about the identities of patients, and explicit rules that not only determine what information is confidential but also prohibit the accumulation and publication of that information.

Commercial Dominance of Clinical Research

Roughly 35 years ago, retiring President Dwight Eisenhower warned Americans about the hidden and growing power of the "military-industrial complex". We are now in an era of dramatic growth of clinical research, but it is an era with an equally dramatic shift in the sponsorship of that research from government to private industry. There is much to welcome from commercial partners in this research, but safeguards against dominance of clinical trials by pharmaceutical or biotechnology firms are desirable. The goals of industry and of investigators do not completely overlap. The scientific goal is the amelioration or cure of MS. While few today will argue that industry goals of increased profit and market share are evil, they are not the goals of clinical research. The difference must be kept clearly in focus.

Conclusion

Scientifically valid and ethical Phase II/III clinical trials can be designed and conducted. The key is to appreciate that a successful clinical trial is a complex co-operative venture. Many different individuals and groups are needed to create and conduct a trial, each with a significant interest in the outcome. A balancing of the differing interests of basic scientists, drug developers, investors, clinical investigators, clinicians, patients and the public at large is always necessary. This means compromise between groups who will not necessarily have the same core values or goals. There is no formula for the successful blending or balancing of these interests, but the external advisory committee for a clinical trial, working from the time of protocol development, can play a critical role in determining how this is achieved.

With every proposed trial, conflicts of interest need to be recognized and dealt with explicitly at each level of study design and execution. The data and safety monitoring committee should be alert to such conflicts and insure that they do not create systematic biases. If this is not done, the effects of these conflicts on the conduct of the research and the interpretation of data, while hidden, may threaten the scientific integrity of the trial and the validity of its conclusions.

While most conflicts will be between different parties, some are between the different roles played by one individual or group. Determining the relative importance of conflicting roles requires individuals to look beyond themselves to the ultimate aim of any trial, the well-being of patients. Subtle and hard to resolve role conflicts are found in the individual who is both clinician and investigator. They are also seen in the individual who is both inventor and tester, or in a company when marketing motives conflict with the need for rigorous product development. More blatant role conflicts, such as occur when individuals or universities act as both investigators and investors, are easier to resolve. These should be forbidden.

Where there are conflicts of interests between two different parties, there must be open appreciation of those conflicts from the start. Since clinical trials begin with a product or a procedure and end with new information about the efficacy or effectiveness of that product or procedure, there must be prior understanding about the ownership of the new information. While the data and safety monitors should assure participant safety and scientific integrity, mechanisms should be established to insure the necessary and appropriate sharing of what is learned. Formal agreements that determine policies regarding ownership of data, access to data, and publication rights should be made in advance. These will tend to maximize the sharing of results, improve the climate of clinical research, and foster more rapid progress toward the goal of a cure for MS.

Finally, the design and conduct of all trials must remain focused on those basic principles formulated into an ethical code earlier in this chapter. The information sought must be new and important. A trial must be able to answer the questions posed only by using human subjects. Benefits from a trial must outweigh possible harms. Research subjects must be chosen fairly and must broadly represent the population for whom treatment is ultimately intended. Individual participants must give genuine informed consent. By understanding and respecting these requirements in their full sense, clinical trials in MS will become models for future trials in all fields of clinical research.

Acknowledgement

The author gratefully acknowledges the sustained interest and support of Donald E. Goodkin, who provided important ideas and usful criticism throughout the preparation of this chapter.

References

Annas GJ, Grodin MA (1992) The Nazi doctors and the Nuremberg Code. Oxford University Press, New York, pp 102–103, 331–342

Beecher HK (1966) Ethics and clinical research. N Engl J Med 274:1354–1360

Clinical Research Subcommittee of the Scientific Issues Committee, American Academy of Neurology (1995) Status of clinical research in neurology. Neurology 45:839–845

Confavreaux C, Paty D (1995) Current status of computerization of multiple sclerosis clinical data for research in Europe and North America: the EDMUS/MS-COSTAR connection. Neurology 45:573–576

Curran WJ (1973) The Tuskegee syphilis study. N Engl J Med 289:730–731

Emanuel E, Steiner D (1995) Institutional conflicts of interest. N Engl J Med 332:262–267

Fischl MA, Richman DD, Grieco MH et al. (1987) The efficacy of azidothymidine (AZT) in the treatment of patients with AIDS and AIDS-related complex. N Engl J Med 317:185–191

Freedman B (1987) Equipoise and the ethics of clinical research. N Engl J Med 317:141–145
Goodkin D, Kanoti G (1994) Ethical considerations raised by the approval of interferon beta-1b for the treatment of multiple sclerosis. Neurology 44:166–170
IFNB Multiple Sclerosis Study Group (1993) Interferon beta-1b is effective in relapsing-remitting multiple sclerosis: I. Clinical results of a multicenter, randomized, double-blind, placebo-controlled trial. Neurology 43:655–661
Kampmeier RH (1972) The Tuskegee study of untreated syphilis. South Med J 65:1247–1251
Kampmeier RH (1974) Final report on the "Tuskegee Syphilis Study". South Med J 67:1349–1353
Katz J (1993) "Ethics and clinical research" revisited: a tribute to Henry K. Beecher. Hastings Cent Rep 23(5):31–39
Munson R (ed) (1992) Intervention and reflection: basic issues in medical ethics, 4th edn. Wadsworth, Belmont, CA, pp 392–394
Noseworthy J, Ebers G, Vandervoort M, Farquhar R, Yetisir E, Roberts R (1994) The impact of blinding on the results of a randomized, placebo-controlled multiple sclerosis clinical trial. Neurology 44:16–20
Rothman DJ (1987) Ethics and human experimentation. N Engl J Med 317:1195–1199
Rothman KJ, Michels KB (1994) The continuing unethical use of placebo controls. N Engl J Med 331:394–398
Spilker B (1991) Guide to clinical trials. Raven Press, New York, pp 124–128
Volberding PA, Lagakos SW, Koch MA et al. (1990) Zidovudine in asymptomatic human immunodeficiency virus infection. N Engl J Med 322:941–949
Whitaker JN, McFarland HF, Rudge P, Reingold, SC (1995) Outcomes assessment in multiple sclerosis clinical trials: a critical analysis. Multiple Sclerosis 1: 37–47
Wittes, J (1994) Monitoring clinical trials: relationships among data monitoring board, sponsor, and investigators [Abstract]. In: Outcomes assessment in multiple sclerosis clinical trials: a critical analysis. A Meeting of the National Multiple Sclerosis Society; 1994 Feb; Charleston, SC

16 The Emergence of Multiple Sclerosis as a "Treatable" Condition: An Historical Perspective

W. Ian McDonald

Introduction

Implicit in the statement that a disease is treatable is the idea that its course can be favourably modified by some kind of intervention. Until recently multiple sclerosis (MS) quite certainly has not been in this category. There is a widespread conviction that it now is, but such convictions have been held before and have proved unfounded. How can we be sure that our present confidence is justified? In this short review I shall trace the evolution of our attempts to treat MS, emphasizing strategies designed to arrest its progress. The development of the complementary and no less important approaches to relieving symptoms lies beyond my present scope.

Early History

The pathology of MS was first depicted nearly 160 years ago (Carswell 1838; Compston 1988) and soon thereafter rudimentary clinical descriptions were appended to pathologic accounts (Cruveilhier 1835–1842). Its relapsing-remitting nature was recognized by Valentiner in 1856. In 1868, Charcot made his magisterial synthesis of his own observations with those of his predecessors, but all that he could say about treatment was "The time has not yet come when such a subject can be seriously considered" (Charcot 1877).

Nevertheless, during this period practising physicians were treating patients with MS, partly to relieve symptoms and partly in the hope of preventing its progression. They used the time-honoured remedies that they had to hand. A diverting account of treatments in vogue in the early part of the last century is provided by Augustus d'Este in the diary of his illness (Firth 1948). His physicians gave him prescriptions (which are recorded in detail) containing salts of various metals such as silver, mercury, copper and iron. Arsenic and iodides were later popular and continued to be used, along with silver and antimony, up to the middle of this century. I still see occasional patients who attended McAlpine's arsenic clinic in the 1950s.

These prescriptions have no discernible rational basis, as Cushny pointed out as long ago as 1910. The experimental effects of arsenic, for example, provided no basis for using it in neurologic disease. The use of silver appeared to derive from the Arabic astrologic system of medicine. The merits of the waters of specific spas were recommended by d'Este's physicians, and those of other spas were still being recommended by Oppenheim (1911) early this century. Though the return of relapses and the later relentless progression of the disease in most of their patients made thoughtful physicians skeptical of the value of their treatments, they often continued to use the regimens by and large inherited from their teachers.

Therapy Based on Theories of Etiology

A new approach appeared in the generation after Charcot as powerful new explanations of disease mechanisms became incorporated into medical thinking. Charcot's idea that the primary process in MS was a hyperplasia of the glia had had no therapeutic implications, but the demonstration that disease could be caused by bacterial infection soon led investigators to try to explain MS in these terms. Not for the last time did eminent practitioners propose a therapeutic approach deriving from an unconvincing interpretation of the disease in fashionable etiologic and pathogenetic terms. Marie wrote in 1895:

> Before concluding this enumeration, a paragraph must be devoted to unnamed infections, so frequent, so little known, I might add so much disregarded. There are no special symptoms at the onset which indicate its existence; fever is known to have occurred, prolonged discomfort with or without gastrointestinal symptoms, occasionally jaundice or pulmonary trouble, nothing else being known about the disease. In such a case, gentlemen, you must not doubt that this is certainly a case of infection, but of such a kind that it has not received any definite clinical name. As regards the patients in whom multiple sclerosis seems to occur from the influence of injury or some other purely physical cause, my conviction is that these cases are also due to infection, but that the infection has passed away completely unperceived, while some less important but more dramatic incident has alone attracted the attention of the patient or those who are with him.

In 1911, Buzzard conjectured that MS might be due to a spirochete and proposed the therapeutic use of salvarsan, an organic arsenical, because of its recent success in treating syphilis. Pathologic observations and claims of transmission to animals, all of which proved to be unfounded, added impetus to the idea (Adams et al. 1924; Gye 1921; Kuhn and Steiner 1917; Marinesco 1919; Siemerling 1918). In 1922, the Association for Research in Nervous and Mental Diseases published the findings of its commission set up to review the present state of knowledge of MS. It emphasized the importance in etiologic studies of distinguishing between exogenous factors, which precipitate relapse, and those that might initiate the disease process. The commission rejected Oppenheim's view that MS was toxic in origin and were cautious about the role of spirochetes. Nevertheless, as in earlier generations, it advised the use of old remedies of iodides, silver and mercury, and neoarsphenamine.

Two years later, Grosz (1924) proposed the use of fever therapy, again based on the assumption of the spirochetal etiology and the success of its use in neurosyphilis. He proposed the use of malaria, but this was not a practical proposition in temperate climates where a variety of alternative regimens were used (see review by Brickner 1935–1936). One involved three-times weekly injections of typhoid vaccine, but because severe reactions were frequent, intramuscular injections of sterile milk were often given instead. The response, however, was scarcely less violent, and Denny-Brown (1952) summed up the position in a later symposium by stating that fever therapy was "seldom beneficial and sometimes disastrous". Though the enthusiasm for a spirochetal etiology declined in the 1930s, I saw one patient treated with an organic arsenical in the 1950s, who died as a result of a catastrophic neurologic reaction to this therapy.

A new infective agent was proposed in 1930: the spherula insularis. This agent had been identified in the cerebrospinal fluid (CSF) of patients with MS (Chevassut 1930). A vaccine was raised against the organism and Purves-Stewart reported spectacular success with it (Purves-Stewart 1930a, b). Zinsser (1930), however, concluded that the observations were artifacts and that the vaccination experiments "judged purely from the immunologist's point of view would be extremely surprising if correct". Carmichael (1931) failed, after a painstaking attempt to repeat the work, to confirm the existence of spherula insularis.

Despite the failure to identify a specific pathogen in MS, a conviction persisted that infection was relevant. Non-specific influences that had so appealed to Marie at the end of the nineteenth century were again in vogue, this time in the form of focal sepsis. The modish use of tonsillectomy and extraction of teeth were accordingly practised extensively and were still thought to have some merit by McAlpine et al. as late as 1955.

The possibility that a viral infection was the initiating event in MS gained increasing attention during the 1960s. At first sight it seemed to be supported by the finding of modestly elevated titres of antibodies against measles (Johnson 1982). It soon became clear, however, that the findings were not specific. Similar elevations of titres of antibodies against several common viruses (sometimes more than one in a single patient) were found in serum and CSF, and similar elevations were found in other chronic inflammatory diseases such as rheumatoid arthritis and systemic lupus erythematosis.

The discovery that some human degenerative neurologic diseases were due to slow viruses gave a new impetus to the viral theories of the etiology of MS, but the failure to obtain confirmed virus isolations from the brains of patients with MS and to transmit the disease to animals eroded confidence in this approach. Nevertheless, a range of antiviral agents was used without convincing benefit. It was in this context that the idea of using the interferons to treat MS first arose, but, as described in Chapter 11, the rationale for continuing to assess them changed during the 1980s to one based on theories of pathogenesis. It is now appropriate to consider this approach.

Therapy Based on Theories of Pathogenesis

Early approaches to treatment did not distinguish between the aim of removing the causative agent and modifying the pathologic consequences of its operation in order to slow or halt progression of the disease. In the 1930s and 1940s, Putnam and his colleagues suggested that the perivenular orientation of plaques was primarily due to thrombosis of the venules and advocated anticoagulant therapy (Putnam 1935; Putnam et al. 1947). Their pathologic observations were not confirmed and anticoagulant therapy proved to be ineffective. Denny-Brown (1952) remarked characteristically, "we have been impressed more by the danger of giving enough dicoumerin to change blood clotting than by its effect on multiple sclerosis".

The ischemic theory of pathogenesis was revived in the 1980s and led to the widespread and uncritical enthusiasm for treatment with hyperbaric oxygen. Again, a beneficial therapeutic effect has not been established (see review by Matthews 1991).

An entirely different approach followed epidemiologic (Swank 1950; Swank et al. 1952) and biochemical (Baker et al. 1963; Sinclair 1956) observations, which were interpreted as indicating the presence of a constitutional defect in lipid metabolism. To compensate, patients were advised to take a diet rich in polyunsaturated fatty acids with or without supplements. Convincing benefit was not obtained (Bates et al. 1989; Paty et al. 1978) and enthusiasm waned as patients deteriorated.

By far the most influential theory of pathogenesis has been that of autoimmunity, based on the histologic similarities between MS and experimental allergic encephalomyelitis, the immune-mediated inflammatory demyelinating disease of the central nervous system induced in a variety of experimental animals by the inoculation of a range of antigens derived from central myelin (Lassmann 1983).

Although the initiating event in the two diseases is certainly different, it nevertheless seemed logical to try to modify the course of events in MS by using agents that had been shown to suppress experimental allergic encephalomyelitis. In principle there have been three main approaches: immunosuppression, induction of tolerance and immune modulation. The earliest was non-specific immunosuppression with cyclophosphamide or azathiaprine, and later with cyclosporin or total lymphoid irradiation (Aimard et al. 1966; Cook et al. 1987; Kappos et al. 1988; Tucker and Kapphahn 1969). At best, these agents, each reviewed in the first edition of this monograph, produced a marginal effect (British and Dutch Multiple Sclerosis Azathioprine Trial Group 1988; Canadian Co-operative Multiple Sclerosis Study Group 1991; Ludkin et al. 1991; Multiple Sclerosis Study Group 1990; Weiner et al. 1984; Wiles et al. 1994). The effects of induction of tolerance using copolymer 1 are reviewed in Chapter 13 of this volume.

This outline of the attempts to MS reveals a common thread. First is the need to treat, leading to: the development of strategies based on an incomplete understanding of etiology and pathogenesis; the enthusiastic promotion of particular treatments and claims for their benefit; and a gradual decline in their use as experience showed that improvement was temporary and represented nothing more than the natural history of the disease. The abandonment of many therapeutic approaches took a generation, and, in the case of arsenic, two.

The realization that the process could be shortened, that conclusions about effectiveness could be made more securely, gradually emerged in the latter part of this century, as the principle of the double-blind placebo-controlled clinical trial was introduced into the study of MS.

The first clearing of the air came when the American Neurological Association set up a commission in 1934 to establish the principles of assessment of treatment in MS. Brickner (1935–1936) summarized its results, emphasizing the importance of careful documentation, classification of clinical subtypes and follow-up at short intervals with recording of changing symptoms and signs.

The next important step was the development by John Kurtzke (1955) of a rating scale to measure the effectiveness of treatment. It was a remarkable achievement and, though it has later been much criticized for combining measures of impairment, disability and handicap (distinctions that were only developed much later), its incompleteness (for example in the assessment of cognitive function, the importance of which has only been appreciated in the past decade) and the coarseness of some of its measures (better measures have still to be developed for the assessment of many functions), it remains central to any clinical trial. It is not that better measures of specific aspects of effects of disease in patients cannot be developed; it is that they have not yet been formulated. Encouraging attempts to do so still require validation, which is an essential prerequisite for their use as an alternative to the Kurtzke system (Whitaker et al. 1995).

An important problem in earlier studies was misdiagnosis. The formulation proposed by Schumacher and his colleagues (1965) at the meeting on MS organized by the the New York Academy of Sciences, represented a wise distillation of the clinical and pathologic knowledge of MS and related diseases at that time. Though restrictive, it provided a reasonably secure basis for selecting patients for clinical trials. The development and validation of investigations in the next generation, including CSF electrophoresis, evoked potentials and imaging, allowed the criteria to be refined (Poser et al. 1983). Though some modification is needed in relation to the progressive forms of MS, the relative certainty of diagnosis can be assigned securely and provide a sound (if not perfect) basis for the selection of patients for clinical trials.

A third ingredient in this progress has been the importance given to calculating the size of clinical trials needed to detect significant differences in relevant endpoints. Here, the data derived from hospital based studies were not useful, but that derived from the population-based sources such as those of Weinshenker et al. (1991b) have led to the realization that many early trials were too small to permit secure conclusions to be drawn (Runmarker & Andersen 1993; Weinshenker et al. 1991a). Current investigations of beta interferon have randomized as many as 700 patients between placebo and actively treated groups.

A similar principle applies to the use of magnetic resonance techniques to study pathologic activity. Here, the numbers may be surprisingly small. Nauta et al. (1994), for example, have calculated that it should be possible to demonstrate a 50% reduction in disease activity with 90% power in just 30 patients in the placebo and actively treated groups after monthly scanning with gadolinium-DTPA enhancement for 7 months.

These principles have been applied with increasing rigour to which considerable impetus has been given by meetings organized by the New York Academy of Sciences in 1965 and 1981, and especially by the National Multiple Sclerosis Society of the United States in 1983 and 1994.

The first clear evidence of success came from the trial of ACTH for the treatment of relapse in 1970 (Rose et al. 1970). There followed a number of trials of immunosuppressant treatment, in which, as already pointed out, convincing benefit was not shown. The publication of the trial of interferon beta-1b in 1993, however, signaled a radical change (IFNB Multiple Sclerosis Study Group 1993; Paty et al. 1993). This demonstrated for the first time an effect of treatment on the course of the disease. The excitment this achievement has engendered is appropriate, not so much for the magnitude of the clinical effect, which is modest (a reduction in relapse rate over 2 years by about one-third; it has no effect on disability), but for the demonstration of the power of the approach. Apparent confirmation has come from trials of interferon beta-1a (Chapter 11, Jacobs et al. 1994) and copolymer 1 (Chapter 13, Johnson 1994), though their status must remain uncertain until the full results are published.

The Present Position

We have arrived at an encouraging position after 152 years of recorded attempts to treat MS pharmacologically (Firth 1948). We have a clinical method, albeit imperfect, time consuming and cumbersome, which is capable of revealing a beneficial effect on the course of MS. In magnetic resonance imaging (MRI) we have a means of detecting pathologic activity, but dangers remain, as the reactions to the interferon trials and the methods used in them attest. It is essential that these dangers are appreciated and avoided in order to continue progress.

The first is that of confusing the significance of endpoints. For example, a reduction in relapse rate does not guarantee a reduction in later disability. Prediction is unreliable because the evidence is conflicting: Weinshenker et al. (1991a), in a large cohort of patients studied for a comparatively short time in relation to the course of MS (1099 patients for 1–12 years) found that the relapse rate in the first 2 years was predictive of later disability, whereas Runmarker and Andersen (1993), in a smaller cohort followed for much longer (308 patients for a minimum of 25 years), found that it was not. The empirical evidence for interferon beta-1b is that in the short term (2 years) disability is unaffected by the modest reduction in relapse rate occurring during that time.

Secondly, pathologic activity as judged by standard MRI is not reliably predictive of later disability, though recent evidence suggests that it may prove to be so for particular groups of patients (Losseff et al. 1995; McDonald et al. 1994). The extent of abnormality on T2-weighted images also correlates poorly with disability. An important factor contributing to these discrepancies is likely to be the lack of specificity of standard magnetic resonance techniques for the different elements of the pathologic process in MS. These methods can readily detect the acute changes associated with the development of a new lesion (or new activity in a pre-existing lesion) and relapse, but they do not discriminate the chronic changes, such as axonal degeneration, which are likely to make an important contribution to irrecoverable deficit (McDonald 1994). New techniques, such as magnetization transfer imaging and magnetic resonance spectroscopy, may do so, but their practical usefulness remains to be determined (Chapter 8).

In planning treatment trials, it is therefore important to expect of MRI only what it can give in the light of present knowledge. Its main current value is as a screening method for putative agents to see whether there is an effect on the acute elements of the pathologic process that would justify the mounting of a major trial with a clinical endpoint. The data being collected in current large scale trials and smaller specifically designed projects should be invaluable in deciding whether and to what extent the standard MRI methods are predictive of clinical outcome and whether newer methods such as magnetisation transfer imaging, diffusion-weighted imaging and proton magnetic resonance spectroscopy are superior.

A third danger is that of early analysis and publication. For example, in the United States Optic Neuritis Study Group's trial the 6-month analysis led to the conclusion that, besides hastening recovery, visual outcome was slightly improved by treatment with high dose intravenous methyl prednisolone (Beck et al. 1992), but, after a further 6 months, the difference between the placebo and actively treated groups had disappeared (Beck and Cleary 1993). The same study also illustrates another danger, that of secondary analysis of trials designed for another purpose. After a follow-up of 2 years, it was reported that the risk of developing MS after optic neuritis was higher in patients treated with oral steroids than in those treated with intravenous methyl prednisolone or placebo (Beck et al. 1993), but, after another year, the difference between the groups was no longer found (Beck 1995) (Chapter 10).

Finally, the danger of producing unreasonable expectations of treatment among patients cannot be overemphasized; disappointment at best, or resentment and anger, follow. The point is cogently made in relation to interferon beta-1b by Mohr et al. (1995), who have illustrated just how difficult it is to convey accurately the limitations of a new treatment as well as the possible benefits, even when dealing with a knowledgeable group of patients.

Conclusion

MS has indeed emerged as a treatable disease after more than a century of endeavor. Progress was initially slow because of the inadequacy of our theories of etiology and pathogenesis, the limited range of therapeutic agents relevant to such ideas as we did have, and the inadequacy of our methods of assessment. Much of this has changed, but we have been lucky too: a treatment introduced as a means of combating a virus that had not been identified turned out to have an effect on the pathogenetic mechanism. The increased understanding of the pathogenesis of MS is suggesting new strategies by which it may be possible favorably to alter the course of disability. I am optimistic that the exploitation of these strategies alone and in combination, using existing methods and the more discriminating methods currently being developed, will lead to more rapid progress.

References

Adams DK, Blacklock JWS, Dunlop EM et al. (1924) An investigation into the pathogenesis of disseminated sclerosis. Q J Med 17:129–150

Aimard G, Girard PF, Raveaou J (1966) Sclérose en plaques et processus d'autoimmunisation: traitement par les antimitotiques. Lyon Méd 215:345–353

Association for Research in Nervous and Mental Diseases (1922) Multiple Sclerosis, vol 2, Hoeber, New York

Baker RWR, Thompson RHS, Zilkha K (1963) Fatty acid composition of brain lecithins in multiple sclerosis. Lancet i:26–27

Bates D, Cartlidge NEF, French JM et al. (1989) A double-blind controlled trial of long chain n-3 polyunsaturated fatty acids in the treatment of multiple sclerosis. J Neurol Neurosurg Psychiatry 52:18–22

Beck RW (1995) The optic neuritis treatment trial: three-year follow-up results. Arch Ophthalmol 113:136

Beck RW, Cleary PA (1993) Optic neuritis treatment trial: one year follow-up results. Arch Ophthalmol 111:773–775

Beck RW, Cleary PA, Anderson MM et al. (1992) A randomised, controlled trial of corticosteroids in the treatment of acute optic neuritis. N Engl J Med 326:581–588

Beck RW, Cleary RA, Trobe JD et al. (1993) The effect of corticosteroids for acute optic neuritis on the subsequent development of multiple sclerosis. N Engl J Med 329:1764–1769

Brickner RM (1935–1936) A critique of therapy in multiple sclerosis. Bull Neurol Inst NY 4:665–698

British and Dutch Multiple Sclerosis Azathioprine Trial Group (1988) Double-masked trial of azathioprine in multiple sclerosis. Lancet ii:179–183

Buzzard EF (1911) The treatment of disseminated sclerosis: A suggestion. Lancet i:98

Canadian Cooperative Multiple Sclerosis Study Group (1991) The Canadian cooperative trial of cyclosphosphamide and plasma exchange in progressive multiple sclerosis. Lancet i:441–446

Carmichael EA (1931) The aetiology of disseminate sclerosis: some criticisms of recent work especially with regard to the 'spherula insularis'. Proc R Soc Med 34:591–599

Carswell R (1838) Pathological anatomy. Illustrations of the elementary forms of disease. Longman, Orme, Brown, Green and Longman, London

Charcot JM (1877) Lectures on diseases of the nervous system (trans. Sigerson G). The New Sydenham Society, London 158

Charcot M (1868) Histologie de le sclérose en plaques. Gazette des Hôpitaux, Paris 141:554–555, 557–558

Chevassut K (1930) Aetiology of disseminated sclerosis. Lancet i:552–560

Compston A (1988) The 150th anniversary of the first depiction of the lesions of multiple sclerosis. J Neurol Neurosurg Psychiatry 51:1249–1252

Cook SD, Devereux C, Troiano R et al. (1987) Total lymphoid irradiation in multiple sclerosis: blood lymphocytes and clinical course. Ann Neurol 22:634–638

Cruveilhier J (1835–1842) Anatomie pathologique du corps humain; descriptions avec figures lithographiées et coloriées; des diverses alterations morbides dont le corps humain est susceptible. Baillière, Paris

Cushny AR (1910) A textbook of pharmacology and therapeutics, 5th edn. Lea and Febiger, Philadelphia, pp 623, 691

Denny-Brown D (1952) Multiple sclerosis: the clinical problem. Am J Med 12:501–509

Firth D (1948) The case of Augustus D'Esté. Cambridge University Press, Cambridge, pp 25–27

Grosz K (1924) Malaria-behandlung der multiplen Sclerose. Jahrbuch Psychiatr Neurol 43:198–214

Gye NE (1921) The experimental study of disseminated sclerosis. Brain 44:213–222

IFNB Multiple Sclerosis Study Group (1993) Interferon beta-1b is effective in relapsing-remitting multiple sclerosis: I. Clinical results of a multicenter, randomized, double-blind, placebo-controlled trial. Neurology 43:655–661

Jacobs L, Cookfaire D, Ludick R et al. (1994) Results of a Phase III trial of intramuscular recombinant beta-interferon as treatment for multiple sclerosis. Ann Neurol 36:259

Johnson KP (1994) Experimental therapy of relapsing-remitting multiple sclerosis with copolymer-1. Ann Neurol 36:S115–S117

Johnson RT (1982) Viral infections of the nervous system. Raven Press, New York

Kappos L, Patzold U, Dommasch D et al. (1988) Cyclosporine versus azathioprine in the long-term treatment of multiple sclerosis: results of the German multicenter study. Ann Neurol 23:56–63

Kuhn P, Steiner G (1917) Über die Ursache der multiplen Sklerose. Med Klin 13:1007–1009

Kurtzke J (1955) A new scale for evaluating disability in multiple sclerosis. Neurology 5:580–583

Lassman H (1983) Comparative neuropathology of chronic experimental allergic encephalomyelitis and multiple sclerosis. Springer-Verlag, Berlin

Losseff N, Kendall BE, Kingsley DPE, Miller DH, McDonald WI, Thompson AJ (1995) Serial magnetic resonance imaging (MRI) in multiple sclerosis (MS): a five year follow up study. J Neurol 242 (Suppl 2):S7

Ludkin PL, Ellison GW, Ghezzi A (1991) Overview of azathioprine treatment in multiple sclerosis. Lancet 338:1051–1055

Marie P (1895) Lectures on diseases of the spinal cord (trans Lubbock M). New Sydenham Society, London 134–136, 153

Marinesco G (1919) Étude sur l'origine et al. nature de la sclerose en plaques. Rev Neurol 35:481–488

Matthews WB (1991) In: Matthews WB (ed) McAlpine's multiple sclerosis, 2nd edn. Churchill Livingstone, Edinburgh pp 251–298

McAlpine D, Compston ND, Lumsden CE (1955) Multiple clerosis. E & S Livingstone, Edinburgh pp 191

McDonald WI (1994) The pathological and clinical dynamics of multiple sclerosis. J Neuropathol Exp Neurol 53:338–343

McDonald WI, Miller DH, Thompson AJ (1994) Are magnetic resonance findings predictive of clinical outcome in therapeutic trials in multiple sclerosis? The dilemma of interferon-beta. Ann Neurol 36:14–18

Mohr DC, Neilley L, Gatto N et al. (1995) Expectations of multiple sclerosis patients initiating Betaseron therapy. Neurology 45 (Suppl 4):139P

Multiple Sclerosis Study Group (1990) Efficacy and toxicity of cyclosporin in chronic progressive multiple sclerosis: a randomised double-blinded placebo-controlled clinical trial. Ann Neurol 27:591–605

Nauta JJP, Thompson AJ, Barkhof F, Miller DH (1994) Magnetic resonance imaging in monitoring the treatment in multiple sclerosis patients: statistical power of parallel groups and crossover designs. J Neurol Sci 122:6–14

Oppenheim H (1911) Text-book of nervous diseases for physicians and students (trans Bruce A). Otto Schulze, Edinburgh (trans 1908 German edn)

Paty DW, Cousin HK, Read S, Adlakha K (1978) Linoleic acid in multiple sclerosis: failure to show any therapeutic benefit. Acta Neurol Scand 58:53–58

Paty DW, Li DKB, the UBC MS/MRI Study Group, and the IFNB Multiple Sclerosis Study Group (1993) Interferon beta-1b is effective in relapsing-remitting multiple sclerosis. II. MRI analysis results of a multicenter, randomized, double-blind, placebo-controlled trial. Neurology 43:662–667

Poser C, Paty D, Scheinberg L et al. (1983) New diagnostic criteria for multiple sclerosis: guidelines for research protocols. Ann Neurol 13:227–231

Purves-Stewart J (1930a) A specific vaccine treatment in disseminated sclerosis. Lancet i:560–564

Purves-Stewart J (1930b) The etiology and treatment of disseminated sclerosis. J Nerv Ment Dis 72:652–660

Putnam TJ (1935) Studies in multiple sclerosis: IV. Encephalitis and sclerotic plaques produced by venular obstruction. Arch Neurol Psychiatry 33:929–940

Putnam TJ, Chiavacci LV, Hoff H et al. (1947) Results of treatment of multiple sclerosis with dicoumarin. Arch Neurol 57:1–13

Rose AS, Cuzma JW, Kurtzke JF et al. (1970) Cooperative study in the evaluation of therapy in multiple sclerosis: ACTH versus placebo; final report. Neurology 20 (Suppl):1–59

Runmarker B, Andersen O (1993) Prognostic factors in multiple sclerosis incidence cohort with 25 years of follow-up. Brain 116:117–134

Schumacher GA, Beebe G, Kibler RF et al. (1965) Problems of experimental trials of therapy in multiple sclerosis; report by the panel on the evaluation of experimental trials of therapy in multiple sclerosis. Ann NY Acad Sci 122:552–568

Siemerling E (1918) Spirochäten in Gehirn eines Falles von multiplen Sklerose. Berl Klin Wochenschr 55:273–274

Sinclair HM (1956) Deficiency of the central fatty acids and atherosclerosis, *etcetera*. Lancet i:381–383

Swank RL (1950) Multiple sclerosis: a correlation of its incidence with dietary fat. Am J Med Sci 220:441–450

Swank RL, Lerstead O, Strjaum A, Backer J (1952) Multiple sclerosis in rural Norway: its geographical and occupational incidence in relation to nutrition. N Engl J Med 246:721–728

Tucker WG, Kapphahn KH (1969) A preliminary evaluation of azathioprine (Imuran) in the treatment of multiple sclerosis. Henry Ford Hosp Med J 17:89–92

Valentiner W (1856) Ueber die Sclerose des Gehirns und Rückenmarks. Deutsche Klinik 8:147–151

Weiner HL, Hauser SL, Hafler DA et al. (1984) The use of cyclophosphamide in the treatment of multiple sclerosis. Ann NY Acad Sci 436:373–381

Weinshenker BG, Rice GPA, Noseworthy JH et al. (1991a) The natural history of multiple sclerosis: a geographically based study: 3. Multivariate analysis of predictive factors and models of outcome. Brain 114:1045–1056

Weinshenker BG, Rice GPA, Noseworthy JH et al. (1991b) The natural history of multiple sclerosis: a geographically based study: 4. Applications to planning and interpretation of clinical therapeutic trials. Brain 114:1057–1067

Whitaker JN, McFarland HF, Rudge P, Reingold SC (1995) Outcomes assessment in multiple sclerosis clinical trials: a critical analysis. Multiple Sclerosis 1:37–47

Wiles CM, Omar L, Swan AV et al. (1994) Total lymphoid irradiation in multiple sclerosis. J Neurol Neurosurg Psychiatry 57:154–163

Zinsser H (1930) In: Purves Stewart J Discussion. The etiology and treatment of disseminated sclerosis. J Nerv Ment Dis 72:652–660

Index